Subfertility, Reproductive Endocrinology and Assisted Reproduction

Subfertility, Reproductive Endocrinology and Assisted Reproduction

Edited by
Jane A. Stewart
Chair British Fertility Society

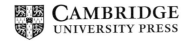

CAMBRIDGE
UNIVERSITY PRESS

University Printing House, Cambridge CB2 8BS, United Kingdom

One Liberty Plaza, 20th Floor, New York, NY 10006, USA

477 Williamstown Road, Port Melbourne, VIC 3207, Australia

314–321, 3rd Floor, Plot 3, Splendor Forum, Jasola District Centre,
New Delhi – 110025, India

79 Anson Road, #06-04/06, Singapore 079906

Cambridge University Press is part of the University of Cambridge.

It furthers the University's mission by disseminating knowledge in the
pursuit of education, learning, and research at the highest international levels
of excellence.

www.cambridge.org
Information on this title: www.cambridge.org/9781107139039
DOI: 10.1017/9781316488294

First published 2019

Printed in the United Kingdom by TJ International Ltd. Padstow Cornwall

A catalogue record for this publication is available from the British Library.

Library of Congress Cataloging-in-Publication Data
Names: Stewart, Jane, MD, editor.
Title: Subfertility, reproductive endocrinology and assisted reproduction /
    edited by Jane Stewart.
Description: Cambridge, United Kingdom ; New York, NY : Cambridge
    University Press, 2019. | Includes bibliographical references and index.
Identifiers: LCCN 2018054577 | ISBN 9781107139039 (hardback : alk. paper)
Subjects: | MESH: Infertility | Reproductive Techniques, Assisted | Endocrine
    System Diseases–complications | Reproductive Medicine–methods
Classification: LCC RG201 | NLM WP 570 | DDC 618.1/78–dc23
LC record available at https://lccn.loc.gov/2018054577

ISBN 978-1-107-13903-9 Hardback

....

Contents

Contents

Contributors

Ali Al Chami
University College London Hospitals, UK

Adam H. Balen
The Leeds Centre for Reproductive Medicine, UK

Harish M. Bhandari
The Leeds Centre for Reproductive Medicine, UK

Debra Bloor
CARE Fertility, UK

Ka Ying Bonnie Ng
University of Southampton, UK

Kate Brian
Infertility Network, UK

Ying Cheong
University of Southampton and Complete Fertility Centre, UK

Maya Chetty
Royal Infirmary of Edinburgh, UK

Meenakshi K. Choudhary
Newcastle upon Tyne NHS Foundation Trust, UK

Rachel Cutting
Sheffield Teaching Hospitals NHS Foundation Trust, UK

Melanie Davies
University College London Hospitals, UK

Andrew A. Dwyer
William F. Connell School of Nursing, Massachusetts & Massachusetts General Hospital, Boston, USA

Janine Elson
Liverpool Women's NHS Foundation Trust, UK

Tarek El-Toukhy
Guy's and St Thomas' Hospital NHS Foundation Trust, UK

Emily Gelson
Addenbrooke's Hospital, UK

Joyce C. Harper
University College London, UK

Kanna Jayaprakasan
Royal Derby Hospital and University of Nottingham, UK

Nick Jones
Human Fertilisation & Embryology Authority, UK

Tulay Karasu
Newcastle upon Tyne NHS Foundation Trust, UK

Narmada Katakam
Genesis Fertility & Laparoscopy Centre, India

Yakoub Khalaf
Guy's and St Thomas' Hospital NHS Foundation Trust, UK

Julia Kopeika
Guy's and St Thomas' Hospital NHS Foundation Trust, UK

Sarah Martins da Silva
Ninewells Hospital, UK

Neil McClure
Queen's University Belfast and Belfast Trust, UK

Kevin McEleny
Newcastle upon Tyne NHS Foundation Trust, UK

Mostafa Metwally
Sheffield Teaching Hospitals NHS Foundation Trust, UK

Asif Muneer
University College London Hospitals, UK

Luciano Nardo
Centre for Reproductive Health, UK

Martine Nijs
Cooper Surgical Fertility and Genomic Solutions, Denmark

Allan A. Pacey
University of Sheffield, UK

Nikoletta Panagiotopoulou
Manchester Fertility, UK

Arie Parnham
The Christie NHS Foundation Trust, UK

Alka Prakash
Cambridge University Hospitals NHS Foundation Trust, UK

Richard Quinton
Newcastle upon Tyne NHS Foundation Trust, UK

Gavin Sacks
IVF Australia and University of New South Wales, Australia

Ertan Saridogan
University College London Hospitals, UK

Ippokratis Sarris
King's College Hospital London and King's Fertility, UK

Karen Schnauffer
Centre for Reproductive Health, UK

Sioban B. SenGupta
University College London, UK

Jane A. Stewart
Newcastle upon Tyne Hospitals NHS Foundation Trust, UK

Sesh K. Sunkara
Guy's and St Thomas' Hospital NHS Foundation Trust, UK

Alison Taylor
Lister Hospital, UK

Shreeya Tewary
University Hospitals Coventry & Warwickshire, UK

Madelon van Wely
Academic Medical Center, University of Amsterdam, The Netherlands

Linsey White
NHS Greater Glasgow and Clyde, UK

Hannah Williams
Ninewells Hospital, UK

Bryan Woodward
X&Y Fertility, UK

Swapna Yesireddy
Nova IVF Fertility, India

The Patient's Perspective

Kate Brian

A good fertility clinic is about more than success rates, and a good fertility specialist has an understanding of fertility problems which goes beyond the clinical aspects of patient care. It is easy to overlook the patient's perspective in the rush to learn about the latest evidence-based scientific developments in fertility treatment, but good quality patient care is not simply a matter of telling patients what you think is best for them and providing that service.

This is something that the UK regulator, the Human Fertilisation and Embryology Authority (HFEA), has recognised. The Authority's 2014 Annual Conference titled 'Putting the patient at the centre of what we do' marked the start of a new strategy to ensure that the patient perspective played a key role in decision-making for the future. The HFEA's plans include making patient views on their experiences at fertility clinics part of the 'Choose a Clinic' website tool which helps patients to find a clinic that is right for them. This means that the way in which patients' needs are met by individual clinics and clinicians in the United Kingdom will become more visible and public.

Although national average success rates for in vitro fertilisation (IVF) in the United Kingdom have risen gradually from 14% in 1991 [1] to 25.8% in 2012 [2], the majority of individual treatment cycles are not successful and the best possible care for patients must involve supporting them through the realities of unsuccessful treatment as well as helping them to pregnancy. The value of emotional support was highlighted by a Danish study of more than 2,000 patients in 2003 which explored the importance of patient-centred care to fertility patients. It concluded, 'A supportive attitude from medical staff and the provision of both medical and psychosocial information and support should be integral aspects of medical care in fertility clinics [3].'

In order to offer patients the best possible care, it is first important to understand how people feel when they arrive at the fertility clinic. In 1997 the UK's National Infertility Awareness Campaign (NIAC), now known as Fertility Fairness, carried out a survey of 980 patients to try to find out more about their experiences of fertility treatment [4]. The results clearly show the emotional impact of fertility problems. Respondents had experienced a wide range of negative emotions, including tearfulness, depression, isolation, anger, inadequacy, guilt, shame and loss of libido. More than half of those who reported very negative feelings had also experienced elation and excitement at times, reflecting the ups and downs of fertility treatment, often described as an 'emotional rollercoaster'. One in three said that their fertility problems had strained their relationship, and worryingly one-fifth of those who responded said that they had experienced suicidal feelings.

The NIAC survey found that feelings of depression and isolation were common to 94% of the fertility patients who responded to the survey. At Infertility Network UK, we regularly hear from patients that they feel lonely and cut off from their friends as a result of their fertility problems. As one female patient explains,

> When we started trying, just a few of our friends had children, but by the time we were doing the IVF everyone had them, and some people had more than one. It wasn't as bad for my husband, but I felt really excluded because all the other women were talking about things I didn't know about, and going to places you couldn't go without a baby [5].

For couples who find themselves unable to conceive, the world around them can appear completely family-orientated and they may feel that it is hard to escape reminders of what they cannot achieve. It can colour every aspect of life, as one female fertility patient explains:

> When I wasn't getting pregnant, I used to wake up and the first few seconds you think, "Oh it's a sunny day," and then all of a sudden the reality would hit you, "hang

on, I am still going through infertility." It was desperately painful and really depressing when everyone around you was pregnant and having babies [6].

Certain times of year such as Christmas, or family events like christenings, can become particularly difficult to deal with. Fertility patients may also put off doing things as they hope that they may be pregnant soon – so applying for a new job or promotion, going away or moving house may be delayed and as time goes on it can start to seem as if an entire life has been put on hold.

As the NIAC survey found, feelings of anger and frustration are a common response, with 84% of those who took part experiencing these emotions. Women often report that they find it difficult to deal with other people's pregnancies and pregnancy announcements, and may then struggle to reconcile the negative emotions pregnancy provokes. A female patient discusses her feelings of jealousy:

Every day I go to work in fear of an announcement about someone being pregnant. I really don't know how I am going to cope with it. I struggle seeing people in the street who are pregnant, I have to not even look at them. I feel like it's turning me into a really horrible person [6].

The sense of time passing can be particularly acute for women who are concerned about their biological clocks, and this is often exacerbated by the feeling that they are left waiting all the time – waiting for appointments, waiting for tests, waiting for results, waiting for treatment. This may add to the frustration, and couples can feel that they are on a conveyor belt and have lost control of their lives, as one female patient explains:

We'd done three cycles consecutively, and by the third one I was like another person... I felt as if I was sitting on the sidelines of my life watching it go by, with absolutely no control over anything. I couldn't play any part in it at all [7].

For some people, this may be the first time they have come up against what appears to be a totally insurmountable problem in their lives.

Infertility does still carry a sense of stigma, and it is easy to underestimate how important childbearing can become to the sense of self for those who are longing to start a family. Both women and men may start to feel that not being able to conceive means that they have somehow failed. The NIAC survey found that 72% of respondents had experienced feelings of inadequacy and 62% felt a sense of guilt or shame. One woman who had been through fourteen full

cycles of IVF treatment unsuccessfully said she was left feeling a complete failure:

Although my brain knows it's not my fault, my heart still says I have failed. I'm sure this is true for lots of women in the same situation. I know it's not true, and I know it's illogical, but a woman who can have children seems a better woman in some way than I am [7].

It is not just the emotional difficulties which couples face that can cause them problems, but more practical financial troubles too. Figures from the HFEA [2] show that just 41% of IVF cycles in the United Kingdom are funded by the National Health Service with the majority of couples paying for their own treatment. At Infertility Network UK, we regularly hear from couples who are borrowing money, building up credit card debt, remortgaging or selling their possessions to pay for treatment. There have even been some attempts to raise funds online following examples from the United States of crowdfunding for IVF [8].

Understanding how patients feel is important if you are to offer the best patient-centred care, and there are some key areas that can cause problems. One of the simplest ways that clinicians can make a difference is by helping to ensure that patients are fully informed about their fertility problems and about any treatment that may be offered to help. Although talking to a patient in a lay-friendly jargon-free manner during consultations is vital, absorbing so much new information can be difficult and it is important to back this up with good written information which people can take away to consider in more depth. Patient information evenings or days can be a helpful way to reinforce the points that you want to ensure patients have understood, and to give wider information about the services you offer.

The Internet is awash with fertility advice, and the best way to ensure that your patients do not get swamped by inaccurate information is to direct them towards reliable sources. You only need to take a brief look at any internet fertility forum to see that fertility patients are using them to ask questions about their fertility and treatments, and patients are offering one another all kinds of medical advice; a quick trawl can find patients advising on issues such as the best protocols for poor responders, dosages of drugs for IVF and whether others should have their levels of Natural Killer Cells tested. This is clearly far from ideal, and yet it happens because patients do not always feel able to access information elsewhere. The better the information they receive from the clinic, the less likely patients are to seek out other opinions elsewhere.

What can make it very difficult for patients is the fact that fertility specialists do not always seem to agree themselves on what is effective treatment. Patients today do not just need to negotiate a path through a treatment cycle but also need to make sense of the different information given by different experts in the field: should they pay extra for time-lapse, embryo glue, immunology testing, endometrial scratch, intralipids. . . ? The list of additions to standard treatment which could possibly boost their chances of success can appear endless, as one patient explains:

> The consultant said "You can decide what sort of treatment you want, these are the costs." It was like, here's the sweet shop and if you have some money, you can have what you like [6].

Getting a second opinion often brings a completely different point of view. For the fertility specialist, perhaps the key question is whether you genuinely believe that any additional treatments you are offering your patients will make a real difference to the outcome of their treatment.

The media is not always helpful to patients either, often focusing on miracle success stories or births to older celebrity mothers which can give a false idea of the chances of fertility treatment success. Anyone concerned about fertility is also bombarded with lifestyle advice about how to improve their fertility – eat more brussels sprouts [9], carrots [10] or raspberries [11], but do not touch bacon [12], use a mobile phone [13], a laptop [14] or get on a bike [15].

What links much of this advice is the suggestion that your fertility is in your own hands, and that you have the power to influence the outcome of your treatment – an idea which is promoted by many of the alternative, complementary or holistic therapists working in the field. Patients may be encouraged to 'take control' of their fertility, to rid themselves of negative thoughts that may be preventing them from conceiving and women are urged to 'visualise' themselves pregnant in order to ensure success. This kind of advice may be particularly attractive to those who have been told that they have unexplained infertility and have been searching for a cause you have failed to identify, but it can be corrosive when treatment does not work as it then leaves patients blaming themselves for an unsuccessful outcome.

There is a plethora of fertility coaches, holistic and complementary therapists pitching their support and advice to patients, and some fertility clinics now offer complementary therapies as part of treatment, with acupuncturists or perhaps hypnotherapists at hand. Patients may welcome this, but it does give credence to the idea that these therapies are evidence-based, and it can be hard for them to say no to additional complementary treatments, as one patient explains:

> We spent so much money, but you get to a stage where you are so desperate that you will try anything. Occasionally I do feel bitter about all the money we spent and all the time we wasted, but at least I can look back and think we tried everything [6].

One other issue that patients often raise is a lack of continuity in fertility treatment; they may find that they always see a different member of staff when they visit the clinic, and have a sense that no one really knows who they are or is keeping an overall track of their treatment. All too often we hear from patients about clinicians who have spent the first five minutes of their appointment time flicking through their notes to brief themselves, or who have asked the patient whether they have had certain tests or treatments; this does not breed confidence in patients for whom the idea of a mix-up in the clinic is a worst nightmare scenario. Spending a few minutes before a patient comes in familiarising yourself with who they are and where they are up to can make all the difference.

It is also important not to forget the stigma that patients can still feel. We know that many patients find it difficult to talk about their fertility problems, and so confidentiality in the clinic is vitally important. Leaving piles of notes with clearly visible names lying out on a desk can be a cause for concern for patients, and limiting the number of staff in the consulting room is something that they appreciate.

Sometimes in the rush to offer the best treatment, there can be a tendency to forget about *how* you offer it, and patients do sometimes feel that clinic staff are not as empathetic as they might be. Delivering bad news can be particularly tricky, but pausing for a moment to consider how it might feel to be on the receiving end of such news and how you would want to be dealt with if it were you may be helpful. No one will get it right all the time, but kindness and sensitivity are often underrated. From a patient perspective, it is the emotional aspects of going through a treatment cycle that can be particularly difficult, as one male patient explains:

> There's all this amazing medical support and yet, in order to do the medical stuff, emotionally you need the constitution of an ox. There's no emotional support [7].

Counselling can help here, but we know that IVF patients say that they are not always asked if they would like to access counselling services by staff at their clinics. When patients are told about counselling, many do not feel that they are made aware of the benefits it can offer. Some patients report that counselling is presented to them as something reserved for those who are unable to cope, when it may be better explained as proactively doing something to help yourself. Counselling is not for everyone, but offering it in a positive light is beneficial as patients may be better able to cope with the emotional ups and downs of a treatment cycle if they are receiving support.

It is worth encouraging patients to look into the support networks offered by the patient charities in the field. Support groups run by the charities offer a unique opportunity to meet other patients who are in similar positions and share emotional experiences, and many of the patient charities have informative websites which list other sources of support and advice.

Making a decision to stop treatment is not easy, and many of those who remain involuntarily childless report that they feel isolated and abandoned and that the clinic has no further interest in helping them once their treatment path has ended. Offering these patients access to a counsellor or referring them to other sources of support can be helpful as they often feel that they need more than they currently receive from their IVF units [16].

Getting patient-centred care right not only makes a huge difference to patients but should be important to clinicians too. Increasingly, performance is not judged solely on clinical success, but also on the patient experience. Contrary to expectations, patient praise is not reserved for clinics with beautiful facilities or those which are always ahead of the curve with the latest cutting-edge treatments – and it is not all about success either. This is what one patient had to say about a clinic where she had had two unsuccessful cycles:

> Sometimes they kept you waiting for hours, but when we did make appointments to see the consultant to discuss things there was so much time given, no sense of being rushed or being pushed out - it was very human, caring and supportive. They put a lot of effort into making things as friendly as possible for people and that makes it feel better [7].

Getting it right for every fertility patient is not an easy task, but by providing as much accurate information as you can, by pointing them in the right direction towards reliable sources of support and advice, by offering counselling and treating them with kindness, it is possible to make a real difference to the experience of what is always going to be a difficult time in a patient's life. What really matters to patients is feeling that a clinic has their best interests at heart, and that is something that everyone can aspire to.

References

(1) A Long Term Analysis of the Human Fertilisation and Embryology Authority Register Data (1991–2006) - HFEA

(2) HFEA Fertility Trends and Figures 2013 - HFEA

(3) L. Schmidt, B. E. Holstein, J. Boivin, H. Sångren and T. Tjørnhøj. Patients' attitudes to medical and psychosocial aspects of care in fertility clinics: findings from the Copenhagen Multi-centre Psychosocial Infertility (COMPI) Research Programme. *Hum. Reprod.* (2003) 18 (3): 628–63.

(4) J. Kerr, C. Brown and A. H. Balen. The experiences of couples who have had infertility treatment in the United Kingdom: results of a survey performed in 1997. *Hum. Reprod.* (1999) 14 (4): 934–8

(5) K. Brian. *The Complete Guide to IVF* (Piatkus, 2009, 2010)

(6) K. Brian. *The Complete Guide to Female Fertility* (Piatkus, 2007, 2010)

(7) K. Brian. *In Pursuit of Parenthood* (Bloomsbury, 1998)

(8) www.mirror.co.uk/news/uk-news/desperate-ivf-couple-crowd-fund-treatment-5178858

(9) www.dailymail.co.uk/health/article-2518129/Eating-Brussels-sprouts-helps-boost-fertility-men-women.html

(10) www.nydailynews.com/life-style/health/carrots-boost-male-fertility-study-article-1.1504019

(11) www.dailymail.co.uk/health/article-2401803/Fertility-How-eating-raspberries-increase-chances-father.html

(12) www.dailymail.co.uk/health/article-2460072/Bacon-harm-mans-fertility.html

(13) www.dailymail.co.uk/news/article-412179/Men-use-mobile-phones-face-increased-risk-infertility.html

(14) http://news.bbc.co.uk/1/hi/ 4078895.stm

(15) www.dailymail.co.uk/health/ article-1337520/Cycling-just-hours-week-damage-mans-fertility.html

(16) V. L. Peddie, E. van Teijlingen and S. Bhattacharya. A qualitative study of women's decision-making at the end of IVF treatment. *Hum. Reprod.* (2005) 20 (7): 1944–51.

Epidemiology of Infertility
An Introduction

Madelon van Wely

1 Prevalence/Incidence of Infertility

Infertility is defined by WHO-ICMART as a disease of the reproductive system defined as the failure to achieve a clinical pregnancy after 12 of more months of regular unprotected sexual intercourse. As all women lose their ability to conceive with age, this definition only holds within the womens' reproductive age-span between the menarche and menopause. On average the woman's fertility is highest in the early and mid-twenties, then slowly declines and drops even faster at 35 years and older.

According to a Scottish study, nearly 20% of couples within their reproductive lifespan failed to conceive within 12 months and 12% failed to conceive within 24 months [1]. A Spanish cross-sectional study found that pregnancy was not achieved within 6, 12 and 24 months of starting to attempt conception in 20%, 11% and 4.4% of women, respectively [2].

Couples that did conceive in the end were apparently not really infertile. In view of the reduced fertility with prolonged time of unwanted non-conception, these couples can better be referred to as subfertile [3].

Couples can most likely be considered infertile when failing to conceive within five years. A worldwide systematic review and meta-analysis concluded that within a period of five years, 1.9% of women aged 20–44 years who wanted to have children were unable to have their first live birth (primary infertility), and 10.5% of women with a previous live birth were unable to have an additional live birth (secondary infertility) [4]. This study found that levels of infertility did not change significantly between 1990 and 2010.

2 You Are Planning to Do a Fertility Study

If you are planning a study in the field of fertility or any other research field, you first need a clear-cut research question. The FINER criteria of Hull and co-authors can help here [5]. Is your study question or aim Feasible, Interesting, Novel, Ethical and Relevant? Does it include a clear-cut outcome? If yes, proceed with your proposal and think with what design your question can most likely be answered. According to the hierarchy of evidence, the most reliable evidence comes from randomised clinical trials, followed by cohorts, case-control studies, cross-sectional studies and case studies.

3 Study Design

Cohorts, cross-sectional and case-control studies have observational designs. Case-control and cross-sectional studies are retrospective in nature, meaning that the study looks backward, that is, data are based on events that have already happened. Cohort studies can also be prospective, meaning that the data was collected from the time point at the start of the cohort on until a certain period of time. A prospective study watches for outcomes, such as the development of a disease, during the study period and relates this to other factors such as suspected risk or protection factors.

For all these observational studies, all efforts should be made to avoid sources of bias such as the loss of individuals to follow up during the study. For retrospective studies, bias and confounding can never be completely controlled for as the database was not specifically made for your question.

Both cohorts and case-control studies can be used to evaluate risk factors and diagnostic tests. Though a cohort is generally a better design than a case-control, for cohorts the outcome of interest should be common; otherwise, the number of outcomes observed will be too small to be statistically meaningful. When the events under study are rare, a case-control study is the better alternative. Cross-sectional studies take a sample of the population (the cross-section) at one time point. This design is well set to determine prevalence and can be used to study associations when development over time is less important. Cross-sectional studies are relatively quick and easy.

A recently published example of a retrospective cohort evaluated the association between vanishing twin syndrome (VTS) and adverse perinatal outcome in 253,000 singleton deliveries [6]. Though statistical analysis included multiple logistic regression models to control for possible confounders, the study was retrospective, that is, data were not collected for this specific question. We will not be sure whether VTS was more often diagnosed in the more complicated pregnancies and more often missed in uncomplicated pregnancies. This is a typical association study. The observed association between VTS and adverse perinatal outcome does not imply that there is a causal relationship.

An example of a case-control study is a recently published study that evaluated whether in a group of women with heart disease (cases) and in healthy women (controls) the second pregnancy was less complicated and resulted in a larger baby [7]. As such cases will be less common, the case-control design is likely to be the most feasible option here.

Observational studies do not try to influence anything but just measure what happened; there is no intervention by the researcher. As a result observational studies never provide information on causation but only on a possible association. In experimental studies, like a controlled clinical trial, the researcher intervenes to change something (e.g., gives some patients a drug) and then observes what happens. As the variables under study are controlled for, we can make conclusions on causation. To evaluate the effectiveness of a new intervention the experimental design needs to be used. A cohort study will not be able to detect a direct relationship between the intervention and treatment success.

For scientific evaluation of treatment, the randomised clinical trial (RCT) is widely accepted as the gold standard. Data from clinical trials are considered to represent the highest level of evidence that can be used to inform about the effectiveness of treatment strategies. The parallel design is the commonest trial design, involving a comparison between two groups, an experimental versus a control group. As this type of trial is the most easily understood by researchers as well as patients, this is the simplest trial design and a lot of examples in fertility, obstetrics and gynaecological research can be given. A trial normally has two arms, one intervention arm and a control

arm. Occasionally a trial may have three arms, for example, aspirin + low molecular weight heparin (LMWH) versus aspirin versus placebo for the treatment of unexplained recurrent pregnancy loss (RPL) [8] or in vitro fertilisation (IVF)–single embryo transfer (SET) versus IVF in a modified cycle versus intrauterine insemination (IUI) in women with unexplained subfertility [9].

There is a great need for well-performed trials in all areas of clinical medicine. With the results of these trials clinicians will be able to make better and more evidence-based decisions about diagnostics and treatment of their patients. 'Evidenced-based medicine' (EBM), defined in 1992 by Gyatt as 'the integration of individual clinical expertise with the best available external evidence from systematic research', is considered the cornerstone of decision-making in current clinical medicine [5].

To make a randomised trial feasible and to increase the quality, issues like recruitment, loss-to-follow-up, power/sample size, randomisation methods, data-collection, statistics and ethics need to have been adequately addressed before starting the trial. Doing a randomised study has costs. It is advisable to work together with other clinical centres as multicentre trials are generally more successfully completed.

4 Presenting and Interpreting the Outcome

4.1 Presenting the Outcome

Both clinician and statistician want to summarise and represent their data as simply as possible. In choosing our effect measure, we require an estimate of risk that is generalisable to a wide variety of circumstances. So, for instance, one might choose a measure because it can be shown to be applicable to patients at different underlying baseline risk; or one might find in a meta-analysis that the measure is approximately constant across different studies.

Let us limit our attention to situations where we wish to summarise the difference between two groups with respect to a binary outcome like occurrence of ovarian hyperstimulation syndrome (OHSS) and pregnancy or live birth. These will have the event rates P_1 and P_2. Imagine a clinical trial with a treated and a control group, with a live birth as the primary outcome. We then decide that P_1 represents the proportion of live births in the treated group and

P_2 represents the proportion of live births in the control group.

The most frequently used effect measures with binary data of this type are as follows:

Risk difference = RD = $P_1 - P_2$

Relative risk = RR = P_1 / P_2

Odds ratio = OR = Odds in group 1 / odds in group 2 = $(P_1/1 - P_1) / (P_2/1 - P_2)$

Number needed to treat = NNT = $1 / (P_1 - P_2)$.

As an example, suppose the live birth rates are $P_1 = 0.4$ and $P_2 = 0.3$ in the treated and control groups, respectively. Then we have the following:

RD = $0.4 - 0.3 = 0.1$;

RR = $0.4 / 0.3 = 1.33$;

OR = $(0.4 / 0.6) / (0.3 / 0.7) = 1.56$;

NNT = $1 / (0.4 - 0.3) = 10$.

Though NNT provides no additional information beyond the RD, while NNT is equal to the reciprocal of RD, it is clinically a very useful effect measure. NNT is a measure of the clinical effort required in order to achieve one additional beneficial outcome in a series of patients.

In randomised or comparative studies, when the outcomes are binary or dichotomous, the clinical effect of a specific treatment is most often reported using both the absolute risk reduction (ARR) and NNT.

Various other strengths and weaknesses pertain to the various effect measures. While RD and RR enjoy greater ease of interpretation, OR has several statistical advantages. For instance, models of constant RR or constant RD can predict risks greater than 100% or less than 0. Such impossible event rates cannot occur if the model is based on OR.

The conclusions from an analysis based on RR can be profoundly influenced by the arbitrary choice of whether risk is expressed in terms of the 'positive' event (e.g., survival) or its 'negative' complement (e.g., death). This problem is avoided with RD or OR. On the other hand the RD is only valid compared to a specific control rate.

For diagnostic studies, case-control studies, studies requiring regression analyses, and when outcomes have more than two levels the OR is the best effect measure.

We should all recognise that measures of risk such as RR and OR are inherently different, and therefore

numerical differences between them should not be surprising. The RR and the OR are comparable only when events are rare. In the field of fertility we usually work with common events like the occurrence of a pregnancy. Do not interpret the OR as if it represents an RR [10]. If necessary, an estimate of the RR can be calculated from the OR.

4.2 Interpreting the Outcome

The findings of a single study, even a well-powered, well-performed trial, should not be considered adequate evidence. There are several examples of subjects where multiple studies had been done and where findings differed. Primarily the results pointed to superiority of one treatment but after even more RCTs no differences were left. To summarise all evidence usually a systematic review and meta-analysis is done.

4.3 Epidemiology of Treatment

IVF was originally developed for women whose tubes were blocked and intracytoplasmic sperm injection (ICSI) was developed for male infertility. These treatments are understandable and are biologically plausible as otherwise these infertile couples will never conceive. The same accounts for women who do no ovulate; ovulation can be induced in these women. But what about the couples with unexplained subfertility, endometriosis and unilateral blocked tube? We all know these couples do have a high chance to conceive naturally. Still these couples are being treated with IUI, IVF and/or ICSI nowadays and largely explain the continuing expansion of the number of ART treatment cycles recorded by European and North American ART registries. We often assume that treatment is better than not offering treatment and we assume that this is what couples want us to do. There is, however, no evidence that these treatments will increase the chance of conception compared to a natural pregnancy. If there is no evidence that treatment helps to improve chances we should not treat.

Prognostic models could help out here. If we can distinguish between couples that benefit from fertility treatment and those that are likely to conceive naturally this can help to offer the best care. The first models look promising – the model of Hunault predicting chance to conceive naturally, is actually being used in the Netherlands. The disadvantage of this model is that it is static. The future in this field lies in dynamic models. These models are able to predict chances over time. If we manage to cooperate, exchange databases and optimise our statistical methods, I believe it will be possible to create models that will help us all.

References

1. Bhattacharya S, Porter M, Amalraj E, Templeton A, Hamilton M, Lee AJ, Kurinczuk JJ. The epidemiology of infertility in the North East of Scotland. *Hum Reprod.* 2009 Dec;24(12): 3096–107.

2. Cabrera-León A, Lopez-Villaverde V, Rueda M, Moya-Garrido MN. Calibrated prevalence of infertility in 30- to 49-year-old women according to different approaches: a cross-sectional population-based study. *Hum Reprod.* 2015 Sep 14. [Epub ahead of print]

3. Gnoth C, Godehardt E, Frank-Herrmann P, Friol K, Tigges J, Freundl G. Definition and prevalence of subfertility and infertility. *Hum Reprod.* 2005 May;20(5):1144–7.

4. Mascarenhas MN, Flaxman SR, Boerma T, Vanderpoel S, Stevens GA. National, regional, and global trends in infertility prevalence since 1990: a systematic analysis of 277 health surveys. *PLoS Med.* 2012;9(12):e1001356.

5. Hulley S, Cummings S, Browner W, Grady, D.; Newman, l. *Designing clinical research.* 3rd edn. Philadelphia (PA): Lippincott Williams & Wilkins; 2007.

6. Evron E, Sheiner E, Friger M, Sergienko R, Harlev A. Vanishing twin syndrome: is it associated with adverse perinatal outcome? *Fertil Steril.* 2015;103(5):1209–14.

7. Gelson E, Curry R, Gatzoulis MA, Swan L, Lupton M, Steer PJ, Johnson MR. Maternal cardiac and obstetric performance in consecutive pregnancies in women with heart disease. *BJOG.* 2015 Oct;122(11):1552–9.

8. Kaandorp, S.P., et al., Aspirin plus heparin or aspirin alone in women with recurrent miscarriage. *N Engl J Med.* 2010;362(17):1586–96.

9. Bensdorp AJ, Tjon-Kon-Fat RI, Bossuyt PM, Koks CA, Oosterhuis GJ, Hoek A, Hompes PG, Broekmans FJ, Verhoeve HR, de Bruin JP, van Golde R, Repping S, Cohlen, BJ, Lambers MD, van Bommel PF, Slappendel E, Perquin D, Smeenk JM, Pelinck MJ, Gianotten J, Hoozemans DA, Maas JW, Eijkemans MJ, van der Veen F, Mol BW, van Wely M. Prevention of multiple pregnancies in couples with unexplained or mild male subfertility: randomised controlled trial of in vitro fertilisation with single embryo transfer or in vitro fertilisation in modified natural cycle compared with intrauterine insemination with controlled ovarian hyperstimulation. *BMJ.* 2015;350:7771.

10. Knol MJ, Duijnhoven RG, Grobbee DE, Moons KGM, Groenwold RHH. Potential misinterpretation of treatment effects due to use of odds ratios and logistic regression in randomized controlled trials. *PLoS One.* 2011;6(6):e21248.

Investigation of Male Infertility

Arie Parnham
Asif Muneer

1 Introduction

Male factor infertility is a contributory factor for approximately 50% of couples that present seeking investigation and treatment for infertility, either in isolation (25%) or in combination with a female factor (25%) [1]. Therefore an accurate and complete investigation of the male partner is essential in assessing all couples with infertility. A significant number of male factors are either reversible or amenable to treatment provided that an accurate assessment and diagnosis is made.

The aims of evaluation, some of which are also mentioned in the American Urological Association (AUA) guidelines are to correctly identify the following:

- Potentially reversible conditions contributing to male infertility either due to obstruction within the reproductive tract or treatment of endocrinopathies
- Irreversible conditions amenable to assisted reproductive techniques using the sperm of the male partner
- Irreversible conditions that are not open to the above, and for which donor insemination or adoption are possible options
- Life- or health-threatening conditions that may underlie the infertility and require medical attention
- Genetic abnormalities that may affect the health of offspring if assisted reproductive techniques are to be employed [2].

2 Definitions

Male factor infertility has a number of definitions, which to the casual or novice investigator can be both confusing and novel. It is important however to have a firm understanding of each term as this underpins the subsequent categorisation of patients and management. Table 3.1 lists common terms employed and their definitions:

3 Causes of Male Factor Infertility

When considering the investigations for male factor infertility it is imperative to have a clear understanding of the potential underlying causes. The causes of male infertility can be broadly categorised as follows:

- Idiopathic
- Congenital or acquired urogenital abnormalities
- Malignancies
- Urogenital infections
- Abberations that impair temperature control such as varicocele
- Endocrine dysfunction
- Genetic abnormalities
- Immunological factors [4].

Idiopathic male infertility is the most commonly found cause with abnormal semen parameters (30–40%). Table 3.2 provides an overview of the frequency of individual disorders as they may occur in a large fertility centre.

4 Timing of Investigation

It is generally agreed that patients should be referred for further investigations if they meet the definition for infertility as defined earlier. However a number of national bodies, including the National Institute of Clinical Excellence (NICE) and the AUA, agree that there are certain circumstances where this can be circumvented. Such circumstances include the following: 1) female partner 36 years old and over; 2) a known clinical cause of infertility or a history of predisposing factors; 3) where treatment is planned that may result in infertility (for example therapy for malignancy); 4) where the couple or individuals question their fertility potential including even in the absence of a partner (AUA only) [2, 7].

Table 3.1 Common terms and definitions based on the WHO 5th edition laboratory manual in 2010[3–5]

Term	Definition
Infertility	Infertility is the inability of a sexually active, non-contracepting couple to achieve spontaneous pregnancy within one year
Primary infertility	When a woman is unable to ever bear a child, either due to the inability to become pregnant or the inability to carry a pregnancy to a live birth, she would be classified as having primary infertility. Thus women whose pregnancy miscarries or whose pregnancy results in a stillborn child, without ever having had a live birth, would present with primary infertility.
Secondary infertility	A woman who is unable to bear a child, either due to the inability to become pregnant or due to the inability to carry a pregnancy to a live birth (following either a previous pregnancy or a previous ability to carry a pregnancy to a live birth) would be classified as having secondary infertility. Therefore those who repeatedly spontaneously miscarry or whose pregnancy results in a stillbirth, or following a previous pregnancy or a previous ability to do so, are then not unable to carry a pregnancy to a live birth would present with secondary infertility. This definition depends on the birth of the first child not involving any assisted reproductive technologies or fertility medications.
Oligozoospermia	$<15x10^6$ spermatozoa per milliliter
Severe Oligozoospermia	$<5x10^6$ spermatozoa per milliliter
Azoospermia	no spermatozoa in the ejaculate (given as the limit of quantification for the assessment method employed)
Asthenozoospermia	$<32\%$ sperm progressively motile
Teratozoospermia	$<4\%$ normal forms on morphology

Table 3.2 [6] Percentage distribution of diagnoses of 12,945 patients attending the Institute of Reproductive Medicine of the University of Munster based on the clinical databank Androbase®. 1,446(=11.2%) of these patients were azoospermic. In the event of several diseases, only the leading diagnosis was included

Diagnosis	Unselected patients N=12,945	Azoospermic patients N=1,446
All	**100%**	**11.2%**
Infertility of (known) possible cause	**42.6%**	**42.6%**
Maldescended testes (current/former)	8.4	17.2
Varicocele	14.8	10.9
Infection	9.3	10.5
Autoantibodies against sperm	3.9	–
Testicular tumour	1.2	2.8
Idiopathic infertility	**30.0**	**13.3**
Hypogonadism	**10.1**	**16.4**
Klinefelter syndrome (47, XXY)	2.6	13.7
XX-male	0.1	0.6
Primary hypogonadism of unknown cause	2.3	0.8
Secondary (hypogonadotrophic) hypogonadism	1.6	1.9
Kallmann syndrome	0.3	0.5

Table 3.2 (cont.)

Diagnosis	Unselected patients N=12,945	Azoospermic patients N=1,446
Idiopathic hypogonadotrophic hypogonadism	*0.4*	*0.4*
Residual after pituitary surgery	*<0.1*	*0.3*
Others	*0.8*	*0.8*
Late onset hypogonadism	*2.2*	*-*
Constitutional delay of puberty	*1.4*	*-*
General systemic disease	**2.2**	**0.5**
Cryopreservation due to malignant disease	**7.8**	**12.5**
Testicular tumour	*5.0*	*4.3*
Lymphoma	*1.5*	*4.6*
Leukaemia	*0.7*	*2.2*
Sarcoma	*0.6*	*0.9*
Disturbances of erection/ejaculation	**2.4**	**-**
Obstruction	**2.2**	**10.3**
Vasectomy	*0.9*	*5.3*
Cystic fibrosis, CBAVD	*0.5*	*3.1*
Others	*0.8*	*1.9*
Gynaecomastia	**1.5**	*0.2*
Y-Chromosomal deletion	**0.3**	**1.6**
Other Chromosomal abberations	**0.2**	**1.3**
Translocations	*0.1*	*0.3*
Others	*<0.1*	*0.3*
Others	**0.7**	**1.3**

5 History and Examination

5.1 History

A thorough history should be taken and should specifically include the following.

5.1.1 Reproductive History

The duration, frequency, timing and success of attempted conception should be noted along with conceptions with previous partners to allow correct characterisation of the infertility and whether or not they meet the definition given earlier. The clinician should attempt to categorise whether the patient or couple is suffering from primary or secondary infertility as this will determine the investigations required

and future options for fertility treatment (See definitions in Table 3.1).

5.1.2 Sexual History

Issues around sexual dysfunction should be explored thoroughly and include erectile dysfunction, premature ejaculation, penile curvature (Peyronie's disease or congenital curvature), changes in libido and orgasmic/ejaculatory function.

The use of contraception and lubricants should be identified as some have been identified as affecting sperm quality [8].

A thorough history should include previous sexually transmitted diseases (STDs) if any and their treatment.

5.1.3 Current General Health

Acute illness can have a profound effect on male fertility and sperm parameters. However, sperm parameters at the time of illness can be normal and only deteriorate several weeks later since the normal human spermatogenesis cycle is 64 days + 5–10 days for epididymal sperm transit.

Symptoms such as headaches, galactorrhea or impairment of the visual fields may be indicative of pituitary lesions.

5.1.4 Childhood Illnesses and Developmental Issues

A number of illnesses in childhood can affect fertility and a careful history combined with examination should identify these patients.

There is ongoing controversy regarding the relevance of a childhood history of unilateral undescended testis (UDT), as, despite having impaired semen parameters in adulthood, the paternity rate of such men is the same as that of men with bilateral descended testes. The same, however, cannot be said for those with bilateral undescended testes [9, 10].

Mumps orchitis, testicular torsion and inguinal surgery are also risk factors for male factor infertility and should be considered in the differential diagnosis.

The onset or delay of puberty can also suggest an endocrinological or genetic basis for male infertility.

5.1.5 Past Medical and Surgical History

Previous genitourinary infections including orchitis, epididymitis, prostatitis or sexually transmitted diseases should be investigated. Post pubertal infection with mumps when associated with orchitis increases the likelihood of male infertility.

Chronic medical conditions can also be associated with infertility. Patients with chronic renal disease diabetes and multiple sclerosis may be infertile and have a higher incidence of erectile dysfunction.

5.1.6 Medications

A number of medications are known to affect fertility and a selection of the common ones is listed in Table 3.3.

5.1.7 Family History

This is covered later in Section 7.3.

Table 3.3 Medications and their effects on male fertility (data from [11])

Class of medication	Effect on male fertility	Example
Alpha-blockers	Ejaculatory dysfunction	Tamsulosin Alfuzosin
Anabolic steroids	Hypogonadism	
Androgens	Inhibited spermatogenesis	Testosterone
Anti-inflammatory	Impaired spermatogenesis	Sulfasalazine
Antiandrogens	Reduced erectile function Reduced libido Suppression of gonadotrophin secretion	Cyproterone Acetate
Antibiotics, antimycotics	Impaired spermatogenesis Hypogonadism	Tetracycline, Chloroquine, Erythromycin, Co-Trimoxazole Gentamicin Ketoconazole
Antidepressants	Effects on spermatogenesis and motility	Imipramine
Antiepileptics	Hypogonadism Effects on spermatogenesis	Carbamazepine Sodium Valporate
Beta blockers	Erectile dysfunction Inhibit sperm motility	Propanolol
Calcium channel blockers	Inhibit sperm motility Inhibit acrosome reaction	Nifedipine Verapamil

Table 3.3 (*cont.*)

Class of medication	Effect on male fertility	Example
Chemotherapy	Impaired spermatogenesis Hypogenadism	Alkylinating agents (Cyclophosphamide) Cisplatin
Dopamine receptor antagonist	Hyperprolactinaemia	Metoclopramide
Gonadotrophin releasing hormone	Hypogonadism	
Histamine receptor blockers	Gonadotoxic Centrally acting effect on reproductive hormones	Cimetidine Ranitidine
Immunosuppressants	Impaired spermatogenesis Hypogonadism Reduced motility	Cyclosporin A Tacrolimus
Opiates	Hypogonadism	Morphine
Retinoid	Impaired spermatogenesis	Isotretinoin

6 Examination

6.1 General Examination

An assessment of the patient's general condition should be documented. Fat distribution, presence of gynaecomastia and hair patterns may be related to underlying hormonal or metabolic abnormalities. Klinefelter's syndrome should be considered in patients who are tall with gynaecomastia and bilateral low volume testes, however they may be phenotypically normal apart from the small volume testicles.

6.2 Genital Examination

This should include both an examination of the penis and scrotum including the scrotal contents.

The penile length should be assessed by measuring the stretched penile length from the symphysis pubis to the coronal sulcus or meatus. A small penis and testes can be a sign of Kallmann's syndrome. Any plaques that may represent Peyronie's disease should be identified and documented as this may cause issues with penetrative intercourse and erectile dysfunction. The urethral meatus should be examined to check for meatal stenosis or hypospadias and the foreskin checked to see if it is easily retractile or if it is phimotic.

The scrotum should be examined in a warm environment and in both the lying and standing positions.

The clinician should proceed in a logical manner starting on one side and completing the examination of one hemiscrotum before moving to the contralateral side. Each structure should be identified and described as below.

6.2.1 Testes

The testes should be examined individually. Two hands should be used with the thumb and forefinger of each being used to isolate and roll over the surface of the testis. Comment should be made on the size, which can be formally assessed using either an orchidometer or callipers. Any masses should be noted as well as the consistency of the testes.

6.2.2 Epididymis

The epididymis should be palpated in a similar manner to the testicles. Dilatation of the epididymis may suggest obstruction, inflammation or infection.

6.2.3 Vas Deferens

The vas deferens should be identified and palpated along its length within the scrotum. A defect in the vas should be palpable after a vasectomy or the vas may be completely absent either unilaterally or bilaterally. Absence of the vas is usually associated with a genetic mutation. Unilateral absence of the vas is associated with an ipsilateral absent kidney whereas bilateral absent vasa, CBAVD (Congenital Bilateral Absence of Vas Deferens) is associated with mutations in the Cystic Fibrosis Transmembrane Regulator gene (CFTR).

6.2.4 Other Cord Structures

The rest of the cord should be examined separately. This should be performed lying and then standing so as to allow comparison and identification of varicoceles.

Large varicoceles are typically described as feeling like a 'bag of worms'; however, they can be more subtle and supplementary manoeuvres such as a Valsalva manoeuvre can be performed to help engorge the incompetent veins within the pampiniform plexus. They typically occur on the left due to the acute insertion of the left gonadal vein into the renal vein. It is therefore worth mentioning out of turn that patients with a left-sided varicocele should undergo ultrasound examination of their abdomen and retroperitoneum as a retroperitoneal process could obstruct the insertion of the gonadal vein (for example a retroperitoneal or renal mass with thrombus).

The grading of varicoceles is shown in Table 3.4.

6.3 Rectal Examination

A rectal examination is selectively used in the evaluation of the infertile male based on the history and clinical examination. The size, symmetry and consistency of the prostate should be assessed. Mildine and Mullerian duct cysts are not usually palpable but can be associated with obstructive azoospermia or severe oligospermia. However, a tender prostate may indicate ongoing prostatitis and enlarged seminal vesicles may indicate obstructive azoospermia or TB.

7 Diagnostic Evaluation

The initial evaluation of the male partner presenting with infertility involves the following:

1. Performing a semen analysis
2. Performing a biochemical assessment of the hypothalamic-pituitary-gonadal axis (HPG) to exclude an underlying endocrinopathy and primary testicular failure

The results of these two investigations will guide subsequent investigation when combined with the clinical history and findings.

7.1 Semen Analysis

The mainstay of initial assessment is a semen analysis. The number of semen analyses that should be performed varies upon different guideline recommendations. The European Association of Urology (EAU) recommend that one semen analysis is sufficient if the sperm parameters are within the normal range and a repeat test should be performed if the test is abnormal. The AUA and NICE recommend two samples. The time separation between the two samples again varies with the AUA recommending at least one month and NICE 3 months if normal and earlier if an abnormality is detected; the rationale for the time separation being that sperm quality varies daily and the normal sperm cycle is 64 +5–10 days.

It is important that the patient is instructed on how to perform and deliver a semen sample.

The semen should be collected 'fresh' through masturbation after 3–4 days abstinence as evidence suggests that the semen volume and parameters can vary depending on the frequency of emission. The sample should be produced preferably on-site at the laboratory to allow prompt analysis but if this is not possible then a sample can be delivered within one hour in order to prevent and reduce secondary abnormalities. All components of the ejaculate should be collected including the pre-ejaculate and thus collection through coitus interruptus is not recommended. Patients can be advised to keep the sterile container in their shirt pocket to mimic the scrotal temperature. It

Table 3.4 Grading of varicoceles[12]

Grading	Description
0 (subclinical)	Not palpable or visible at rest or during valsalva. Demonstrated on Doppler Ultrasound studies.
I	Palpable on valsalva only
II	Palpable at rest but not visible
III	Palpable and visible at rest

is also possible to collect the semen sample using specially designed condoms that have no spermicidal qualities.

The semen sample should be analysed by an accredited laboratory to ensure standardisation of measurement and reporting. The WHO laboratory manual for the examination of human semen and sperm-cervical mucus interaction is the standard for such analysis [3]. The 'normal' values were revised by the WHO in the 5th edition laboratory manual in 2010. The new values changed from the previous reference ranges as for the first time semen analyses were included from multiple countries. Prior to this latest update, reference values were based on the experience of investigators who had studied healthy men with an unknown time to pregnancy (TTP).

For the current guidelines, data was collected on 1953 semen samples across 7 countries and 3 continents [5, 13–17]. Data was only collected from labs that used the standardised WHO methods of semen analysis and patients that had a TTP of less than 12 months. Time to pregnancy was defined as the number of months (or cycles) from stopping contraception to achieving pregnancy [3]. The reference values are based on the 5th centile.

Interestingly the new values compared to previous iterations would suggest a decline in global male fertility, although this could be a function of improved quality control of laboratory analysis and the difference in the type and quality of data previously alluded to.

The analysis of the semen sample, as in pathology, involves a macroscopic and microscopic assessment.

Macroscopically the semen sample should be assessed for liquefaction, appearance, viscosity, volume and pH (normal values are given in Table 3.5).

Semen should liquefy within 60 minutes to a homogenous grey opalescent colour.

Table 3.5 Percentage contribution of different areas of male reproductive tract to total semen volume

Location	Percentage contribution
Testes	2–5%
Seminal vesicle	65–75%
Prostate	25–30%
Bulbourethral glands	<1%

The importance or relevance of viscosity is unconfirmed. It is tested by drawing up a sample of semen into a 1.5 mm pipette. The semen is then allowed to drop from the pipette and the thread measured. A length greater than 2 cm is considered as abnormally viscous.

The normal semen volume is >1.5 mls. A low volume may indicate either an obstruction at the level of the ejaculatory ducts or retrograde ejaculation. A post ejaculatory urine sample can be submitted to look for sperm in cases where retrograde ejaculation is suspected and the vasa are palpable. A volume consistently less than 1 ml requires further investigation using a transrectal ultrasound to investigate whether ejaculatory duct obstruction is present.

The pH of the semen sample should be greater than 7.2. It is worth considering that different parts of the male reproductive tract contribute varying amounts to the ejaculate and the overall acidity or alkalinity (see Table 3.5). The vast majority of the semen volume derives from secretions from the seminal vesicles and prostate. The pH of the prostatic secretions is generally acidic whilst the seminal vesicle secretions are alkaline due to the presence of fructose. Therefore, in cases where the semen pH and volume are low, the level of obstruction is likely to be at the ejaculatory duct either due to ejaculatory duct obstruction or absent or atrophic seminal vesicles such as is associated with CBAVD.

Microscopic assessment of semen is performed under a light microscope using a wet prep. The semen is assessed for the parameters detailed in Table 3.6.'

7.1.1 Total Sperm Count and Concentration

The total sperm count and concentration correlate well with TTP and pregnancy rates [18].

7.1.2 Total Motility

Sperm are classified as being either motile or immotile. Those sperm deemed motile can be further characterised as progressive (i.e., moving in a linear direction or large circle) or non-progressive.

In Kallmann's syndrome and necrospermia (see vitality) complete immotility can be a common finding.

7.1.3 Vitality

Vitality is the measure of the sperm intact membrane. It is expressed as a percentage and, as referred to earlier, is important in assessing immotile sperm to diagnose necrospermia.

7.1.4 Morphology

The morphology of sperm is a subjective assessment. A number of classifications exist; however the most commonly used are the Kruger and WHO criteria.

7.1.5 Leucocytes

The presence of more than 106 leucocytes per ml may indicate a genitourinary tract infection. Consequently the patient should be appropriately screened for a urinary tract infection (including prostatitis) or an undiagnosed sexually transmitted disease.

7.1.6 Anti-sperm Antibodies (ASA)

Under normal circumstances the seminiferous tubules are immunologically isolated from the body's immune surveillance. Consequently there should be no anti-sperm antibodies (ASA). However, the immune privileged status can be compromised by obstruction, surgery, trauma, undescended testes, infection and varicoceles resulting in the presence of IgG and IgA in the serum, seminal plasma or bound to the spermatozoa. The creation of anti-sperm antibodies can lead to reduced motility and agglutination as well as death of the spermatozoa. The relevance of ASA in serum is undefined and many investigators have suggested that it is the presence of ASA attached to the spermatozoa which accounts for the infertility. A number of assays exist including the following:

- Gelatin agglutination test (GAT)
- Tray agglutination test (TAT) – detects antibodies in patients serum or seminal plasma
- The mixed anti-globulin reaction (MAR test) – detects antibodies on patients spermatozoa

Table 3.6 WHO lower reference limits (5th centiles and their 95% confidence intervals) for semen characteristics [3]

Parameter	Lower reference limit
Semen volume (ml)	1.5 (1.4–1.7)
Total sperm number (10^6 per ejaculate)	39 (33–46)
Sperm concentration (10^6 per ml)	15 (12–16)
Total motility (PR+NP, %)	40 (38–42)
Progressive motility (PR, %)	32 (31–34)
Vitality (live spermatozoa, %)	58 (55–63)
Sperm morphology (normal forms, %)	4 (3.0–4.0)
Other consensus threshold values	
pH	≥ 7.2
Peroxidase-positive leukocytes (10^6 per ml)	<1.0
MAR test (Motile spermatozoa with bound particles, %)	<50
Immunobead test (motile spermatozoa with bound beads, %)	<50
Seminal zinc (µmol/ejaculate)	$\geq$**2.4**
Seminal fructose (µmol/ejaculate)	$\geq$**13**
Seminal neutral glucosidase (mU/ejaculate)	$\geq$**20**

7.2 Biochemical Assessment of the Hypothalamic-Pituitary-Gonadal (HPG) Axis

Biochemical assessment of the HPG should be performed when the semen parameters are found to be abnormal. Typically this comprises an early morning testosterone concentration, follicle stimulating hormone (FSH) and luteinising hormone (LH) concentrations and prolactin.

It is important to understand the underlying pathophysiology of the HPG axis so as to allow correct identification of any abnormalities. (See Figure 3.1)

Spermatogenesis and production of testosterone is controlled by the anterior pituitary gland, which secretes both LH and FSH in a pulsatile fashion in response to gonadotrophin- releasing hormone (GnRH). GnRH is synthesised in neurosecretory neurons in the median eminence of the hypothalamus and released into the hypophyseal portal system.

FSH promotes spermatogenesis by binding to specific FSH receptors on the Sertoli cells. LH stimulates testosterone production from Leydig cells. Both LH and FSH indirectly and directly maintain normal spermatogenesis. Testosterone directly inhibits the production of FSH and LH through negative feedback on both the hypothalamus and the pituitary gland. Sertoli cells also produce a substance called inhibin (a glycoprotein), which negatively influences the production of FSH.

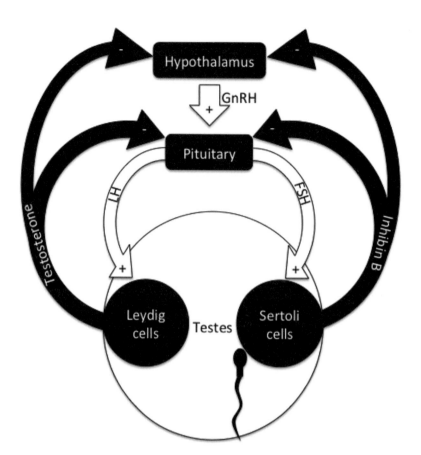

Figure 3.1 Hypothalamic-pituitary-gonadal axis (HPG)

Prolactin is also produced by the pituitary gland and appears to have a direct inhibitory effect on GnRH release.

The measurement of serum testosterone is a complex area. Briefly, the majority of testosterone is bound to sex hormone–binding globulin (SHBG) and albumin with only 2% being classed as 'free testosterone'. The amount of free testosterone available is influenced by a number of factors including age, nutrition and chronic disease states. The measurement of free and bioavailable testosterone, although possible, is an expensive and complex process. Equations exist that allow an estimate to be made and require the albumin, SHBG and total testosterone levels to be measured. Consequently most people use total testosterone for convenience.

Testosterone is secreted in a pulsatile circadian rhythm with levels reaching a peak in the morning, hence the need to perform laboratory measurements at this time; otherwise, the clinician runs the risk of a falsely lowered value.

The normal value for total testosterone depends very much on the population the patient derives from; however, a value of above 12 nmol/l is considered to be normal and 8–12 nmol/l is borderline.

Hypogonadism can be classified as primary (hypergonadotrophic) hypogonadism, secondary (hypogonadotrophic) hypogonadism and target organ resistance. The results of the biochemical assessment can help classify and guide the diagnosis (see Table 3.7).

7.2.1 Kallmann Syndrome

Kallmann syndrome results in primary hypogonadotrophic hypogonadism due to the failure of the hypothalamus to secrete GnRH. This syndrome is generally autosomal dominant and is characterised by a delay in the onset of puberty and often small testes and penis.

Patients with Kallmann syndrome characteristically are anosmic (loss of sense of smell).

Table 3.7 Hypogonadism biochemical findings and potential diagnoses[19]

Hypogonadism	FSH	LH	Testosterone	Causes
Primary	↑↑	↑	↓	Anorchia, UDT, Klinefelter's syndrome, Y-microdeletions, chromosomal abnormalities, trauma, torsion, iatrogenic, exogenous factors, systemic diseases, testicular tumour, varicocele, idiopathic
Secondary	↓	↓	↓	Idiopathic, Kallmann's syndrome, tumours of the diencephalon, hypothalamus, pituitary, empty sella syndrome, granulomatous illness, base of skull fractures, ischaemic or haemorrhagic lesions of the hypothalamic region, hyperprolactinaemia, drugs, radiotherapy
Target organ resistance	↑ →	↑ →	↑→	Testicular feminisation, Reifenstein syndrome

7.3 Genetic Testing

Men presenting with infertility are more likely to have some underlying genetic abnormality compared to fertile men. In fact, the frequency of chromosomal abnormalities increases with the severity of testicular deficiency such that men with counts <5 million/mL have a 10-fold increase in incidence compared to the general population [20, 21].

Genetic testing has two distinct roles: 1) to identify those individuals with an identifiable genetic underlying cause for their infertility; 2) to allow informed counselling regarding the potential inheritance of said abnormality to potential future offspring.

The most common genetic abnormalities associated with male factor infertility are 1) cystic fibrosis, 2) chromosomal abnormalities and 3) Y-chromosome microdeletions.

The EAU guidelines recommend that a standard karyotyping should be offered to all men with <10 x 10^6/ml spermatozoa and Yq microdeletion testing if <5 x 10^6/ml spermatozoa [4].

The AUA suggest that CFTR testing should be used in couples where the male partner has bilateral absent vasa. Karyotyping should be performed on all patients with non-obstructive azoospermia and oligozoospermia (<5 million/mL) [2].

7.3.1 Cystic Fibrosis

Cystic fibrosis is inherited in an autosomal recessive manner and is attributed to a defect in the cystic fibrosis transmembrane conductance regulator (CFTR) protein located on chromosome 7p. The most common abnormalities are ΔF508-CFTR followed by R117H and W1282X; however, many more have been described (>1500) and are listed on the CFTR database [22, 23]. It is impractical to test for all of these and consequently only the most common are analysed based on local genetic profiling. The right number is yet to be defined and laboratories may vary in the number they test for.

The CFTR protein marshals Cl⁻ and H_2O and a defect in this leads to respiratory (chest infections), pancreatic and gastrointestinal sequelae.

CBAVD is associated with cystic fibrosis and therefore these patients and consequently partners should undergo genetic counselling and testing. When considering intracytoplasmic sperm injection (ICSI) in couples with CFTR carrier status, care must be taken to counsel them appropriately. If both male and female carry the gene, then their offspring have a 25% chance of cystic fibrosis and CBAVD. If the female is negative for common mutations, there is a 0.4% chance of being a carrier of an unknown mutation [4].

7.3.2 Chromosomal Abnormalities

A number of chromosomal abnormalities have been recognised that are associated with male infertility. As alluded to earlier, the chance of having a genetic abnormality increases with the degree of infertility.

The most common genetic abnormality seen in the infertility clinic is Klinefelter's syndrome (KS) which occurs in 1 in 600 male births. It is characterised by the addition of an X chromosome (47XXY).

Table 3.8 Genetic abnormalities

	Genetic abnormality	Karyotype	Frequency	Inheritance
Klinefelter's syndrome	47XXY	Muscle weakness, increased height and gynaecomastia	1 in 600	Not inherited
Kallmann's syndrome	Kalig-1, ANOS-1 Chromosome X	Anosmia	1 in 10,000–86,000	X-linked recessive pattern
XYY syndrome	47XYY	Normal	1 in 1,000	Not inherited
XX male	46XX (one or both contain SRY gene due to unequal crossing over between X and Y in meiosis in the father)	Atrophic testes and feminisation	1 in 100,000	Rarely if misplaced onto another chromosome other than the X chromosome
Androgen insensitivity syndrome	Androgen receptor on X chromosome	Spectrum of phenotypes from females to phenotypic males with azoospermia	1 in 20,000	X-linked recessive pattern
5-alpha reductase syndrome	Chromosome 2p23 SRD5A2	Wide spectrum of phenotypes, but characteristically there is virilisation of a phenotypic female at puberty.	rare	autosomal recessive pattern
Noonan's syndrome	PTPN11 gene SOS1 gene RIT1 gene RAF1 gene KRAS gene	broad forehead, drooping eyelids and a wider-than-usual distance between the eyes, heart defects	1 in 1000–2500	Autosomal dominant pattern
Down's syndrome	Trisomy 21	Mental impairment and characteristic facies	1 in 1,000	Rarely

Patients with Klinefelter's syndrome can have a variable phenotype which can include muscle weakness, increased height and gynaecomastia. They often have a raised FSH, normal LH and normal or reduced total plasma levels. Small volume testicles are a feature and on histological examination of the testes, they usually exhibit sclerotic tubules and scarce spermatozoa.

Other genetic abnormalities that may be found are listed in Table 3.8.

7.3.3 Y-chromosome Microdeletions

Microdeletions on the Y-chromosome were first described in 1976 by Tiepolo and Zuffardi [24].

They are the most frequent genetic cause of oligozoospermia and azoospermia [25, 26]. Approximately 10–15% of men with azoospermia and 7–10% of men with severe oligozoospermia will have a Y-microdeletion [27].

There are three microdeletions that are commonly tested: AZFa, AZFb and AZFc.

On histological examination of patients with an AZFa microdeletion, there is a lack of germ cells or sertoli cell–only syndrome. AZFb microdeletions demonstrate spermatogenic arrest and AZFc a spectrum of spermatogenic arrest post meiosis, azoospermia and oligozoospermia [27].

The chances of finding sperm in men with AZF microdeletions at microdissection Testicular Sperm

Extraction (m-TESE) was investigated by a group in the United States [28]. They found that only men with complete AZF-c mutations had sperm found at m-TESE (56%). Those men with AZF-a, AZF-b, AZF-b+c and AZF-a+b+c had a 0% chance of finding sperm at m-TESE.

Individuals with an AZF mutation must be counselled appropriately that their male offspring will carry the defect, although the extent of its effects are not predictable.

7.4 Imaging

A number of imaging modalities have been used in the investigation of male factor infertility. The role of each is detailed below.

7.4.1 Transrectal Ultrasound

Transrectal ultrasound (TRUS) uses a probe with a 7 MHz frequency. It affords excellent views of the seminal vesicles and ejaculatory ducts and can aid in the diagnosis of obstruction at the level of the latter. Patients with the following findings should therefore undergo TRUS: low semen volume, low semen pH, azoospermia, absent fructose and palpably enlarged vas deferens. Accepted normal values for the width of each are: seminal vesicle ≤ 1.5 cm and the ejaculatory duct ≤ 2.3 mm. A TRUS may also identify an absence of vas or atrophic seminal vesicles as in those patients with CBAVD, a congenital abnormality such as Mullerian duct cysts or Wolffian duct abnormalities.

7.4.2 Ultrasound of Testes

An ultrasound of the testicles can provide useful information to the clinician. An assessment of the testicular volume can be made along with excluding any intratesticular lesion such as malignancies, which are more common in patients with infertility. Further rete testis, epididymal and vas dilatation may be detected indicating more proximal obstruction.

Doppler flow analysis may be performed to confirm the clinical diagnosis of a varicocele and spermatic venous reflux may be detected in the absence of a clinical varicocele.

7.4.3 Vasography

With the increasing use of ultrasound, vasography is less commonly used. It is employed in situations where the diagnosis of obstruction is unclear and should only be performed in specialist centres where microsurgical reconstruction is performed. As it is performed by delivering the testes, it is often combined with a testicular sperm extraction (TESE) or m-TESE such that sperm can be stored for future use if any obstruction cannot be resolved or is absent.

7.4.4 Magnetic Resonance Imaging (MRI)

MRI has been used extensively in the imaging of the prostate for other conditions such as prostate cancer. Its ability to discern structures within soft tissues makes it ideal for identifying and characterising developmental cysts and other prostate, seminal vesicle and ejaculatory duct disorders.

8 Conclusion

A thorough history accompanied by careful and directed investigation is paramount when considering the infertile male. Further investigations are guided by the hormone profile and semen analysis. It is essential to fully investigate the male patient for reversible causes for male infertility.

8.1 Key Points

- A full history and focussed examination can often identify the underlying cause for male factor infertility.
- A correctly performed semen analysis is essential in determining further investigations.
- Male semen parameters are based on the 2010 WHO laboratory manual for the examination and processing of human semen.
- Assessment of the hypothalamic-gonadal-axis involves an early morning total testosterone, follicle stimulating hormone, luteinising hormone and prolactin.
- Genetic testing is indicated in patients with $<10 \times 10^6$ /ml spermatozoa and Yq microdeletion testing if $<5 \times 10^6$ /ml spermatozoa.
- Bilateral absent vasa should alert the clinician to the possibility of cystic fibrosis.
- Imaging can help establish a diagnosis based on the investigations above. Common imaging

modalities include: transrectal and testicular ultrasound, magnetic resonance imaging and vasography

- The presence of ejaculatory duct obstruction or vasal and epididymal obstruction are all potentially reversible causes of male infertility.

References

1. Tielemans, E., et al., Sources of bias in studies among infertility clients. *Am J Epidemiol*, 2002. 156(1): 86–92.

2. Jarow, J., Sigman, M., Kolettis, P.N., Lipshultz, L.R., McClure, R.D., Nangia, A.K., Naughton, C.K., Prins G.S., Sandlow, J.I., Schlegel, P.N.MD. The optimal evaluation of the infertile male: Best practice statement. 2011 [cited 2018 29/11/2018] Available from: www.auanet.org/guidelines/male-infertility-optimal-evaluation.

3. World Health Organization, *WHO Laboratory Manual for the Examination and Processing of Human Semen*. 5th edn. 2010, Geneva: World Health Organization. xiv, 271 p.

4. Jungwirth, a., Diemer, T., Dohle, G.R., Giwercman, A., Kopa, Z., Krausz, C., Tournaye, H., European Association of Urology guidelines on male infertility. 2017 [cited 2018 29/11/2018] Available at: http://uroweb.org/wp-content/uploads/17-Male-Infertility_2017_web.pdf.

5. Cooper, T.G., et al., World Health Organization reference values for human semen characteristics. *Hum Reprod Update*, 2010. 16(3): 231–45.

6. Tüttelmann, F., Nieschlag, E., *Classification of Andrological Disorders,* in *Andrology,* E. Nieschlag, Hermann, B.M., Nieschlag, S., eds. 2010, Berlin: Springer-Verlag Berlin Heidelberg. p. 90.

7. Fertility problems: assessment and treatment [CG156]. 2013 [cited 2016 13/01/2016]; Available from: www.nice.org.uk/guidance/cg156/chapter/recommendations - investigation-of-fertility-problems-and-management-strategies.

8. Agarwal, A., et al., Effect of vaginal lubricants on sperm motility and chromatin integrity: a prospective comparative study. *Fertil Steril*, 2008. 89(2): 375–9.

9. Lee, P.A., et al., Paternity after bilateral cryptorchidism. A controlled study. *Arch Pediatr Adolesc Med*, 1997. 151(3): 260–3.

10. Miller, K.D., Coughlin, M.T., Lee, P.A., Fertility after unilateral cryptorchidism. Paternity, time to conception, pretreatment testicular location and size, hormone and sperm parameters. *Horm Res*, 2001. 55(5): 249–53.

11. Inci, K., Gunay, L.M., *Exogenous Medication or Substance-Induced Factors,* in *Male Infertility. Contemporary Clinical Approaches, Andrology, ART & Antioxidants*, S.J. Parrekattil, Agarwal, A., eds. 2012, New York: Springer-Verlag. p. 297–306.

12. WHO, *WHO Manual for the Standardized Investigation, Diagnosis abd Management of the Infertile Male*. 2000, Cambridge: Cambridge University Press.

13. Stewart, T.M., et al., Associations between andrological measures, hormones and semen quality in fertile Australian men: inverse relationship between obesity and sperm output. *Hum Reprod*, 2009. 24(7): 1561–8.

14. Slama, R., et al., Time to pregnancy and semen parameters: a cross-sectional study among fertile couples from four European cities. *Hum Reprod*, 2002. 17(2): 503–15.

15. Swan, S.H., et al., Geographic differences in semen quality of fertile U.S. males. *Environ Health Perspect*, 2003. 111(4): 414–20.

16. Jensen, T.K., et al., Regional differences in waiting time to pregnancy among fertile couples from four European cities. *Hum Reprod*, 2001. 16(12): 2697–704.

17. Haugen, T.B., Egeland, T., Magnus, O. Semen parameters in Norwegian fertile men. *J Androl*, 2006. 27(1): 66–71.

18. Spira, A., Epidemiology of human reproduction. *Hum Reprod*, 1986. 1(2): 111–15.

19. Eberhard Nieschlag, E., Behre H.M., Nieschlag, S., *Andrology*. 3rd edn. 2010, Berlin: Springer-Verlag Berlin Heidelberg.

20. Clementini, E., et al., Prevalence of chromosomal abnormalities in 2078 infertile couples referred for assisted reproductive techniques. *Hum Reprod*, 2005. 20(2): 437–42.

21. Vincent, M.C., et al., Cytogenetic investigations of infertile men with low sperm counts: a 25-year experience. *J Androl*, 2002. 23(1): 18–22; discussion 44–5.

22. Chillon, M., et al., Mutations in the cystic fibrosis gene in patients with congenital absence of the vas deferens. *N Engl J Med*, 1995. 332(22): 1475–80.

23. De Braekeleer, M., Ferec, C., Mutations in the cystic fibrosis gene in men with congenital bilateral absence of the vas deferens. *Mol Hum Reprod*, 1996. 2(9): 669–77.

24. Tiepolo, L., Zuffardi, O., Localization of factors controlling spermatogenesis in the nonfluorescent portion of the human Y chromosome long arm. *Hum Genet*, 1976. 34(2): 119–24.

25. Vogt, P.H., et al., Human Y chromosome azoospermia

factors (AZF) mapped to different subregions in Yq11. *Hum Mol Genet*, 1996. **5**(7): 933–43.

26. Krausz, C., Degl'Innocenti, S., Y chromosome and male infertility: update, 2006. *Front Biosci*, 2006. **11**: 3049–61.

27. Krausz, C., McElreavey, K., Y chromosome and male infertility. *Front Biosci*, 1999. **4**: E1–8.

28. Hopps, C.V., et al., Detection of sperm in men with Y chromosome microdeletions of the AZFa, AZFb and AZFc regions. *Hum Reprod*, 2003. **18**(8): 1660–5.

Chapter 4

Female Fertility
An Overview

Emily Gelson
Alka Prakash

1 Introduction

Infertility is defined as the inability to conceive naturally after one year of regular unprotected intercourse. Most couples do not have absolute infertility but subfertility with a reduced chance of conception in each cycle due to one or more factors. Subfertility has major clinical and social implications and affects approximately thirteen to fifteen per cent of couples worldwide. In the United Kingdom, one in six to seven couples complain of infertility. Half of these couples will conceive either spontaneously or with relatively simple advice or treatment. However, eight per cent of the population remain subfertile and require more complex treatment with assisted reproductive techniques (ART) [1].

The incidence of female subfertility is rising and varies from ten to twenty per cent. On one hand lifestyle changes such as delayed child bearing, increasing weight, alcohol intake and smoking have a negative impact on fertility but on the other hand modern medicine has increased life expectancy for severe illnesses such that women with complex co-morbidities are now surviving to the child-bearing age and requiring help with conception. The causes of female subfertility are ovulation failure, tubal damage, endometriosis, uterine abnormalities, psychosexual disorders or a combination of the above, but equally may be unexplained.

2 Evaluation of the Subfertile Female

2.1 History and Examination

The assessment of infertility requires a detailed history from the patient and her partner. Examination should include measurement of body mass index (BMI), assessment for signs of endocrine disorders and a pelvic examination (Box 4.1).

3 The Impact of Lifestyle Factors on Female Fertility

3.1 Age

A woman's age is one of the most important determinants of her fertility. Up to twenty-five years of age the cumulative conception rate is sixty per cent at six months and eighty-five per cent at one year. By the age of thirty-five years the cumulative conception rate is half of this [2]. The incidence of genetic abnormalities and miscarriage also increases with advancing age. The chance of a live birth after ART also varies with the woman's age, with the chance of a live birth significantly decreased after thirty-five years of age and less than fifteen per cent above the age of forty years [3].

3.2 Weight

Fecundity has been found to be lower at extremes of BMI in women trying to conceive spontaneously and with assisted conception. Time to pregnancy is increased among obese women compared to women of normal weight and the chance of conception falls with increasing BMI. Being underweight (BMI less than twenty) is also associated with reduced fecundity among nulliparous women.

3.2.1 Obesity

Obesity is now a common problem in women of reproductive age. The relationship between obesity and subfertility is well documented and obesity is known to be associated with anovulation, irregular menstrual cycles, miscarriage and adverse pregnancy outcomes. The mechanisms responsible for these effects are however complex, multifactorial and still not fully understood. Some of the factors that may contribute include insulin resistance, hyperandrogenaemia and changes in leptin, adipokine and steroid concentrations [4].

Box 4.1 History, examination and investigations in women presenting with infertility

History

- Age
- Duration of infertility
- Frequency and any difficulty with intercourse
- Menstrual history

  . Menarche
  . Menstrual cycle length
  . Duration of menstrual blood loss
  . Dysmenorrhea
  . Oligomenorrhoea or amenorrhoea
  . Intermenstrual bleeding

- Surgical history

  . Previous abdominal or pelvic surgery

- Medical history

  . Thyroid disease
  . Chronic illness
  . Previous chemo or radiotherapy

- Obstetric history

  . Number of previous pregnancies, including miscarriages, ectopic pregnancies and termination of pregnancy

- Gynaecological history

  . Cervical smear history
  . Previous pelvic infection and STI
  . Previous contraceptives duration and type

- Drug history
- Family history

  . Genetic defects
  . Birth defects
  . Medical disorders

- Tobacco and marijuana smoking
- Alcohol intake
- Caffeine intake

Examination

- Body Mass Index
- Fat and hair distribution
- Thyroid nodules or enlargement
- Galactorrhea
- Signs of androgen excess
- Abdominal masses or tenderness
- Pelvic examination

Investigations

- Early follicular phase LH/FSH
- Mid-luteal progesterone
- HSG/HyCoSy

- Rubella status
- Screen for chlamydia
- HIV/Hep B/Hep C (prior to ART)

A number of hypotheses have been developed to explain the effect of obesity on female fertility by studying the outcomes of obese women undergoing ART and animal models of obesity. Obese women undergoing ART are less likely than women of normal weight to achieve a clinical pregnancy due to decreased clinical pregnancy rate, increased early pregnancy loss and reduced live birth rates [5]. Whether obesity affects fertility through poorer oocyte or embryo quality, impairment in embryo implantation or a combination of these factors is unknown.

It is evident that weight loss among overweight and obese women improves fertility. The British Fertility Society recommends that ART should not be recommended in women with a BMI greater than thirty. Even a small weight loss in anovulatory, obese, subfertile women results in improved ovulation, pregnancy rate and pregnancy outcome. However, the effect of weight loss in overweight and obese women with regular menstrual cycles is still unclear. Bariatric surgery may be considered in women with a BMI of forty or higher (or thirty-five and above with sleep apnoea/diabetes/cardiac disease); however, there is limited evidence about its effect on fertility. Data from observational studies suggest it improves menstrual regularity, ovulation and thus fertility [6]. To avoid nutritional deficiencies, pregnancy should be delayed for one to two years following surgery.

3.2.2 Underweight

Being underweight and having extremely low amounts of body fat are associated with ovarian dysfunction and subfertility. The risk increases in women with a BMI less than seventeen by affecting the hypothalamo-pituitary-ovarian axis and causing hypogonadotroph-ism that leads to a down stream hypogonadism. In general, weight gain restores ovulatory function and consequent fertility.

3.3 Smoking

Female smokers have an increased risk of infertility compared to non-smokers. This is due to reduced ovarian function and reserve and altered hormone levels with higher FSH and lower luteal progesterone. There is also evidence of impaired tubal oocyte pick up and transport of the fertilized embryo within the oviduct [7]. Women trying to conceive should be advised to stop smoking and be referred for smoking cessation counselling.

3.4 Alcohol

High alcohol consumption is associated with subfertility. This is thought to be due to hormonal fluctuations leading to increased oestrogen and reduced FSH levels and thus reduced ovulation [8]. Women trying to conceive either naturally or through ART should be advised to limit alcohol intake or not drink alcohol at all.

3.5 Caffeine

Excessive caffeine consumption (greater than five hundred milligrams per day) has been associated with increased time to pregnancy, increased risk of miscarriage and stillbirth. While the exact mechanism by which caffeine affects fertility is unknown, it may be related to caffeine causing reduced oocyte and embryo quality [9]. Women with subfertility should be advised to limit caffeine consumption although the exact safe threshold remains unclear.

3.6 Existing Illnesses

Many pre-existing illness can have an impact on female fertility; common examples include Turner's syndrome, severe renal, hepatic, respiratory and cardiac disease, diabetes and the effects of cancer treatment. These patients require careful pre-pregnancy counseling and consideration prior to ART.

Both clinical and subclinical hypo and hyperthyroidism are associated with subfertility and recurrent miscarriage. In women with hypothyroidism, maintaining serum TSH levels below 2.5 mU/l pre-conceptually may be associated with improved fertility [10].

4 Investigation and Management of Female Subfertility

4.1 Tubal Factor

The Fallopian tube is the site for fertilization and not only needs to be patent but also function effectively as damage to the tubes can effect sperm transport, oocyte pick up and fertilization and transport of the embryos to the uterus.

Tubal factor infertility is caused by tubal obstruction, endosalpingeal destruction and peri-adenexal adhesions. Pelvic inflammatory disease (PID) secondary to *Chlamydia trachomatis* is the most common etiology representing greater than fifty per cent of cases. One episode of PID increases the rate of subsequent infertility by eight per cent; two or three episodes increase it further by twenty and forty per cent respectively. Other infective causes of tubal disease are *Neisseria gonorrhoeae*, *Actinomyces isrealli* (a rare complication of intrauterine devices) and in the developing world, genital tuberculosis. The other potential causes of tubal disease are complicated appendicitis, endometriosis, previous ectopic pregnancy and congenital abnormalities.

Distal tubal obstruction is the most common site of tubal disease. It is caused by salpingitis secondary to any pelvic inflammatory condition namely infection, endometriosis, appendicitis and abdomino-pelvic surgery. Mid-tubal obstruction is usually iatrogenic from tubal sterilization. Proximal tubal obstruction occurs in only fifteen per cent of women. It can be due to salpingitis isthmica nodosa (nodular thickening of the tunica muscularis of the isthmic portion of the Fallopian tube), mucus plugs, endometriosis, tubal polyps or congenital tubal obstruction.

Before tubal patency is assessed, both semen analysis and assessment of ovulation should occur. Women without co-morbidities should be offered a hysterosalpingography (HSG) or hysterosalpingo-contrast-sonography (HyCoSy) as a screening test for tubal patency. In women with a history of PID, previous ectopic pregnancy or symptoms suggestive of endometriosis, a laparoscopy and dye should be offered. Salpingoscopy and falloposcopy allow direct visualization of the internal tubal mucosa but are not used in routine practice.

The main determinants for the prognosis of pregnancy in women with tubal disease are the severity, the site and the nature of the disease. There are two therapeutic options: tubal surgery or ART. Reconstructive tubal surgery aims to correct damage to the Fallopian tube and restore the normal anatomical relationship between the fimbriae and ovary.

Counselling patients with tubal infertility regarding corrective surgery versus ART is complex and requires a number of considerations [11]. The advantages of tubal surgery are that it involves a single procedure, it is usually minimally invasive, patients may attempt conception every month without further intervention and may conceive more than once. They also avoid the complications of ART. However, the disadvantages are the risks of the procedure, the surgical expertise required and the increased risk of ectopic pregnancy. Several patient factors are important and include maternal age, ovarian reserve, prior fertility and the site and extent of disease.

The advantage of ART is the improved per cycle success rates and reduced invasive surgery. However the disadvantages are the need for frequent hormonal injections, monitoring, risks of multiple pregnancy and ovarian hyperstimulation syndrome. A recent Cochrane review comparing the probability of a live-birth following tubal surgery compared with expectant management or in vitro fertilization (IVF) in the context of tubal infertility (regardless of grade of severity) was inconclusive due to a lack of randomized control trials [12].

4.1.1 Tubal Surgery Prior to ART

Numerous studies have shown that hydrosalpinges have a detrimental effect on IVF success rates thought to be due the direct embyrotoxic effects of the fluid from within the hydrosalpinx. Randomized control trials have shown that laparoscopic salpingectomy in women with hydrosalpinges prior to IVF improves IVF success rates. A recent Cochrane review concluded that laparoscopic salpingectomy or occlusion should be considered for all women with a hydrosalpinx prior to IVF treatment [13]. The couple should be counselled regarding tubal pathology and be given the option of treating the hydrosalpinx. However, the possible effects of surgery on the ipsilateral ovary and the reduced chance of spontaneous conception post treatment should also be considered.

4.2 Ovarian Factors

Ovulation disorders account for twenty to thirty per cent of female subfertility. Ovulation is a complex process that requires a functioning hypothalamo-pituitary-ovarian axis, responsive target organs and interrelated feedback mechanisms. Ovulatory dysfunction can result from interruption at any point along the hypothalamo-pituitary-ovarian axis. It is usually assessed by mid luteal serum progesterone levels or urinary LH detection during the ovulatory LH surge. The causes of ovulatory dysfunction can be classified using the WHO classification (Box 4.2) [14].

Box 4.2 WHO classification of ovulatory disorders

WHO Classification	Description	Findings	Aetiology
Group 1	Hypogonadotrophic hypogonadism	Estradiol low FSH low LH low	Low BMI, anorexia, excessive exercise, Kallman syndrome, Sheehan syndrome
Group 2		Estradiol normal FSH normal LH normal	PCOS
Group 3	Hypergonadotrophic hypogonadism	Estradiol low FSH high LH high	X-chromosomal abnormalities (Turner syndrome, FMR-1 pre-mutation, Fragile X syndrome) 46 XY Gonadal dysgenesis, primary ovarian insufficiency
	Hyperprolactinemic anovulation	Estradiol low FSH normal LH normal High prolactin	Stress, pituitary prolactinoma

4.2.1 Causes of Ovulatory Dysfunction

4.2.1.1 WHO I

Hypogonadotrophic hypogonadism may arise from decreased hypothalamic secretion of gonadotrophin releasing hormone (GnRH) or a pituitary that is unresponsive to the effects of GnRH. The potential causes are outlined in Box 4.2. A fall in GnRH leads to a fall in the secretion of gonadotrophins. Patients will present with primary or secondary amenorrhea and the diagnosis is based on a detailed history and the presence of low follicular stimulating hormone (FSH), luteinizing hormone (LH) and estradiol levels with a normal serum prolactin. A negative response to progestin challenge is seen.

In WHO type I ovulatory disorders treatment of fertility is dependent on the cause. Weight gain should be encouraged in women with a BMI less than nineteen and strenuous exercise should be moderated. Pulsatile GnRH analogues are appropriate where pituitary function is normal whilst pituitary deficiency requires gonadotrophin therapy.

4.2.1.2 WHO II

PCOS is the most common cause of ovulatory dysfunction. It is classified using the Rotterdam ESHRE/ASRM [5] consensus group diagnostic criteria that states that PCOS can be diagnosed when two of the following criteria are met:

1. Oligomenorrhea or amenorrhea
2. Clinical and/or biochemical signs of hyperandrogenism
3. Polycystic ovaries (12 or more follicles in each ovary measuring 2–9mm in diameter and/or increased ovarian volume)

Fertility treatment in PCOS involves weight loss in obese patients. Induction of ovulation is the first line treatment when weight is normal and clomifene citrate is the mainstay treatment in this setting. Aromatase inhibitors have been used for ovulation induction in women with PCOS with the advantage that they do not suppress the effects of oestrogen on the uterus and cervix with the potential to achieve higher pregnancy rates. Two large studies have shown no increased risk of minor or major congenital malformations or cardiac abnormalities in newborns after usage of Letrozole for ovulation induction [16, 17]. Indeed, a Cochrane review demonstrated that Letrozole appears to improve live birth and pregnancy rates in subfertile women with anovulatory PCOS,

compared to clomiphene citrate. However, the quality of the evidence was low and hence should be regarded with some caution due to possible bias in study methods and publication [18]. Second line treatment options for women who fail to ovulate with maximum doses of clomifene include gonadotrophin stimulation and laparoscopic ovarian drilling. ART is the final step in women who fail to conceive despite successful ovulation induction.

Metformin is an insulin-sensitizing agent that reduces hyperinsulinaemia and suppresses the excessive ovarian production of androgens. A recent Cochrane review has demonstrated that when metformin is used in women with PCOS as a co-treatment during ART, no improvement in live birth rate is seen. However, clinical pregnancy rates are improved and the risk of ovarian hyperstimulation syndrome is lower [19].

4.2.1.3 WHO III

Premature ovarian insufficiency (POI) is an uncommon cause of ovulatory dysfunction affecting one per cent of women before the age of forty years. The diagnosis is based on elevated serum FSH and LH levels with a low serum estradiol. The cause may be identified with a thorough history and careful examination followed by baseline and secondary investigations. Fertility treatment for women with WHO type III ovulatory disorder involves pregnancy with oocyte or embryo donation.

4.2.2 Treatment of Functional Ovarian Cysts prior to ART

The coincidental finding of a simple ovarian cyst during pelvic ultrasound in the assessment of female subfertility is common. Previous research has suggested a relationship between the presence of simple ovarian cysts prior to controlled ovarian hyperstimulation for IVF and poor outcome during IVF. However, a recent Cochrane review of three randomized control trials comparing cyst aspiration versus conservative management demonstrated no difference in the clinical pregnancy rate, mean number of follicles recruited or mean number of oocytes collected. The authors concluded that there is insufficient evidence to recommend cyst aspiration prior to IVF particularly in view of the requirement for anaesthesia, extra cost, psychological stress and risk of surgical complications [20].

4.3 Uterine Infertility

Uterine abnormalities account for 10 per cent of female subfertility. The cause may be congenital or acquired and can have an impact on the ability to conceive (naturally or through IVF) or to sustain a pregnancy.

The diagnosis of uterine pathology can be made using pelvic ultrasound, HSG or saline infusion sonography (SIS). Pelvic ultrasound performed in the secretory phase has a high specificity and sensitivity for detecting uterine abnormalities. When available a three-dimensional ultrasound scan (USS) offers highly accurate imaging of the uterus and other pelvic anatomy. HSG provides information about the contours of the endometrial cavity or the presence of any complex communications but has a low sensitivity (fifty per cent) and cannot look at external contours of the uterus. Hysteroscopy gives an accurate assessment of the uterine cavity but its role as a routine investigation in subfertility or prior to ART is presently debatable and under review. MRI when indicated is an excellent technique for the detailed evaluation of the uterus.

4.3.1 Congenital Abnormalities

The prevalence of congenital abnormalities of the genital tract in the subfertile female population is eight per cent [21]. They result from a defect in the development or fusion of the paired mullerian ducts.

4.3.1.1 Septate Uterus

The septate uterus is the most common type of congenital abnormality of the female genital tract. The degree of septation varies from partial to complete and the septum may be muscular or fibrous. Women with a septate uterus have reduced conception rates and increased risk of first trimester miscarriage, preterm birth and fetal mal-presentation. The surgical treatment option to dissect a uterine septum is hysteroscopic metroplasty. Based on limited evidence, the National Institute for Health and Care Excellence (NICE) has stated that this procedure has a role in the management of recurrent miscarriage, to reduce the risk of miscarriage and preterm delivery. However, its role in the treatment of primary subfertility or prior to ART is not clear [22]. To determine this, further investigation with large randomized control trials are required.

4.3.2 Acquired Abnormalities

4.3.2.1 Endometrial Polyps

Endometrial polyps are localized hyperplastic overgrowths of the endometrium, the large majority of which are benign. They can range in size, number and may be sessile or pedunculated. Diagnosis can be made with pelvic ultrasound, a uterine filling defect on HSG or direct visualization during hysteroscopy. The association between the presence of an endometrial polyp and subfertility is unclear. It is plausible, however, that an endometrial polyp may disturb sperm and embryo transport, implantation and endometrial receptivity. Several studies have looked at the effect of endometrial polyps on pregnancy rates after ART. Pre-treatment polypypectomy has shown to improve intrauterine insemination pregnancy rates but the effect on IVF pregnancy rates is less clear [23]. In unexplained fertility polypectomy increases spontaneous pregnancy rates. Although the evidence is lacking, polypectomy prior to infertility treatment is often recommended.

4.3.2.2 Adhesions

Intrauterine adhesions can cause partial or incomplete obliteration of the uterine cavity resulting in menstrual abnormalities, amenorrhea, pelvic pain, subfertility or recurrent pregnancy loss. Hysteroscopic adhesiolysis improves fertility and reduces pregnancy loss however recurrence is a potential complication. Several methods have been proposed to reduce this risk and include the copper coil, estradiol therapy, intrauterine balloon stenting, foley catheter insertion and hyaluronic acid [24]. The patient needs to be counselled regarding the potential for obstetric complication (preterm delivery, placenta accreta and uterine dehiscence).

4.3.2.3 Fibroids

Fibroids are the most common benign uterine tumour with a prevalence of twenty to fifty per cent in women aged thirty-five to fifty years. Their size and location determine their effect on female fertility. Sub-mucous fibroids have a significant impact on implantation, their presence leading to a significant reduction in live birth rates [25]. Subserous fibroids do not appear to have an impact on female fertility. The hysteroscopic resection of submucous fibroids of type 0 and type 1 [26] has been shown to be safe and effective in the control of menstrual disorders. There is currently a paucity of evidence from randomized control trial on the effect of hyteroscopic resection of fibroids on unexplained subfertility and outcomes of ART [27]. The question of whether intra-mural fibroids need to be removed to improve fertility remains a matter of ongoing debate and should be considered on an individual basis.

4.4 Endometriosis

Endometriosis is defined as the presence and proliferation of endometrial-like tissue outside the uterus, usually on the pelvic peritoneum, ovaries or rectovaginal septum. Clinical features include pelvic pain, dyspareunia and infertility. On examination there may be tenderness or nodules on the uterosacral ligaments and rectovaginal septum with a fixed retroverted uterus and tender enlarged ovaries. Diagnosis is made with pelvic USS, MRI or laparoscopy.

In women who present with subfertility and minimal or mild endometriosis, following a full assessment of other potential causes of subfertility, expectant management can be offered dependent on age and duration of infertility. Surgical excision of mild to moderate endometriosis improves pregnancy rates compared to diagnostic laparoscopy alone [28]. Suppression of ovarian function (by means of hormonal contraceptives, GnRH analogues or danazol) does not produce an improvement in pregnancy rates compared to expectant management and should not be offered for this indication alone.

4.4.1 Treatment of Endometriosis prior to ART

Women with endometriosis are often ultimately offered ART. In cases of severe endometriosis, the evidence is not clear as to whether surgical excision or ablation of endometriosis prior to ART improves outcome. Ovarian cystectomy for endometriomas should only be offered if there is a doubt in diagnosis or if it is interfering with follicular access for oocyte retrieval. Couples should be counselled about the risk of reduced ovarian function after surgery and the possibility of oophorectomy. In women with previous ovarian surgery the decision to proceed with surgery is more complex and should be carefully considered [29].

Adenomyosis is found in a proportion of women with subfertility, particularly those with endometriosis or with symptoms of menorrhagia and dysmenorrhea. It can be diagnosed with MRI or pelvic ultrasound. Whether the presence of adenomyosis has a negative impact on fertility or the success of assisted conception is not clear. The proposed mechanisms for it doing so are impaired mechanism of uterine contractility, thereby disrupting sperm transport and/or implantation or an altered uterine environment. There are currently no fertility-sparing treatments of proven effectiveness for women with adenomyosis and subfertility.

5 Conclusion

Female factors are a common cause of subfertility, which are often multifactorial and may be related to lifestyle. There is a socio-cultural trend in delaying childbirth that has a strong impact on the outcome of fertility treatment at a later age. Several controversies still exist regarding the diagnostic modalities and management of women with subfertility and further studies are required to clarify these dilemmas. On the positive side, the advances in scientific techniques, specifically in ART, allow hope to couples and have increased the success rates in all infertility programmes.

References

1. Boivin J, Bunting L, Collins JA, Nygren KG. International estimates of infertility prevalence and treatment-seeking: potential need and demand for infertility medical care. *Hum Reprod* 2007; **22**: 1506–1512.

2. Wood JW. *Oxford Reviews of Reproductive Biology.* New York, Oxford University Press. 1989.

3. www.hfea.gov.uk/docs/ FertilityTreatment2012Trends Figures.PDF

4. Dag Z. Impact of obesity on infertility in women. *J Turk Ger Gynecol Assoc.* 2015; **16**(2): 111–117.

5. Maheshwari A, Stofberg L, Bhattacharya S. Effect of overweight and obesity on assisted reproductive technology —a systematic review. *Hum.*

Reprod. Update 2007; **13**(5): 433–444.

6. Maggard M *et al.* Pregnancy and fertility following bariatric surgery: a systematic review. *JAMA.* 2008; **300**(19): 2286–2296.

7. Zeinab H, Zohreh S, Samadaee GK. Lifestyle and outcomes of assisted reproductive techniques: a narrative review. *Glob J Health Sci.* 2015; 7(5): 41418.

8. Eggert J, Theobald H, Engfeldt P. Effects of alcohol consumption on female fertility during an 18-year period. *Fertil Steril.* 2004; **81**: 379–383.

9. Wilcox A, Weinberg C, Baird D. Caffeinated beverages and decreased fertility. *Lancet* 1988; **2**: 1453–1456.

10. Jefferys A, Vanderpump M, Yasmin E. Thyroid dysfunction and reproductive health. *Obstet Gynec.* 2015; **17**: 39–45.

11. Practice Committee of the American Society of Reproductive Medicine. Role of tubal surgery in the era of assisted reproductive technology: a committee opinion. *Fertil Steril.* 2015; **103**(6): e37–43.

12. Pandian Z, Akande VA, Harrild K, Bhattacharya S. Surgery for tubal infertility. *Cochrane Database Syst Rev.* 2008; Issue 3. Art. No.: CD006425. doi:10.1002/14651858.CD006415.pub2

13. Johnson N et al., Surgical treatment for tubal disease in women due to undergo in vitro fertilisation. *Cochrane Database Syst Rev.* 2010; Issue 1. Art. No.: CD002125. doi:10.1002/14651858.CD00215.pub3

14. ESHRE Capri Workshop Group. Health and fertility in World Health Organization group 2 anovulatory women. *Hum Reprod Update.* 2012; **18**(5): 586–599

15. The Rotterdam ESHRE/ASRM-sponsored PCOS consensus workshop. Revised 2003 consensus on diagnostic criteria and long-term health risks related to polycystic ovary syndrome (PCOS). *Hum. Reprod.* 2004; **19** (1): 41–47.

16. Tulandi T, Martin J, Al-Fadhli R, Kabli N, Forman R, Hitkari J, Librach C, Greenblatt E, Casper RF. Congenital malformations among 911 newborns conceived after infertility treatment with letrozole or clomiphene citrate. *Fertil Steril.* 2006; **85**(6): 1761.

17. Forman R, Gill S, Moretti M, Tulandi T, Koren G, Casper R. Fetal safety of letrozole and clomiphene citrate for ovulation induction. *J Obstet Gynaecol Can.* 2007; **29**(8): 668.

18. Franik S, Kremer JAM, Nelen WLDM, Farquhar C. Aromatase inhibitors for subfertile women with polycystic ovary syndrome. *Cochrane Database Syst Rev.* 2014; Issue 2. Art. No.: CD010287. doi:10.1002/14651858.CD010287.pub2

19. Tso LO, *et al.* Metformin treatment before and during IVF or ICSI in women with polycystic ovary syndrome. *Cochrane Database Syst Rev.* 2014; Issue 11. Art. No.: CD006105. doi: 10.1002/14651858.CD006105.pub2

20. McDonnell R, Marjoribanks J, Hart RJ. Ovarian cyst aspiration prior to in vitro fertilization treatment for subfertility. *Cochrane Database Syst Rev.* 2014; Issue 12. Art. No.: CD005999. doi: 10.1002/14651858.CD005999.pub2

21. S Saravelos, K Cocksedg, Tin-Chiu Li. Prevalence and diagnosis of congenital uterine anomalies in women with reproductive failure: a critical appraisal. *Hum Reprod Update.* 2008; **14**(5): 415–429.

22. NICE (2015). Hysteroscopic Metroplasty of a uterine septum for primary infertility. Access www.nice.org.uk/guidance/ipg509/resources/guidance-hysteroscopic-metroplasty-of-a-uterine-septum-for-primary-infertility-pdf

23. Perez-Medina T, Bajo-Arenas J, Salazar F, Redondo T, Sanfrutos L, Alvarez P, Engels V. Endometrial polyps and their implication in the pregnancy rates of patients undergoing intrauterine insemination: a prospective, randomized study. *Hum Reprod.* 2005; **20**: 1632–1635.

24. Conforti A, Alviggi C, Mollo A, De Placido G, Magos A. The management of Asherman syndrome: a review of literature. *Reproductive Biology and Endocrinology: RB&E.* 2013; **11**: 118.

25. Pritts E, Parker W, Olive D. Fibroids and infertility: an updated systematic review of the evidence. *Fertil Steril.* 2009; **91**: 1215–1223.

26. Wamsteker, K, Emanuel, MH, and de Kruif, JH Transcervical hysteroscopic resection of submucous fibroids for abnormal uterine bleeding: results regarding the degree of intramural extension. *Obstet Gynecol.* 1993; **82**: 736–740.

27. Bosteel J, Kasius J, Weyers S, Broekmans FJ, Mol BW, D'Hooghe TM. Hysteroscopy for treating subfertility associated with suspected major uterine cavity abnormalities. *Cochrane Database Syst Rev.* 2015; Issue 2. Art. No.: CD009461. doi: 10.1002/14651858.CD009461.pub3.

28. Brown J, Farquhar C. Endometriosis: an overview of Cochrane Reviews. *Cochrane Database Syst Rev.* 2014; Issue 3. Art. No.: CD009590. doi: 10.1002/14651858.CD009590.pub2.

29. Dunselman *et al.* ESRHE guideline: management of women with endometriosis. *Hum Reprod.* 2014 Mar; **29**(3): 400–412.

Chapter 5

Unexplained Infertility

Melanie Davies
Ali Al Chami

1 Size of the Problem

It is estimated that infertility affects 1 in 7 heterosexual couples trying for a child in the United Kingdom. The main causes of infertility are as follows [Figure 5.1]:

- Unexplained (25%)
- Ovulatory disorders (25%)
- Tubal factor (20%)
- Male factor (30%)
- Uterine or peritoneal disorders (10%)[1]

The high proportion of couples with 'unexplained infertility' in this review from 2013 differs little from Hull's classic publication in 1985 [2], even though there has been immense progress in reproductive technology in the interim.

Fertility problems may not be due to a single factor; in about 40% of cases, disorders are found both in the man and woman.

2 Definition of Unexplained Infertility

The term 'subfertility' is preferable to 'infertility' since few individuals have absolute sterility. Subfertility is usually defined as the inability to conceive after one year of regular unprotected intercourse. This definition is based on the cumulative chance of conception [3][Figure 5.2]. Healthy couples trying to conceive have a 25% chance of conception in the first cycle, 20% in the second, though this falls month-by-month as the most fertile couples achieve pregnancy [4] [Figure 5.3]. By the end of the first year, 85% of couples will have conceived.

If the remaining couples are followed up, half of them will conceive in the second year. Thus these couples could not have had any major fertility problem; they may have been unlucky rather than infertile.

It follows that, in offering fertility investigations promptly after a year, we would expect to find no

causes of subfertility

Fig. 5.1 Causes of subfertility (based on NICE 2013) [1]

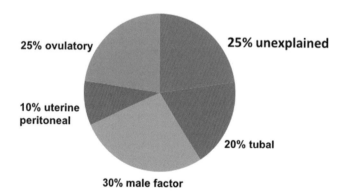

derived from **NICE 2013**

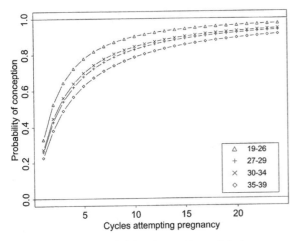

Fig. 5.2 Cumulative probability of conceiving a clinical pregnancy by the number of menstrual cycles attempting to conceive for women in different age categories (assuming intercourse occurs at a frequency of 2 times/week). Prospective cohort study of 782 women recruited through 7 European centres (with permission) [3]

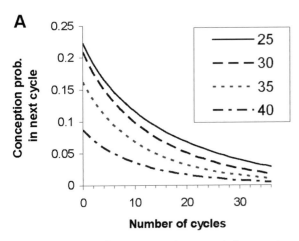

Fig. 5.3 Probability of conceiving on the next cycle for a couple who have not yet conceived; shown for female ages of 25, 30, 35 and 40 at the start of the attempt to conceive [4]

significant problem in up to half of the couples. They will be labelled as having 'unexplained' infertility and their prognosis is good. The standard recommendation to investigate at a year allows 'triage' of couples who will need intervention from those who can be reassured.

Unexplained infertility is a diagnosis of exclusion. Infertility is unexplained when the results of standard fertility evaluation are normal. These tests include a semen analysis, assessment of ovulation and tubal patency.

Practitioners should be aware of the limitations of these tests and consider carefully other factors before assigning a diagnosis of genuinely unexplained infertility. 'Unexplained' infertility may actually be 'undiagnosed'.

3 Factors Influencing Fecundity

Female age is a major determinant of fecundity. The cumulative probability of conceiving a clinical pregnancy declines with age as shown in Figure 5.2. Between ages 25 and 30 the overwhelming majority of couples are of high fertility, and only a very small proportion are sterile. However, fecundity drops by the time female age reaches 35 and markedly by 40. The probability of conception in the first cycle falls to below 10% in women of 40 [Figure 5.3]. The same trend affects success rates from treatment. Investigations should therefore be offered earlier to older women, that is, at 6 months if aged over 35.

Currently in the United Kingdom, the average age of women at childbirth is 30 years [5] and demographic changes make age-related subfertility increasingly common.

Other factors that influence conception rates include smoking and obesity, which is increasingly important.

4 Diagnostic Tests

4.1 Male Factor

The assessment of male fertility relies on the semen analysis. Semen analysis results should be compared with the World Health Organization reference values [6]. These values were generated after analyzing a large bulk of data from published studies of recent fathers with time to pregnancy of less than 12 months. These fertile men had a wide range of semen parameters, and the calculated fifth centile was accepted as being the appropriate lower reference for normality. The reference range does not provide a 'cut-off value' to categorize men as infertile or fertile; semen parameters should be seen as a continuum.

Semen parameters within the reference range do not guarantee fertility. The prognostic value of semen components is influenced by frequency of sexual activity, the function of accessory sex glands and other unrecognized conditions. Besides, the semen analysis itself does not account for putative sperm dysfunctions such as immature chromatin or fragmented DNA. Therefore, the reference limits should not be over-interpreted to distinguish fertile from subfertile men.

4.2 Ovarian Function

Women undergoing investigations for infertility are usually offered a blood test to measure serum progesterone in the mid-luteal phase of their cycle to confirm ovulation. However, it is debatable whether this adds value to the fertility assessment, as a low value is usually due to mistimed sampling rather than anovulation. A regular menstrual cycle is a good indicator of ovulation, and many women now use home testing to confirm the luteinizing hormone (LH) surge. Moreover, proof of ovulation does not indicate egg quality, nor does it predict ovarian reserve or the likely ovarian response to gonadotrophin stimulation in any future fertility treatment. Infertility that is apparently unexplained warrants a more comprehensive assessment of ovarian function.

Female age is the best initial predictor of fertility potential. Follicle stimulating hormone (FSH), antral follicle count (AFC) and anti-Mullerian hormone (AMH) are generally the tests used to assess ovarian reserve.

FSH measurement is widely used as a marker of ovarian reserve but has serious limitations. FSH varies throughout a woman's cycle and measurement must therefore be standardized by sampling in the early follicular phase. Moreover, FSH fluctuates from cycle to cycle, and these fluctuations become wider as ovarian reserve diminishes. Persistently raised FSH is a late marker of ovarian insufficiency. FSH should not be used independently as an exclusion criterion for low ovarian reserve in unexplained infertility. It is suitable as a screening test for counselling purposes and further diagnostic steps are needed.

The number of small antral follicles, sized 2–10 mm, in both ovaries as measured by ultrasound is clearly related to reproductive age and could well reflect the size of the remaining primordial follicle pool. Before the age of 37, the mean yearly decline of AFC is 4.8% compared with 11.7% thereafter [7]. AFC does not appear to provide added predictive value beyond AMH [8]. It may well be used as a screening test for possible 'poor responders' but not as a solitary test to exclude low ovarian reserve in unexplained infertility. Moreover, it is relatively

expensive, requiring transvaginal ultrasound by a skilled operator.

AMH appears to be a more stable predictor of ovarian reserve as it does not fluctuate significantly through the menstrual cycle and is not operator-dependent. One should be aware of the different laboratory assays in use and interpret the results in the context of the woman's age and history. It is not uncommon to see discrepancy between AMH and FSH where, without the result of low AMH, the subfertility would otherwise be unexplained.

4.3 Tubal Factor

Confirmation of tubal patency is the last in the triumvirate of standard investigations for subfertility. Hysterosalpingography (HSG) and Hysterosalpingo-contrast sonography (HyCoSy) are considered as first-line tests for tubal patency. Both are substitutes for laparoscopy which is widely accepted as the gold standard for diagnosing tubal occlusion and other pelvic pathology.

A systematic review with meta-analysis studied the diagnostic accuracy of HSG and HyCoSy in comparison with laparoscopy [9]. In nine studies all patients underwent HSG in addition to HyCoSy and laparoscopy allowing direct comparison of accuracy. The estimates of sensitivity and specificity were 0.95 (95% CI:0.78–0.99) and 0.93 (95% CI:0.89–0.96) for HyCoSy and 0.94 (95% CI:0.74–0.99) and 0.92 (95% CI:0.87–0.95) for HSG respectively. In conclusion, HyCoSy performs similarly to HSG. However, the technique of HyCoSy has the advantage of visualizing the ovaries, myometrium and the fallopian tubes in a single study; this can yield relevant findings such as polycystic ovarian morphology or suspected endometriosis.

Patent fallopian tubes on HSG or HyCoSy do not confirm that ovum pick-up will occur. HSG has almost no value in the detection of peritubal adhesions [10]. In a study to assess the value of laparoscopy in 265 subfertile women with normal HSG, 51% of laparoscopies were normal, whereas 49% had abnormal findings including endometriosis, adnexal adhesions, subserosal fibroids, ovarian neoplasms and salpingitis isthmica nodosa [11]. A history of dysmenorrhoea or dyspareunia increased the likelihood of detecting endometriosis from 41% to 64% and 69% respectively. The presence of both symptoms increased the likelihood to 83%. A careful history and pelvic examination is crucial before selecting the best test to confirm tubal patency.

5 Undiagnosed Subfertility

Diagnostic tests currently available are not exhaustive. Other subtle causes that have been proposed as underlying unexplained infertility include: tubal abnormal peristaltic or cilial activity, altered cervical mucus, genetic abnormalities, cytological abnormalities in oocytes, abnormal secretion of endometrial proteins, abnormalities in uterine perfusion and contractility, altered cell mediated immunity or abnormal T-cell and natural killer activity, abnormal follicle growth or reduced growth hormone sensitivity. Many of these abnormalities have been found in couples of normal fertility and proposed correction of the abnormality has not always been shown to improve fertility.

A balance needs to be struck between thorough and speculative investigation, accepting that subtle causes of subfertility may not be detectable, and moving on to management of the situation.

6 Prognosis of Unexplained Infertility

As stated earlier, about half of the couples who do not conceive in the first year will achieve a pregnancy in the second year. It is important to consider treatment in this context; it should offer a significant benefit compared to natural conception rates with expectant management. The main factors determining the chance of natural pregnancy are the woman's age and the duration of infertility. If the couple present after more than three years of unexplained infertility, and particularly after five years, the prognosis is significantly worse [Figure 5.4].

7 Management of Unexplained Infertility

7.1 Expectant Management

Expectant management may be the best advice for couples who have a short duration of subfertility, are young (under 35) and have genuinely unexplained delay in conception. As explained earlier, their prognosis is good, and assisted conception offers no great advantage over natural conception in the next 6–12 months. They will avoid the small but real risks of invasive treatment and the associated costs [12].

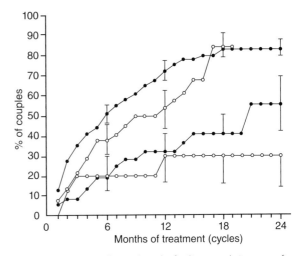

Fig. 5.4 Prognosis of unexplained infertility: cumulative rates of spontaneous conception in relation to duration of infertility. From [2] with permission

7.2 Lifestyle Changes

Couples often ask what they can do to maximize their fertility. Evidence-based advice aligns with common sense:

- Vaginal intercourse every two to three days optimizes the chance of pregnancy.
- Cigarette smoking may reduce fertility in the female partner. Smoking is also associated with reduced semen quality. Couples who smoke should be offered referral to a smoking cessation programme to support their efforts to stop smoking.
- Excessive alcohol consumption is detrimental to semen quality. The Department of Health states that men should not regularly drink more than 3 to 4 units of alcohol a day.
- Men and women with BMI of 30 kg/m^2 or more are likely to take longer to conceive and should be advised on weight loss

7.3 Complementary Therapies

There is a lack of evidence on complementary therapies as the sole treatment for unexplained infertility. They are often used as an adjunct to assisted reproductive treatments; there are no published randomized controlled trials (RCTs) on the effectiveness of using Chinese herbal medicines, but a systematic review was performed to determine the effectiveness of acupuncture [13]. Fourteen trials (a total of 2670 subjects) studied were included in meta-analysis; the results provided no evidence of benefit from the use of acupuncture during assisted conception.

7.4 Ovarian Stimulation

Over the past decades, controlled ovarian hyperstimulation (COH), with or without intrauterine insemination (IUI), has been widely used in the treatment of unexplained infertility. Both clomiphene citrate (CC) and gonadotrophins have been used for stimulation. The effectiveness of CC has been demonstrated in treatment of subfertility associated with infrequent or irregular ovulation; however, the physiologic effects and clinical benefits in ovulatory women with unexplained infertility are less clear. It used to be thought that CC boosts fertility by correcting subtle defects in ovarian function. However, it has an anti-oestrogenic effect on cervical mucus and endometrial development. Bhattacharya and colleagues reported no statistically significant difference in live birth rate when CC was compared with expectant management (OR 0.79, 95% confidence intervals 0.45 to 1.33) [14]. A Cochrane review incorporating this study reported no evidence that CC without IUI was more effective than no treatment or placebo for clinical pregnancy (OR 1.03, 95% CI 0.64 to 1.66; P=0.91) [15]. A further subgroup analysis of two RCTs in this review reported that CC with human chorionic gonadotrophin and without IUI was not more effective than no treatment or placebo (OR 1.66, 95% 0.58–4.80; p=0.35). In light of these findings, the current NICE recommendation [1] is not to offer oral ovarian stimulation agents to women with unexplained infertility.

7.5 Intrauterine Insemination (IUI)

IUI is less invasive and less expensive than in vitro fertilization (IVF); however, unstimulated IUI is unlikely to offer superior live birth rates compared with expectant management [14]. Stimulated IUI is more common in clinical practice. A meta-analysis of 4 RCTs, involving 396 couples with unexplained infertility, showed a significant increase in live birth following IUI with ovarian stimulation compared with IUI in a natural cycle (OR 2.07, 95% CI 1.22–3.5) [16]. However, safety concerns were raised by the increased multiple pregnancy rate (reported in these studies between 10 and 40%) and occasional cases of ovarian hyperstimulation syndrome.

The efficacy and side-effects of different treatment protocols prior to IUI have been evaluated by several studies. A Cochrane review compared gonadotrophins with anti-oestrogens in pooled data from 7 trials involving 556 couples [17]. The clinical pregnancy rates were significantly higher with gonadotrophins (OR 1.76, 95% CI 1.16–2.66). This result is not very robust in the context of unexplained infertility because of differences between studies that included couples using donor sperm, single women, or couples where protected intercourse was necessary due to HIV status of one of the couples. The multiple pregnancy rate was 10% in both groups. The use of high-dose gonadotrophins seems to lead to more multiple pregnancies without improving pregnancy rates significantly; mild stimulation protocols combined with strict cancellation criteria reduces the rate of multiple pregnancy per cycle and couple.

In an attempt to compare IUI with stimulation against expectant management, Steures and colleagues randomly assigned 253 couples to have either IUI with controlled ovarian stimulation (gonadotrophin) or expectant management for six months [18]. There was no beneficial effect of IUI with COH (relative risk 0.85, 95% CI 0.63–1.1). This was the only trial identified by NICE that was methodologically adequate for inclusion in NICE guidance, hence their recommendation 'do not routinely' use IUI in unexplained infertility [1].

7.6 IVF

IVF is widely used to treat prolonged unexplained infertility. It is considered effective although expensive, invasive and associated with risks including ovarian hyperstimulation syndrome and multiple pregnancy. Pandian and colleagues performed a systematic review to compare IVF to expectant management [19]. Only one RCT of 51 couples was identified [20]. The live birth rate per woman was significantly higher with IVF (45.8%) than expectant management (3.7%) (odds ratio (OR) 22.00, 95% CI 2.56–189.37).

The same Cochrane review compared IVF with IUI + SO in couples with unexplained infertility [19]. The live birth rate did not differ significantly between the groups among treatment-naive women (OR 1.09, 95% CI 0.74–1.59, 2 RCTs, 234 women) but was significantly higher with IVF in a large RCT which randomized women pretreated with three unsuccessful cycles of IUI + clomiphene citrate (OR 2.66, 95%

CI 1.94–3.63, 1 RCT, 341 women). These three studies could not be pooled due to high heterogeneity. There was no significant difference in multiple pregnancy rate or ovarian hyperstimulation syndrome between the two treatments. The implication of these findings is that couples who have already failed treatment with IUI should be offered IVF.

A recent RCT in the Netherlands compared different modalities of assisted conception: 602 couples, a mixed population with unexplained or mild male factor infertility, were randomized to IUI with controlled ovarian hyperstimulation (6 cycles in a 12-month period) or IVF in a modified natural cycle (6 cycles) or IVF using single embryo transfer (3 cycles with subsequent frozen-thaw cycles)[21]. The primary outcome was the birth of a healthy child resulting from a singleton pregnancy conceived within 12 months after randomization. This occurred in 47% after IUI with COH, 43% after IVF in a modified natural cycle, and 52% of couples undergoing IVF with single embryo transfer. Both forms of IVF were non-inferior to IUI. Multiple pregnancies did not differ significantly between groups, all were <10%. This RCT may have a potential impact on any future systematic review.

8 Conclusion

In conclusion, there is no clear advantage in any particular type of assisted conception for couples with unexplained infertility, and indeed the benefits of assisted conception relative to expectant management remain uncertain. Practitioners should therefore take an individualized approach to management of unexplained subfertility, taking into account the duration of infertility, the age of the female partner and the couple's wishes.

References

1. National Institute for Health and Care Excellence. Fertility: Assessment and treatment for people with fertility problems. NICE Clinical Guideline CG156. Published February 2013. www.nice.org.uk/guidance/cg156/resources/fertility-problems-assessment-and-treatment-pdf-35109634660549

2. Hull MG, Glazener CM, Kelly NJ, Conway DI, Foster PA, Hinton RA, Coulson C, Lambert PA, Watt EM, Desai KM. Population study of causes, treatment, and outcome of infertility. *BMJ* (Clin Res Ed) 1985; 291: 1693

3. Dunson DB, Baird DD, Colombo B. Increased infertility with age in men and women. *Obstet Gynecol.* 2004; 103: 51–56

4. Sozou PD, Hartshorne GM. Time to pregnancy: a computational method for using the duration of non-conception for predicting conception. *PLoS ONE* 2012; 7(10): e46544.

5. www.ons.gov.uk/ons/rel/vsob1/characteristics-of-Mother-1-england-and-wales/2013/stb-characteristics-of-mother-1-2013.html

6. Cooper TG, Noonan E, Von Eckardstein S, Auger J, Baker HW, Behre HM, Haugen TB, Kruger T, Wang C, Mbizvo MT et al. World Health Organization reference values for human semen characteristics. *Hum Reprod Update* 2010; 16(3): 231–245

7. Scheffer GJ, Broekmans FJ, Dorland M, Habbema JD, Looman CW, te Velde ER. Antral follicle counts by transvaginal ultrasonography are related to age in women with proven natural fertility. *Fertil Steril.* 1999; 72(5): 845–851

8. Nelson SM, Fleming R, Gaudoin M, Choi B, Santo-Domingo K, Yao M. Antimüllerian hormone levels and antral follicle count as prognostic indicators in a personalized prediction model of live birth. *Fertil Steril.* 2015; 104(2):325–332

9. Maheux-Lacroix A, Boutin A, Moore L, Bergeron M-E, Bujold E, Laberge P, Lemyre M, Dodin S. Hysterosalpingosonography for diagnosing tubal occlusion in subfertile women: a systematic review with meta-analysis. *Hum Reprod.* 2014; 29: 953–963

10. Mol BW, Swart P, Bossuyt PM, van Beurden M, van der Veen F. Reproducibility of the interpretation of hysterosalpingography in the diagnosis of tubal pathology. *Hum Reprod.* 1996; 11(6): 1204–1208

11. al-Badawi IA, Fluker MR, Bebbington MW. Diagnostic laparoscopy in infertile women with normal hysterosalpingograms. *J Reprod Med*, 1999; 44(11): 953–957

12. Kersten FA, Hermens RP, Braat DD, Hoek A, Mol BW, Goddijn M, Nelen WL, Improvement Study Group. Overtreatment in couples with unexplained infertility. *Hum Reprod.* 2015; 30(1):71–80

13. Cheong Y, Nardo LG, Rutherford T, Ledger W. Acupuncture and herbal medicine in *in vitro fertilisation*: a review of the evidence for clinical practice. *Hum Fertil (Camb).* 2010; 13(1): 3–12

14. Bhattacharya S, Harrild K, Mollison J, Wordsworth S, Tay C, Harrold A, McQueen D, Lyall H, Johnston L, Burrage J, Grossett S, Walton H, Lynch J, Johnstone A, Kini S, Raja A, Templeton A. Clomifene citrate or unstimulated intrauterine insemination

compared with expectant management for unexplained infertility: pragmatic randomised controlled trial. *BMJ.* 2008; 337: a716

15. Hughes E, Brown J, Collins JJ, Vanderkerchove P. Clomiphene citrate for unexplained subfertility in women. *Cochrane Database Syst Rev.* 2010; Issue 1. Art. No.: CD000057. doi: 10.1002/14651858.CD000057.pub2

16. Veltman-Verhulst SM, Cohlen BJ, Hughes E, Heineman MJ. Intrauterine insemination for unexplained subfertility. *Cochrane Database Syst Rev.* 2012; Issue 9. Art. No.: CD001838. doi: 10.1002/14651858.CD001838.pub4

17. Cantineau AEP, Cohlen BJ. Ovarian stimulation protocols (anti-oestrogens, gonadotrophins with and without GnRH agonists/antagonists) for intrauterine insemination in women with subfertility. Copyright © 2011 The Cochrane Collaboration

18. Steures P, van der Steeg JW, Hompes PG, et al. Intrauterine insemination with controlled ovarian hyperstimulation versus expectant management for couples with unexplained subfertility and an intermediate prognosis; a randomised clinical trial. *Lancet.* 2006; 368: 216–221

19. Pandian Z, Gibreel A, Bhattacharya S. In vitro fertilisation for unexplained subfertility. *Cochrane Database Syst Rev.* 2012 Apr 18; Issue 4. Art. No.: CD003357

20. Hughes EG, Beecroft ML, Wilkie V, Burville L, Claman P, Tummon I, Greenblatt E, Fluker M, Thorpe K. A multicentre randomized controlled trial of expectant management versus IVF in women with Fallopian tube patency. *Hum Reprod.* 2004; 19(5):1105–1109

21. Bensdorp AJ, Tjon-Kon-Fat RI, Bossuyt PMM, Koks CAM, Oosterhuis GJE, Hoek A et al. Prevention of multiple pregnancies in couples with unexplained or mild male subfertility: randomised controlled trial of in vitro fertilisation with single embryo transfer or in vitro fertilisation in modified natural cycle compared with intrauterine insemination with controlled ovarian hyperstimulation. *BMJ* 2015; 350:g7771

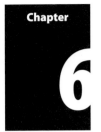

Chapter

6

Overview of Management of Male Infertility

Mostafa Metwally
Swapna Yesireddy

1 Introduction -The Male Infertility Epidemic

Male infertility is becoming a worldwide epidemic. Data suggest that there has been a constant decline in semen parameters throughout the decades of the 20th century with the mean sperm count ranging around 60 million sperm per ml in the late 1930s and dropping down to around 40 million sperm per ml in the late 1970s [1]. More recent data from the Human Fertilisation and Embryology Authority suggests that male factor infertility is the sole cause of couple infertility in around 30% of cases and in a further 10% of cases there is a combination of male and female factors. This means that in just under one half of couples seen in a typical infertility clinic setting there will be a male factor and hence the importance of thorough investigation and management of the male partner. The exact cause for this decline in male infertility is largely unknown but may be due to various environmental factors or lifestyle changes such as smoking and obesity [2].

This chapter will examine the underlying causes of male factor infertility with a brief description of the background theory underlying sperm production. It will also aim to provide a clinical approach to the management of male factor infertility appropriate for both secondary and tertiary care clinicians.

2 Clinical Approach to Management of Male Infertility

Male fertility problems can be classified based on the semen analysis into two main categories. The first is when no sperm is seen in the ejaculate (**azoospermia**) and the second category is when sperm are present but of suboptimal quality. This may be due to a low sperm count (**oligozoospermia**), low sperm motility (**teratozoospermia**), poor sperm morphology (**asthenozoospermia**) or a combination of two or more of these problems. Azoospermia should be differentiated from aspermia, which is the absence of semen during ejaculation, which is either due to retrograde ejaculation into the urinary bladder or due to obstruction of the outflow tract. We will approach these two problems separately.

2.1 Azoospermia

Azoospermia is defined as the absence of sperm in the ejaculate. A second sample is always necessary to confirm the diagnosis. The diagnosis of the cause starts with a firm understanding of the different compartments responsible for sperm production. The first of these compartments is the hypothalamus and pituitary gland. The second is the testicle containing Leydig and Sertoli cells. The third compartment is the outflow tract (ejaculatory ducts) with contributions from the prostate gland and seminal vesicles.

2.1.1 Compartment 1: Hypothalamus and Pituitary (Hypogonadotrophic Hypogonadism)

This is the top compartment involved in spermatogenesis. The hypothalamus and pituitary gland affect spermatogenesis through producing FSH and LH, influencing the Sertoli and Leydig cells. Consequently the hypothalamic-pituitary compartment is assessed through measurement of the following hormones: FSH, LH, testosterone and sex hormone binding globulin (SHBG) in addition to prolactin and imaging in certain cases where a pituitary tumour is suspected. Clinical conditions that can affect this compartment include the following:

(i) Congenital conditions such as Kallman syndrome; this is due to a congenital defect in the arcuate nucleus where the GnRH producing neurones failed to migrate from olfactory bulb. The olfactory bulb is also affected leading to anosmia.

(ii) Suppression of gonadotrophin production through exogenous sources (anabolic steroids and exogenous testosterone therapy) or endogenous sources such as in cases of congenital adrenal hyperplasia [3].

(iii) Traumatic conditions such as surgical removal of the pituitary gland.

(iv) Neoplastic conditions leading to destruction of the pituitary gland such as pituitary macroadenomas or extra pituitary tumours compressing the pituitary gland, or microadenomas producing prolactin (prolactinomas).

(v) The use of anabolic steroids and testosterone supplements. This is becoming a growing problem with increased use of so-called exercise-enhancing supplements and bodybuilding products many of which can be purchased over the internet. The use of these products can lead to suppression of the hypothalamus and pituitary gland with suppression of sperm and testosterone production.

2.1.2 Compartment 2: The Testicle

Two types of cells in the testicle are of interest to sperm production; the first is the Sertoli cell which lines the seminiferous tubules and is important for the process of spermatogenesis. Circulating FSH influences Sertoli cells while the second type of cells, Leydig cells, located within the interstitial tissue of the testicles are influenced by LH and are responsible for the production of testosterone. The testicular compartment produces both testosterone and sperm. Production of both is important in the assessment of this compartment and they do not necessarily go hand in hand. Damage to the testicular compartment may be either primary as a result of testicular failure (hypergonadotrophic hypogonadism) or secondary as a result of a defect in the hypothalamic-pituitary compartment (hypogonadotrophic hypogonadism). Hence to fully assess this compartment, the products of both the testicles (testosterone and sperm) and the hypothalamus/ pituitary (LH and FSH) need to be assessed together. Additional tests such as genetic testing are necessary depending on the suspected aetiology.

A number of conditions can affect the testicle:

(i) Congenital conditions such as testicular dysgenesis or chromosomal anomalies such as Klinefelter syndrome (47 XXY).

(ii) Traumatic conditions such as direct trauma, torsion or surgical removal of the testicle as a result of testicular cancer.

(iii) Inflammatory conditions such as mumps epididymo-orchitis.

(iv) Sertoli cell–only syndrome is a condition where the tubules are lined with only Sertoli cells with absence of spermatogenic cells. Since Leydig cells are normal, LH and testosterone levels will be normal. Despite normal Sertoli cells, inhibin production is decreased, leading to increased FSH levels. Most cases of Sertoli-only syndrome are idiopathic and characterised by complete absence of germ cells due to failure of migration of the germ cells from the primitive yolk sac [4].

2.1.3 Compartment 3: The Outflow Tract

The outflow tract includes the vas deferens and contributing secretions from the seminal vesicles and prostate. Problems associated with this compartment will lead to obstructive azoospermia characterised by a normal hormonal profile (normogonadotrophic hypogonadism). Assessment of the outflow tract is conducted through thorough examination of the semen analysis (e.g., absence of fructose and acidic pH in cases of the seminal vesicles obstruction) and imaging techniques such as MRI, vasography and rectal ultrasound. Factors affecting this compartment include the following:

(i) Congenital conditions such as congenital absence of the vas, commonly associated with mutations of the cystic fibrosis gene.

(ii) Traumatic conditions such as surgical trauma during hernia operations and other types of scrotal surgery and most commonly as a result of previous vasectomy.

(iii) Inflammatory conditions such as mumps epididymitis or chlamydia.

2.1.4 Clinical Workup for Azoospermia

Clinical evaluation should be conducted in a comprehensive and systematic way starting with the history and examination. In fact, a provisional diagnosis is often reached on the basis of history and examination alone. History should include a thorough enquiry regarding history of trauma, hernia operations, and torsion of the testicle, testicular tumours, undescended testicle, mumps, smoking and the use of exercise-enhancing products, steroids or other medical

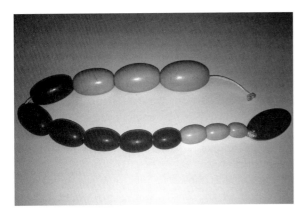

Fig. 6.1 Orchidometer

treatments (chemotherapy/radiotherapy). Examination of the testicle should include the size and consistency. Often an orchidometer (Figure 6.1) is used to objectively evaluate the size of the testicle. A normal testicle should be around 15 mls in size with firm consistency. Testicular size correlates with sperm production and in many cases testicular failure can be diagnosed at this stage through finding a small soft testicle. Examination should also include the spermatic cord, the epididymis and the vas. Per rectal examination usually conducted by the urologist can reveal cystic distension of the seminal vesicles in cases of seminal vesicle obstruction and can also reveal problems with the prostate. Semen analysis can also be very helpful in establishing a diagnosis, apart from focussing on sperm count, morphology and motility, other aspects may be equally important including the presence of a low volume in cases with ejaculatory duct obstruction, low fructose and acidic pH may also be associated with seminal vesicle obstruction [5].

History, examination and gonadotrophin levels will then allow classification into one of the three categories of hypogonadism and can then direct further testing.

2.1.4.1 Hypergonadotrophic Hypogonadism (Primary Testicular Failure): FSH and LH Will Be Elevated along with Normal/Low Testosterone Levels

Further tests should be directed towards genetic testing including screening for aneuploidies (e.g., Klinefelter syndrome, 47 XXY), translocations and Y chromosome microdeletions. Y chromosome microdeletions are present in about 10% of cases of non-obstructive azoospermia and are of particular interest from a prognostic point of view. Three main types of microdeletions can affect the azoospermia factor (AZF) regions present on the long arm of the human Y chromosome AZFa, AZFb and AZFc [6]. The chances of surgical sperm recovery are negligible in patients with AZFa and AZFb complete microdeletions whilst those with AZFc usually will have a successful surgical sperm recovery [7].

2.1.4.2 Normogonadotrophic Hypogonadism (Obstructive Azoospermia): FSH, LH and Testosterone Levels Are Normal

Further testing should include cystic fibrosis screening, particularly in men with congenital bilateral absence of the vas. The commonest CF mutation associated with abnormal sperm production abnormality is the Δ-F508 mutation. The finding of a CF mutation in the male partner indicates testing the female partner. If both carry a CF mutation then in vitro fertilisation / intracytoplasmic sperm injection (IVF/ICSI) with preimplantation genetic diagnosis can be offered. Radiological investigations are necessary before surgical intervention to correct an obstruction and include vasography, MRI scan and transrectal ultrasound.

2.1.4.3 Hypogonadotrophic Hypogonadism (Hypothalamic-Pituitary Disorders, Secondary Testicular Failure): FSH and LH Will Be Inappropriately Normal or Low with Low Testosterone Levels

Further investigations should be directed towards any abnormalities in the hypothalamic-pituitary axis. This includes estimation of prolactin levels along with checking other anterior pituitary hormones and appropriate pituitary imaging. Endocrinology referral may be appropriate.

2.1.5 Treatment of Azoospermia

2.1.5.1 Hypergonadotrophic Hypogonadism (Primary Testicular Failure)

Treatment will depend on whether sperm is present or absent in the testicular tissue and/or the epididymis. Therefore the first step is to offer surgical sperm recovery. If sperm is detected, then the couple can proceed with IVF/ICSI treatment, if no sperm is found then the couple will need to be counselled regarding alternative treatments such as treatment with donor sperm or adoption.

Techniques of Surgical Sperm Recovery Surgical sperm recovery can be achieved from either the epididymis (PESA, percutaneous epididymal sperm aspiration) or from the testicle. In men with non-obstructive azoospermia, sperm are usually retrieved from the testicular biopsy. There are different methods for obtaining sperm from the testicle, the least invasive is known as TESA (testicular sperm aspiration). This involves the insertion of a fine needle into the testes to aspirate a small amount of tissue, different areas in the testicle can be sampled and provided tubules are seen in the specimen, sperm can usually be extracted. In order to increase the yield of tissue retrieved from the testicle, an open testicular biopsy can be used (TESE, testicular sperm extraction). Both these procedures can be performed under a local anaesthetic and are minimally invasive. Several techniques have been used to improve sperm yield using these procedures, including perivascular nerve stimulation and testicular aspiration under ultrasound guidance. Unfortunately none of these techniques are, as yet, supported by good quality evidence [8].

In a further attempt to improve sperm yield, a technique known as Micro TESE may be used which involves surgical sperm extraction from the testicle using the surgical microscope. The use of optimal magnification can allow the surgeon to explore and sample areas where sperm are likely to be found after dissecting the seminiferous tubules. The technique also allows minimal testicular trauma and maximises exposure. Micro TESE can offer higher success rates than conventional TESE [9]. Furthermore, Micro TESE has been reported to successfully result in sperm extraction in over 60% of men with Klinefelter syndrome [10].

Predictors of Success of Surgical Sperm Recovery
Several indices have been used to predict the success of surgical sperm recovery. Perhaps one of the most important, as previously discussed, is testing for the type of AZF microdeletion if present. Other biochemical indicators include FSH, AMH and inhibin. Testicular volume has also been suggested to correlate with the success of surgical sperm recovery. Unfortunately none of these tests has been shown to be a good predictor. In one study, men with FSH levels of 31–45 still had around a 60% chance of having surgical sperm recovery [11]. A further study comparing AMH, inhibin and testicular volume showed no significant advantage for any of these over the other in predicting success of surgical sperm recovery. All of them had a poor sensitivity and specificity [12].

2.1.5.2 Normogonadotrophic Hypogonadism (Obstructive Azoospermia)

Treatment of men with obstructive azoospermia is usually through surgical sperm recovery followed by ICSI. In men with obstructive azoospermia, sperm is usually recovered from the epididymis (PESA). This involves the insertion of a small fine needle to aspirate semen from the epididymis and a local anaesthetic. Adequate samples can usually be stored for later usage in repeated cycles.

Occasionally, however, men may opt for surgical correction of the obstruction. This would require referral to a urologist and radiological investigation and imaging will be required to determine the exact site of the obstruction and the feasibility of surgical correction. The most commonly encountered, surgically correctable obstruction is reversal of vasectomy. Counselling for either surgical correction or ICSI would depend on many factors including other associated female factors such as age and the presence of tubal and/or ovarian disorders.

2.1.5.3 Hypogonadotrophic Hypogonadism (Secondary Testicular Failure)

Treatment in these cases is easily achieved by replacement of the deficient hormones, that is, FSH and LH. HCG is often prescribed alone or in combination with FSH. Treatment will need to be prolonged in order to initiate and then maintain sperm production. Sperm counts should be expected to increase gradually over a period of 1–2 years. It is important to take into consideration other fertility factors such as the female age. In a couple where the female age is approaching the point where there may be a significant decline in oocyte number and quality, or where there was an associated tubal or ovarian factor, it may not be appropriate to wait for a normal sperm count. In such cases, once sperm production is initiated, sperm can be retrieved through the ejaculate and used for treatment with ICSI or IVF depending on the sperm count.

Perhaps one of the most important but often missed causes of hypogonadotrophic hypogonadism is the use of so-called exercise-enhancing and bodybuilding supplements containing androgenic-anabolic steroids and/or testosterone. Some of these can also have a direct effect on sperm morphology and function [13]. This is easily diagnosed through detailed history and a hormone profile showing low gonadotrophins but normal to high testosterone

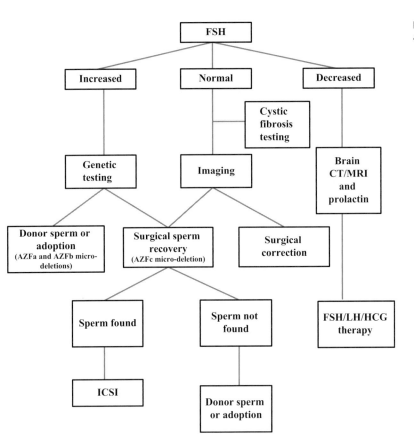

Fig. 6.2 Flowchart for management of azoospermia

levels. Treatment in this case is by simply stopping the offending agent and this will usually result in spontaneous resumption of spermatogenesis. A flowchart for management of azoospermia is seen in Figure 6.2.

3 Suboptimal Sperm Quality

This is the more commonly encountered semen abnormality in a clinical setting and involves suboptimal sperm parameters affecting the sperm count, motility, morphology or a combination of any of these factors. Many of the factors mentioned previously that can manifest by azoospermia (primary or secondary testicular failure) may manifest in suboptimal semen quality rather than azoospermia depending on the severity of the condition. However, often the cause is not identified and is termed idiopathic. In addition, there are several other possible mechanisms and underlying causes.

(i)   **Oxidative stress:** Oxidative stress may be a result of excessive generation of reactive oxygen species (ROS), decreased activity of

antioxidants or a combination of both [14]. Reactive oxygen species are essential for normal sperm function, however elevated levels of ROS can, on the other hand, be associated with abnormal sperm production and decreased fertilisation potential [15]. Oxidative stress can affect sperm mitochondrial adenosine triphosphate (ATP) production, affect sperm morphology and motility and cause DNA fragmentation [16,17]. Oxidative stress can be induced by exposure to environmental toxins, smoking and obesity. Even mild infections can also lead to oxidative stress. A recent study has shown that low level leukocytospermia, defined as presence of $<1 \times 10^{\wedge 6}$ WBC per ml, can result in increased production of reactive oxygen species, hence impairing sperm function [18].

(ii)   **Lifestyle factors:** Obesity has been shown to be associated with decreased male fertility. The increased prevalence mirrors the steady decline in sperm quality over the last decades suggesting a strong association [19]. This may be due to several mechanisms including oxidative stress, DNA damage and increased scrotal temperature impairing spermatogenesis [20]. Furthermore, in obese males, an increase in aromatase activity will lead to an increased peripheral conversion of androgens to oestrogen [20]. Studies have indeed shown a linear decline in serum parameters associated with an increase in the severity of obesity [21]. The biochemical markers of obesity have also been correlated with abnormal semen quality, where increased serum cholesterol and phospholipids have been shown to be associated with a lower percentage of sperm with intact acrosome and with increased sperm morphological abnormalities [19]. Studies have also shown that the adverse effect of obesity on sperm DNA fragmentation can be reversed with an improvement in lifestyle factors and a decrease in BMI [22]. Other lifestyle factors that can affect sperm quality through increased sperm DNA fragmentation include cigarette smoking and alcohol consumption [23].

(iii) **Varicocele:** The prevalence of varicocele is around 11.7% in men with normal semen parameters and 25.4% in men with abnormal semen and attending for fertility treatment [24]. Varicocele can lead to impaired spermatogenesis through several possible mechanisms: (a) heat related stress, (b) hypoperfusion leading to hypoxia (c) oxidative stress and (d) hormonal imbalances [25]. The question as to whether or not varicoceles should be treated to treat infertility remains a matter of debate. One meta-analysis found that for palpable varicoceles, spontaneous pregnancy was nearly three times more likely to occur with varicocelectomy compared to no treatment [26]. However, this study was associated with relatively high heterogeneity making the evidence less reliable. Similar findings come from a Cochrane review that showed that in couples with otherwise unexplained infertility the chance of conception was increased by varicocele treatment. However again the authors demonstrated a high degree of statistical heterogeneity amongst included studies and

consequently emphasised the poor quality of the existing evidence [27]. The decision to treat a varicocele should therefore be individualised and only be considered when clinically palpable in men with otherwise unexplained infertility and where assisted conception treatment is not a desirable option.

3.1 Treatment of Men with Suboptimal Semen Quality

Treatment will depend on a number of factors including the severity of the condition and presence of other factors in the female partner. Generally speaking in those with mild to moderate abnormalities, treatment will be in the form of either intrauterine insemination (IUI) with or without ovarian stimulation or IVF. Severe cases should be investigated in a manner similar to that described for azoospermia to determine whether the testicular insufficiency is primary or secondary and whether there is an underlying cause (FSH/LH, prolactin, testosterone, genetic testing and CF screening). Severe cases are treated by IVF with or without ICSI depending on the degree of severity. Adjuvant treatments have also been advocated and will be briefly discussed.

3.1.1 IUI Versus IVF

Whether to proceed directly with IVF or to have a trial of IUI for mild to moderate male factor infertility is a matter of debate and the decision should be individualised. IUI does have a modest success rate compared to IVF and other factors need to be taken into consideration, particularly the female partner's age, duration of infertility, previous parity, availability of funding and the patient's wishes and values. A Cochrane review showed that in male infertility, IUI with ovarian stimulation was no different from timed intercourse with ovarian stimulation [28]. However, only three studies were included in this meta-analysis with significantly high level of heterogeneity and hence the results should be interpreted with caution.

3.1.2 Adjuvant Treatments

Several treatments have been advocated in the past including the use of anti-oestrogens, bromocriptine, testosterone and aromatase inhibitors, none of these have been shown to improve fertility outcomes and

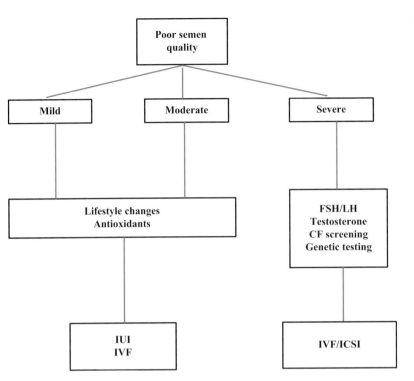

Fig. 6.3 Flowchart for management of suboptimal semen quality

their use should not be recommended. Furthermore and since the effect of antisperm antibodies on fertility is uncertain, the use of steroids is not advocated for treatment in men with antisperm antibodies [29].

Antioxidants, however, do have a potential place in the management of male subfertility in view of the increasing awareness of the importance of oxidative stress in male fertility. Indeed a Cochrane review has shown that antioxidants may improve success rates for couples going through IVF treatment, however, only a few studies were included and there is yet uncertainty regarding the best antioxidant and appropriate dosage [30].

Finally, when investigating male fertility the importance of coital dysfunction should not be underestimated and should always be explored during history taking. Erectile dysfunction, in many cases, is due to psychosexual problems and can be helped with appropriate psychosexual counselling. Medical treatments such as sildenafil can also easily remedy many erectile problems. Retrograde ejaculation can be treated by retrieval of sperm from the urine with appropriate precautions (alkalisation of the urine) and used for IVF/ICSI. In men with sphincter neurological damage such as in paraplegia, electro ejaculation or vibrostimulation can also be used to retrieve sperm, again to be used in assisted conception. A flowchart for management of azoospermia is seen in Figure 6.3.

To conclude, there is an increasing prevalence of male factor infertility and hence it is important that all clinicians involved in the fertility management are fully aware of the magnitude and the impact of the problem. Diagnosis is often simple when directed by a solid understanding of the underlying process of sperm production. A thorough history and examination cannot be underestimated and together with estimation of gonadotrophin levels will often result in a definitive diagnosis which would then allow appropriate management and referral on to tertiary care for surgical intervention or assisted conception as appropriate.

References

1. Jensen TK, Carlsen E, Jorgensen N, Berthelsen JG, Keiding N, Christensen K, et al. Poor semen quality may contribute to recent decline in fertility rates. *Hum Reprod*. 2002;17(6):1437–40.

2. HFEA. Fertility facts and figures. 2008.

3. Speiser PW, Azziz R, Baskin LS, Ghizzoni L, Hensle TW, Merke

DP, et al. Congenital adrenal hyperplasia due to steroid 21-hydroxylase deficiency: an Endocrine Society clinical practice guideline. *J Clin Endocrinol Metab.* 2010;95(9):4133–60.

4. Anniballo R, Ubaldi F, Cobellis L, Sorrentino M, Rienzi L, Greco E, et al. Criteria predicting the absence of spermatozoa in the Sertoli cell-only syndrome can be used to improve success rates of sperm retrieval. *Hum Reprod.* 2000;15(11):2269–77.

5. WHO. *WHO laboratory manual for the examination and processing of human semen.* Fifth ed. 2010.

6. Navarro-Costa P, Plancha CE, Goncalves J. Genetic dissection of the AZF regions of the human Y chromosome: thriller or filler for male (in)fertility? *J Biomed Biotechnol.* 2010;2010:936569.

7. Hopps CV, Mielnik A, Goldstein M, Palermo GD, Rosenwaks Z, Schlegel PN. Detection of sperm in men with Y chromosome microdeletions of the AZFa. *AZFb and AZFc regions. Hum Reprod.* 2003;18(8):1660–5.

8. Van Peperstraten A, Proctor ML, Johnson NP, Philipson G. Techniques for surgical retrieval of sperm prior to intra-cytoplasmic sperm injection (ICSI) for azoospermia. *Cochrane Database Syst Rev.* 2008; Issue 2. Art. No.: CD002807.

9. Tiseo BC, Hayden RP, Tanrikut C. Surgical management of nonobstructive azoospermia. *Asian J Urol.* 2015;2.

10. Ozveri H, Kayabasoglu F, Demirel C, Donmez E. Outcomes of micro-dissection TESE in patients with non-mosaic Klinefelter's Syndrome without hormonal treatment. *Int J Fertil Steril.* 2015;8(4):421–8.

11. Ramasamy R, Lin K, Gosden LV, Rosenwaks Z, Palermo GD, Schlegel PN. High serum FSH levels in men with nonobstructive azoospermia does not affect success of microdissection testicular sperm extraction. *Fertil Steril.* 2009;92(2):590–3.

12. Goulis DG, Tsametis C, Iliadou PK, Polychronou P, Kantartzi PD, Tarlatzis BC, et al. Serum inhibin B and anti-Mullerian hormone are not superior to follicle-stimulating hormone as predictors of the presence of sperm in testicular fine-needle aspiration in men with azoospermia. *Fertil Steril.* 2009;91(4):1279–84.

13. Fronczak CM, Kim ED, Barqawi AB. The insults of illicit drug use on male fertility. *J Androl.* 2012;33(4):515–28.

14. Morielli T, O'Flaherty C. Oxidative stress impairs function and increases redox protein modifications in human spermatozoa. *Reproduction.* 2015;149(1):113–23.

15. Ko EY, Sabanegh ES, Jr., Agarwal A. Male infertility testing: reactive oxygen species and antioxidant capacity. *Fertil Steril.* 2014;102(6):1518–27.

16. Gvozdjakova A, Kucharska J, Dubravicky J, Mojto V, Singh RB. Coenzyme Q(1)(0), alpha-tocopherol, and oxidative stress could be important metabolic biomarkers of male infertility. *Dis Markers.* 2015;2015:827941.

17. Muratori M, Tamburrino L, Marchiani S, Cambi M, Olivito B, Azzari C, et al. Investigation on the origin of sperm DNA fragmentation: role of apoptosis, *Immaturity and Oxidative Stress.* Mol Med. 2015;21:109–22.

18. Agarwal A, Mulgund A, Alshahrani S, Assidi M, Abuzenadah AM, Sharma R, et al. Reactive oxygen species and sperm DNA damage in infertile men presenting with low level leukocytospermia. *Reprod Biol Endocrinol.* 2014;12:126.

19. Schisterman EF, Mumford SL, Chen Z, Browne RW, Boyd Barr D, Kim S, et al. Lipid concentrations and semen quality: the LIFE study. *Andrology.* 2014;2(3):408–15.

20. Shukla KK, Chambial S, Dwivedi S, Misra S, Sharma P. Recent scenario of obesity and male fertility. *Andrology.* 2014;2(6):809–18.

21. Eisenberg ML, Kim S, Chen Z, Sundaram R, Schisterman EF, Buck Louis GM. The relationship between male BMI and waist circumference on semen quality: data from the LIFE study. *Hum Reprod.* 2014;29(2):193–200.

22. Faure C, Dupont C, Baraibar MA, Ladouce R, Cedrin-Durnerin I, Wolf JP, et al. In subfertile couple, abdominal fat loss in men is associated with improvement of sperm quality and pregnancy: a case-series. *PLoS One.* 2014;9(2): e86300.

23. Anifandis G, Bounartzi T, Messini CI, Dafopoulos K, Sotiriou S, Messinis IE. The impact of cigarette smoking and alcohol consumption on sperm parameters and sperm DNA fragmentation (SDF) measured by Halosperm((R)). *Arch Gynecol Obstet.* 2014;290(4):777–82.

24. WHO. The influence of varicocele on parameters of fertility in a large group of men presenting to infertility clinics. World Health Organization. *Fertil Steril.* 1992;57(6):1289–93.

25. Sheehan MM, Ramasamy R, Lamb DJ. Molecular mechanisms involved in varicocele-associated infertility. *J Assist Reprod Genet.* 2014;31(5):521–6.

26. Marmar JL, Agarwal A, Prabakaran S, Agarwal R, Short RA, Benoff S, et al. Reassessing the value of varicocelectomy as a treatment for male subfertility with a new meta-analysis. *Fertil Steril.* 2007;88(3):639–48.

27. Kroese AC, de Lange NM, Collins J, Evers JL. Surgery or embolization for varicoceles in subfertile men. *Cochrane*

Database Syst Rev. 2012; Issue 10. Art. No.: CD000479.

28. Bensdorp AJ, Cohlen BJ, Heineman MJ, Vandekerckhove P. Intra-uterine insemination for male subfertility. *Cochrane*

Database Syst Rev. 2007; Issue 4. Art. No.: CD000360.

29. NICE. Fertility problems: assessment and treatment; NICE guidelines [CG156]. 2013.

30. Showell MG, Mackenzie-Proctor R, Brown J, Yazdani A, Stankiewicz MT, Hart RJ. Antioxidants for male subfertility. *Cochrane Database Syst Rev.* 2014; Issue 12. Art. No.: CD007411.

Chapter

7

Semen Analysis and Sperm Function Tests

Hannah Williams
Sarah Martins da Silva

1 Semen Analysis

Semen analysis is a fundamental part of male fertility investigation. Samples are produced by masturbation, ideally in a private room nearby to the andrology laboratory or submitted within one hour if produced off-site. The ejaculate should be collected in a wide-mouthed, clean, glass or plastic container, from a batch confirmed to be non-toxic to spermatozoa. Patients should be given clear instructions about collection of their sample. To ensure consistency and reliable interpretation of results, there should be a minimum of two days and maximum of seven days abstinence (1), and the complete sample should be collected. Loss of the first portion of the ejaculate, which mainly comprises sperm-rich prostatic fluid, may significantly affect sperm count and concentration.

The *World Health Organisation (WHO) Laboratory Manual for the Examination and Processing of Human Semen* (fifth edition) was published in 2010 and includes standardised methods for semen analysis, sperm preparation and cryopreservation, as well as laboratory quality assurance and quality control (1). Routine assessment of semen includes visual and microscopic inspection, viscosity, volume, pH, presence of round cells or anti-sperm antibodies, sperm count, motility and morphology.

Semen volume is almost entirely made up of secretions from the accessory organs, mainly the prostate and seminal vesicles. Volume is best measured by weighing the sample in its container, then subtracting the weight of the empty container. Volume can be calculated from the sample weight, using the assumption that the density of semen is 1g/ml (2). Semen volume may also be measured using a volumetric pipette, although this is only accurate to the degree of markings on the pipette itself. Viscous samples or presence of bubbles in the semen may cause inaccuracies in volume measurement.

Semen pH is measured using colorimetric pH test strips, and reflects contributions from accessory gland secretions. Seminal vesicle secretions are alkaline and prostatic secretions are acidic. Consensus opinion suggests that semen pH should be no lower than 7.2.

Sperm count is assessed using a haemocytometer (a thick glass microscope side with a rectangular indentation that creates a chamber). Semen is diluted in a known concentration of water to render sperm immobile. By counting the number of cells in a specified volume, the overall concentration can then be calculated.

Sperm motility is assessed by analysis of at least 200 sperm. Motility is described as progressively motile (PR), non-progressively motile (NP) and immotile.

Vitality testing is used to determine if immotile sperm are alive or dead and is indicated when sperm motility is less than 40%. There are two approaches commonly used. The dye exclusion assay relies on the ability of live sperm to resist absorption of certain dyes, which penetrate and stain nonviable sperm. Trypan blue and Eosin Y stains are commonly used. After staining, spermatozoa are smeared on a glass slide and air dried, so cannot be used in treatment. The hypo-osmotic swelling (HOS) test also evaluates the functional integrity of the plasma membrane of the spermatozoa. Under hypo-osmotic conditions, influx of fluid causes the sperm tail to coil and swell, and thus identifies live cells. This method does not damage or kill spermatozoa and can be used to identify viable immotile sperm for intracytoplasmic sperm injection (ICSI) (3).

Morphology is arguably the most contentious element of diagnostic semen analysis. The variable morphology of human spermatozoa makes standardised assessment very challenging, however, evidence supports a relationship between in vivo fertilisation and the percentage of normal forms in a sample (strictly defined and/or using computer-aided assessment of morphology) and therefore justifies attempts to assess and record. Optionally, *Teratozoospermia index (TZI)* can be calculated by recording individual abnormalities identified in head, neck and midpiece, tail (principle piece) and excess cytoplasm (4). The total number of abnormalities recorded is divided by the number of spermatozoa with one or more defects to calculate TZI, and is significant if >1.5.

Anti-sperm antibodies (ASAs) may cause cell death, immobilisation of spermatozoa or create agglutinated clumps of moving sperm, thus impeding passage through cervical mucus, defective zona binding and fertilisation. Agglutination specifically refers to motile spermatozoa sticking to each other. ASAs may be IgG or IgA, although IgA are acknowledged to be of greater clinical significance. There are two direct tests for ASAs: the mixed agglutination reaction test (MAR test), which is performed using fresh semen, and the immunobead-binding assay (IB), which uses prepared sperm. There are currently no reference values for antibody-bound spermatozoa in the MAR test of semen from fertile men. Pending further evidence, the WHO manual consensus opinion recommends >50% motile spermatozoa with adherent particles to be considered clinically significant.

The WHO laboratory manual also includes revised reference values for human semen characteristics (5). These values were derived from semen analysis characteristics from men with a known time to pregnancy (TTP) of less than 12 months. Retrospective and prospective semen analysis data was collected and included 1953 samples from 5 studies, performed in 8 countries across 3 continents. Inclusion criteria were stringent and laboratory methods standardised, resulting in creation of a cohort of fertile men representative of a global population. The data was used to generate one-sided lower reference limits (5th centile), which are used as current criteria to define male fertility (Table 7.1).

If the result of the first semen analysis is abnormal, a repeat confirmatory test should be offered, ideally after three months to allow for a cycle of spermatogenesis. However, if a significant abnormality is identified (azoospermia, severe oligozoospermia), then the repeat test should be undertaken sooner. The nomenclature describing semen analysis abnormalities is shown in Box 7.1. Descriptive terms

Table 7.1 Normal values for semen parameters, according to WHO (2010)

Parameter	Lower reference limit
Semen volume (ml)	1.5
Total sperm number (10^6 per ejaculate)	39
Sperm concentration (10^6 per ml)	15
Total motility (PR + NP, %)	40
Progressive motility (PR, %)	32
Vitality (live spermatozoa, %)	58
Sperm morphology (normal forms, %)	4
Other consensus threshold values	
pH	>7.2
MAR test (motile spermatozoa with bound particles, %)	<50

Box 7.1 Nomenclature describing abnormal semen analysis parameters

Azoospermia	**No sperm in ejaculate**
Oligozoospermia	Total number / concentration of sperm below reference limit
Asthenozoospermia	% progressive motile sperm below reference limit
Teratozoospermia	% morphologically normal sperm below reference limit
Oligoasthenozoospermia	Total number / concentration of sperm and % progressive motility below reference limit
Oligoteratozoospermia	Total number / concentration of sperm and % normal morphology below reference limit
Asthenoteratozoospermia	% progressive motile sperm and % normal morphology below reference limit
Oligoasthenoteratozoospermia	Total number / concentration of sperm, % progressive motility and % normal morphology below reference limit

are used in combination where more than one abnormality is present.

2 Sperm Function Tests

Although semen analysis represents the cornerstone of male fertility investigation, it is a quantitative, rather than qualitative, test and does not evaluate sperm function. The journey of the human sperm in vivo includes penetration through viscous cervical mucus and negotiation of the uterus and oviduct to the site of fertilisation. Mammalian sperm also undergo a series of cellular changes, termed capacitation, to acquire the ability to fertilise. Only capacitated spermatozoa can penetrate the cumulus, undergo acrosome reaction, penetrate the zona pellucida, bind to the oocyte and achieve fertilisation.

Sperm function tests aim to examine various functional attributes of spermatozoa. However, lack of standardised methods, or available laboratory kit, generally limits their widespread use. Initial promise commonly fades because wider use reveals a more subjective endpoint than anticipated, or inadequate sensitivity and/or specificity, or that it is relevant to only a few selected cases and therefore of limited utility. Furthermore, cut-off values tend to be unclear and may be affected by measurement uncertainty. Moreover, sperm function tests may not help clinical management or improve success, or may simply identify a problem that has no effective treatment.

The *post-coital test* examines functional sperm motility by examining the ability of spermatozoa to penetrate cervical mucus. Timing is critical, due to the varying composition of the cervical mucus during the course of the menstrual cycle. The couple are advised to have intercourse around the predicted time of ovulation, and then attend the fertility clinic 9–12 hours later. Cervical mucus is aspirated for analysis, and presence or absence of motile sperm within the mucus is determined. Post-coital testing is no longer practised widely, mainly due to logistical difficulties, but also because it has no predictive value on pregnancy rate.

An alternative approach, based on the *Kremer penetration test*, involves the use of an artificial viscous media to replicate cervical mucus at the correct menstrual cycle phase. One per cent methylcellulose is used as an accepted surrogate for cervical mucus or cumulus complex (6). This sperm penetration assay is not widely used for clinical purposes, but remains a key tool in the research laboratory for assessing sperm function.

Computer aided sperm analysis (CASA) uses negative phase contrast to identify and track the motility and kinematics of individual spermatozoa, in either semen or prepared sperm samples. CASA systems have evolved greatly over the past 40 years, although the basic concepts for identifying sperm and their motion characteristics have changed little. Each system comprises a high power microscope, with image capture and computer analysis software, and uses mathematical algorithms to compute detailed movement variables. Kinematics measured by CASA systems are listed below, and illustrated in Figure 7.1.

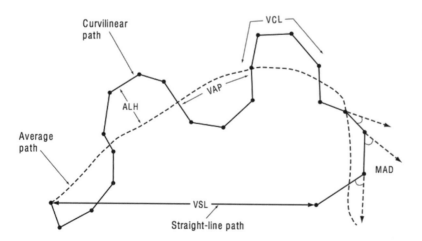

Fig. 7.1 Standard terminology for sperm motility characteristics measured by CASA systems

1. VCL, curvilinear velocity (Pm/s): Time-averaged velocity of a sperm head along its actual curvilinear path.
2. VSL, straight-line velocity (Pm/s): Time-averaged velocity of a sperm head along the straight line between its first and last detected position.
3. VAP, average path velocity (Pm/s): Time-averaged velocity of a sperm head along its average path.
4. ALH, amplitude of lateral head displacement (Pm): Magnitude of lateral displacement of a sperm head about its average path, either expressed as a maximum or an average.

Note that different CASA instruments compute ALH using different algorithms, so values may not be comparable between systems.

5. LIN, linearity: The linearity of a curvilinear path, VSL/VCL.
6. WOB, wobble: A measure of oscillation of the actual path about the average path, VAP/VCL.
7. STR, straightness: Linearity of the average path, VSL/VAP.
8. BCF, beat-cross frequency (Hz): The average rate at which the curvilinear path crosses the average path.
9. MAD, mean angular displacement (degrees): The time-averaged absolute values of the instantaneous turning angle of the sperm head along its curvilinear trajectory.

CASA can also calculate the concentration of sperm within a sample. CASA is useful as it eliminates the variation between individual assessors of semen motility and concentration. However, the computer cannot distinguish between sperm and other cells or debris of a similar size, thus counting them as non-motile sperm. CASA is available in some assisted reproduction technology (ART) centres, but the extent of use and reliance ranges widely; its main use is within a research setting.

Hyaluronic binding assay. Hyaluronan is the major component of the cumulus complex surrounding the oocyte. The ability of spermatozoa to bind to hyaluronic acid (HA) is a biochemical marker of spermatozoa maturity, morphology and DNA integrity. *Hyaluronic binding assay* (HBA slides; Origio) can be used to predict fertilisation ability of sperm in in vitro fertilization (IVF) cycles and distinguish sperm samples suitable for IVF or ICSI (7). Viewed on a microscope, sperm bound to HA on a slide are distinguished by beating tails with heads that make no progressive movement. Low HBA score (65% or less) suggests that ICSI patients would benefit from HA sperm diagnostics and selection to improve clinical pregnancy rate and reduce pregnancy loss (PICSI dish; Origio), although it is notable that the HBA slide and PICSI dish manufacturer has funded the only published study to date.

The *hemizona / zona pellucida (ZP) assay* involves the use of the human ZP, the glycoprotein coat surrounding the oocyte, to assess sperm-ZP binding. Half of the ZP is incubated with sperm from the male partner, whilst the other half is incubated with sperm from a proven fertile sperm donor. Significant discrepancies between the numbers of partner or donor sperm bound to the ZP could indicate an inability of the partner sperm to bind to the oocyte. However this technique requires a regular supply of human ZP, which could, in theory, be obtained from oocytes surplus to IVF treatment, but in reality are not readily available. Specificity of sperm, which only binds to human ZP, further limits the use of this technique, and as such is not routinely used. Alternatively, induced *acrosome reaction (AR) assays* are also predictive of fertilisation outcome. The acrosome reaction is induced by contact with the ZP in vivo, and results in release of acrosomal enzymes. Calcium ionophore is commonly used to induce AR in vitro.

Sperm penetration assay, also known as *sperm capacitation index* or *zona-free hamster oocyte penetration assay* utilises golden hamster oocytes, which are unusual in that removal of their ZP results in loss of species specificity to egg penetration. This test measures the ability of sperm to undergo capacitation, fuse with the oocyte membrane and decondense the sperm head resulting in the formation of the male pronucleus (8). The *acrosin assay* is an indirect assessment of sperm penetrating capability. Acrosin, a sperm acrosomal serine protinase, is involved in triggering of AR, binding of sperm to the ZP and is important for fertilisation. Measurement of acrosin is thought to correlate with sperm binding to and penetration of ZP.

DNA damage. The sperm nucleus lacks protection against oxidative stress and is vulnerable to oxidation-mediated DNA damage. DNA fragmentation may be increased in infertile male spermatozoa(9), and poorer DNA integrity can impact on success of ART and contribute to a higher risk of miscarriage(10). Sperm DNA damage can be assessed by a variety of approaches: sperm chromatin structure assay (SCSA), sperm chromatin dispersion test (SCD), terminal deoxynucleotidyl transferase-mediated deoxyuridine triphosphate-nick end labelling (TUNEL) and Comet Assays.

SCSA is probably the most robust method of evaluating DNA damage, although test results may be inconclusive for men with severe oligozoospermia ($<1x10^6$/ml). Acid pH conditions unwind double-stranded (ds) DNA. Acrinine orange binds to DNA and fluoresces green with ds DNA (non-denatured) and red with single-stranded (ss) DNA (denatured). Fluorescence detection is by flow cytometry, with results expressed as % DNA fragmentation index (DFI). Current data show a significant reduction in probability of successful pregnancy (spontaneous conception or ART) when DFI above 30%, albeit that this is a statistical threshold rather than absolute value. In addition to DFI, SCSA also identifies a fraction of sperm with high DNA stainability (HDS). HDS sperm are considered to contain immature chromatin and abnormal nuclear proteins. Samples with HDS above 15% may have lower rates of fertilisation with IVF, but not ICSI (www.scsadiagnostics.com).

SCD has been developed as a commercially available kit and uses chromatin staining and conventional bright-field microscopy to identify ss and ds DNA breaks in human sperm (Halosperm;(11)). This method uses acid denaturation and detergent lysis to remove protamines and histones. The unravelled DNA without damage produces a large halo, whereas fragmented DNA results in a small or no halo. The kit is simple and turnaround time is fast, however, interpretation is subjective.

TUNEL assay detects ds and ss DNA breaks present in spermatozoa using fluorescein-labelled dUTP nucleotides (12). Fluorescence or bright-field microscopy, or flow cytometry, can be used to measure the percentage of cells with labelled DNA. It can be performed with low numbers of sperm, but assay protocols are labour-intensive, variable and not specifically designed for human spermatozoa. Thresholds are non-standardised.

Comet assay measures small pieces of DNA that are free to move out of individual sperm. Alkaline conditions denature DNA to reveal ss and ds DNA breaks, whereas mostly ss DNA breaks are revealed under neutral conditions. Electrophoresis results in the migration of broken strands towards the anode, forming a comet tail when observed under fluorescence microscope. The relative fluorescence in the tail compared with its head serves as a measure of the level of DNA damage (13). The test is sensitive and can be performed on low numbers of sperm, but requires complicated imaging software, and there are variable assay protocols and unclear thresholds.

Sperm DNA damage testing is now available commercially, although not currently approved or recommended in clinical guidelines. The different tests measure slightly different aspects of sperm DNA damage, and concerns also remain regarding reliability and reproducibility. More frustratingly, rather than identifying sperm with low levels of DNA damage to select for ICSI, sperm DNA damage tests destroy the sperm studied, and thus render them clinically unusable. There are no agreed-upon clinical thresholds, although current consensus is DNA fragmentation index greater than 30% is clinically significant. High levels of sperm DNA damage may be amenable to lifestyle modification, correction of varicocele and/or anti-oxidant treatment, such as high dose vitamin C (1000 mg), but this is also controversial (14).

Oxidative stress occurs when the production of potentially destructive reactive oxygen species (ROS), such as oxygen ions, free radicals and peroxides, exceeds natural antioxidant defences. It is a common pathology, seen in 30–80% of infertile men (15). Oxidative stress is thought to have a dual mechanism of action, causing damage not only to DNA (16) but also to the sperm membrane, resulting in decrease in sperm motility and a reduced ability to fertilise the oocyte. ROS can be measured using cellular probes coupled with flow cytometry to detect chemiluminescence. Fresh semen or sperm suspensions are incubated with a redox-sensitive light-emitting probe, such as luminol, and light emission is then measured over time. However, the clinical value of semen ROS determination is unproven, and there are no established semen ROS cut-off values that can be used to predict reproductive outcomes.

Proteomics allows comparison of sperm protein expression by normal (fertile) and infertile men. It may be possible to identify molecular targets crucial to fertilisation and implicated in sperm dysfunction, such as phospholipase C zeta, CatSper, ADAMs and Izumo, but is currently an experimental technique.

Summary

Diagnostic semen analysis is the first step to identify male factor subfertility, however it neither measures the fertilising potential of spermatozoa nor the complex changes that occur in the female reproductive tract in vivo. Furthermore, diagnostic semen analysis techniques are often subjective, and results may vary between laboratory staff. Sperm function tests aspire to predict functional capabilities of spermatozoa, and success of fertilisation in vitro, but many lack clinical utility to date.

References

1. *World Health Organisation. Laboratory Manual for Examination and Processing of Human Semen.* 5th edn. 2010.

2. Auger J, Kunstmann JM, Czyglik F, Jouannet P. Decline in semen quality among fertile men in Paris during the past 20 years. *The New England Journal of Medicine.* 1995 Feb 2; 332(5):281–5. PubMed PMID: 7816062.

3. Jeyendran RS, Van der Ven HH, Rachagan SP, Perez-Peleaz M, Zaneveld LJ. Semen quality and in-vitro fertilization. *The Australian & New Zealand Journal of Obstetrics & Gynaecology.* 1989 May;29 (2):168–72. PubMed PMID: 2803129.

4. Menkveld R, Wong WY, Lombard CJ, Wetzels AM, Thomas CM, Merkus HM, et al. Semen parameters, including WHO and strict criteria morphology, in a fertile and subfertile population: an effort towards standardization of in-vivo thresholds. *Human Reproduction.* 2001 Jun; 16(6):1165–71. PubMed PMID: 11387287.

5. Cooper TG, Noonan E, von Eckardstein S, Auger J, Baker HW, Behre HM, et al. World Health Organization reference values for human semen characteristics. *Human Reproduction Update.* 2010 May-Jun;16(3):231–45. PubMed PMID: 19934213.

6. Ivic A, Onyeaka H, Girling A, Brewis IA, Ola B, Hammadieh N, et al. Critical evaluation of methylcellulose as an alternative medium in sperm migration tests. *Human Reproduction.* 2002 Jan;17(1):143–9. PubMed PMID: 11756379.

7. Pregl Breznik B, Kovacic B, Vlaisavljevic V. Are sperm DNA fragmentation, hyperactivation, and hyaluronan-binding ability predictive for fertilization and embryo development in in vitro fertilization and intracytoplasmic sperm injection? *Fertility and Sterility.* 2013 Apr;99(5):1233–41. PubMed PMID: 23290739.

8. Hwang K, Lamb DJ. The sperm penetration assay for the assessment of fertilization capacity. *Mol Biol.* 2013;927:103–111.

9. Irvine DS, Twigg JP, Gordon EL, Fulton N, Milne PA, Aitken RJ. DNA integrity in human spermatozoa: relationships with semen quality. *Journal of Andrology.* 2000 Jan–Feb; 21(1):33–44. PubMed PMID: 10670517.

10. Robinson L, Gallos ID, Conner SJ, Rajkhowa M, Miller D, Lewis S, et al. The effect of sperm DNA fragmentation on miscarriage rates: a systematic review and meta-analysis. *Human Reproduction.* 2012 Oct; 27(10):2908–17. PubMed PMID: 22791753.

11. Fernandez JL, Muriel L, Rivero MT, Goyanes V, Vazquez R, Alvarez JG. The sperm chromatin dispersion test: a simple method for the determination of sperm DNA fragmentation. *Journal of Andrology.* 2003 Jan-Feb;24(1):59–66. PubMed PMID: 12514084.

12. Sailer BL, Jost LK, Evenson DP. Mammalian sperm DNA susceptibility to in situ denaturation associated with the presence of DNA strand breaks as measured by the terminal deoxynucleotidyl transferase assay. *Journal of Andrology.* 1995 Jan–Feb;16(1):80–7. PubMed PMID: 7768756.

13. Collins AR. The comet assay for DNA damage and repair: principles, applications, and limitations. *Molecular Biotechnology.* 2004 Mar;26(3):249–61. PubMed PMID: 15004294.

14. Showell MG, Mackenzie-Proctor R, Brown J, Yazdani A, Stankiewicz MT, Hart RJ. Antioxidants for male subfertility. *The Cochrane Database of Systematic Reviews.* 2014 Dec 15;Issue 12. PubMed PMID: 25504418.

15. Tremellen K. Oxidative stress and male infertility–a clinical perspective. *Human Reproduction Update.* 2008 May–Jun; 14(3):243–58. PubMed PMID: 18281241.

16. Shiva M, Gautam AK, Verma Y, Shivgotra V, Doshi H, Kumar S. Association between sperm quality, oxidative stress, and seminal antioxidant activity. *Clinical Biochemistry.* 2011 Mar;44(4):319–24. PubMed PMID: 21145315.

Chapter

8

Assessment of Fallopian Tube Patency

Ka Ying Bonnie Ng
Ying Cheong

1 Introduction

Fallopian tubes make vital portals for the transfer of gametes and the early conceptus, and were named after Gabrielis Fallopius (Italy, 1423–1562) who first described the structures. Reinier De Graaf (1641–1673), however, was the first to understand the function of the Fallopian tubes. The Fallopian tubes were described as

> The trumpets or tubes . . . are two in number either side of the uterus. Where they originate, at the fundus, they are quite narrow. . . As they pass through the substance of the uterus and for some distance outside they proceed in a straight course, gradually widening. When, however, they have attained an appreciable size, they curve perceptibly more and more and proceed, bending from side to side or twisting like vine-tendrils. In this way they get half way round the "testicles" at a distance from them.

It is estimated that one in six couples requires investigation and treatment of subfertility, and tubal factors account for about 14% of causes of infertility in women. The prevalence tends to be higher in India due to higher rates of unrecognised pelvic inflammatory disease and tuberculosis.

Alongside the investigation of tubal patency, the results of semen analysis and investigations to assess ovulation should be performed. Tubal blockage can involve either the proximal part (closest to the uterus), mid part or distal part (furthest from the uterus). The Fallopian tube is a dynamic and complex structure, and hence, it is important to understand that demonstration of tubal patency does not always correspond to tubal function. The combination of coordinated neuromuscular activity, cilial action and endocrine secretions are required for successful tubal function.

Compromised tubal damage can occur with any external or internal injury, hindering the normal transport of gametes. Causes of tubal disease include pelvic infection, endometriosis and previous abdominal surgery. Endometriosis, the presence of endometrial tissue occurring outside the uterine cavity causing peritoneal lesions, accounts for about 5% of female infertility.

An 'ideal' or 'gold standard' test for tubal patency would be sensitive (i.e. all true positives would be identified by a positive test result and a negative test result would rule out disease in all those without the disease) and specific (i.e. the test result would only be positive in women with the disease). There are many tests available in the assessment of tubal disease and this reflects the fact that there is no 'ideal' test; none yield perfect accuracy and predictive values. They are also subject to operator expertise and potential intraoperative or technical complications.

2 Methods of Assessing Fallopian Tube Patency

A comparison of the various tubal assessment methods is shown in Table 8.1.

2.1 Hysterosalpingography (HSG)

HSG is the radiographic evaluation of the uterus and Fallopian tubes; its main use is in assessing the whole tube, condition of the tubal lumen and site of block. It is useful in diagnosing endometrial and Mullerian abnormalities including congenital anomalies, leiomyomas, synechiae, polyps, tubal occlusion, salpingitis isthmica nodosum (also known as diverticulosis of the Fallopian tube), hydrosalpinx and peritubal adhesions.

An analgesic (e.g. NSAIDs) or antispasmodic medication may be given to the patient prior to the procedure to reduce lower abdominal cramping and chances of tubal spasm. HSG is usually performed in the early follicular phase; this avoids the possibility of pregnancy and facilitates maximum uterine visibility

Table 8.1 Table comparing the various tubal assessment tests –: No, +: Yes

	HSG	HyCoSy	Lap and dye	Falloposcopy	Salpingoscopy	CAT
Gold standard – diagnostic and therapeutic	-	-	+	-	-	-
Widely available	+	-	+	-	-	-
Assess tubal patency	+	+	+	+	+	-
Assess tubal function	-	-	-	-	-	-
Learning curve	+	++	+	+++	+++	+
Cost	++	++	+++	++	++	+
Requires general anaesthetics	-	-	+	+/-	+/-	-
Outpatient procedure	+	+	–	+/-	+/-	+
Blood test	-	-	-	-	-	+
Ultrasound scan performed at the same time	-	+	-	-	-	-
Research only	-	-	-	+	+	+/-
Ascending Infection risk	+	+	+	+	+	-
Procedure associated discomfort	++	++	+	++	++	-

as the endometrium is thin in the proliferative phase. Patients are tested for chlamydia prior to undergoing HSG as pelvic infection is a contraindication; if required, prophylactic antibiotics are given.

HSG is performed with the patient in the lithotomy position on the fluoroscopy table and aseptic precautions apply. A speculum exposes the cervix, and the vagina and cervix are cleaned using antiseptic solution. A tenaculum is used to grasp the anterior lip of the cervix, an HSG cannula is introduced and stabilised in the cervix. A very small amount of radiopaque contrast solution, warmed to body temperature, is introduced through the cannula into the uterus. The filling of the solution in the uterine cavity and passage through the Fallopian tubes, including its spill from the fimbrial end is observed and captured in the form of X-rays. Clear intraperitoneal spill must be demonstrated. If spill is not demonstrated, rotating the patient from side to side or gentle abdominal pressure may increase likelihood of intraperitoneal dispersion. It has been suggested that the use of intravenous smooth muscle relaxants such as terbutaline and prostaglandins may help to relieve spasm. Figure 8.1 shows a normal HSG.

Both proximal and distal tubal blockage can be recognised in HSG. Proximal tubal blockage caused by salpingitis isthmica nodosa (SIN), also referred to as tubal diverticulosis, has a characteristic honeycomb appearance. There are multiple small diverticular collections of contrast protruding from the lumen into the wall of the isthmic portion of the Fallopian tube (Figure 8.2). White flecks of contrast material often persist at the site of suspected blockage even in the post drainage X-ray. In tuberculous salpingitis, there may be a similar calcification appearance; however, calcification of the uterus, ovaries and lymph nodes can also be present. The aetiology of SIN is unknown, but it is probably a post-infectious reaction. Distally obstructed tubes might have small club-shaped ends on HSG, representing the presence of hydrosalpinges. However, in most cases, distal tubal obstruction is detected by proximal filling with dye, but no spillage of dye into the peritoneum.

HSG is widely used for tubal evaluation in women presenting with subfertility and is a fairly accurate and easy way of identifying proximal tubal damage. The whole procedure is very quick, taking about 3–5 minutes. It is generally very safe and fairly cheap.

The risks associated with HSG include potential reaction to the iodine containing radiopaque contrast. The most common complication is cramping at the time of contrast injection. Premedication, minimising

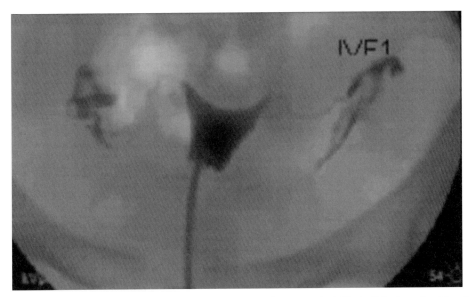

Fig. 8.1 Normal Hysterosalpingogram showing cannulation of contrast, which fills the Fallopian tubes. There is free spillage of contrast from the patent tubes.

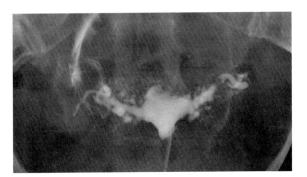

Fig. 8.2 Salpingitis ismica nodosa (SIN) on hysterosalpingogram. This is an inflammatory, probably post-infectious disease of the Fallopian tubes characterised by multiple diverticula. SIN may be associated with tubal obstruction and increased risk of ectopic pregnancy.

cervical trauma and a consideration to the emotional state of the patient may increase the tolerance of the procedure. Pelvic infection is a complication affecting 1–3% of women having HSG; prophylactic antibiotics should be given to those with risk factors for pelvic infection detected in the clinical history or examination. The procedure also exposes women to radiation, and as it is done in a radiology setting, the patient and operator may feel uncomfortable or embarrassed. Retrospective review of the images is only possible if the procedure is recorded in real time.

A meta-analysis of three studies gave pooled estimates of HSG sensitivity as 0.65 (95% CI 0.50–0.78)

and specificity as 0.83 (95% CI 0.77–0.88) [1]. Because of HSG's low sensitivity, it is of limited use for detecting tubal obstruction, but its high specificity makes it a useful test for ruling out tubal obstruction. A high false positive rate is a problem; the diagnosis of peritoneal adhesions based on HSG findings are unreliable and proximal tubal 'occlusions' may be due to transient tubal spasms (20% of cases), amorphous debris collections or minimal adhesions (40% of cases) [2]. Results from one review suggested that HSG may be used as a screening test for couples with no history of pelvic infection and if the test is abnormal, laparoscopic assessment should be performed [3].

The potential therapeutic effect of tubal flushing at HSG has been under speculation for more than 50 years. Historically, a variety of agents have been used to 'flush' the Fallopian tubes. At HSG, a water-soluble contrast media (WSCM) or oil-soluble contrast media (OSCM) is used. A Cochrane review collected evidence from 13 randomised controlled trials [4]. This review showed that women having OSCM tubal flushing had a higher rate of pregnancy and live birth compared to women with no intervention; evidence suggests that for subfertile women, the chance of an ongoing pregnancy will be increased from 17% without intervention to between 29 to 55% with intervention. Despite positive effects on pregnancy rates, extravasation of OSCM into the pelvic cavity has potentially serious adverse effects such as lipogranuloma formation, which occurs if there is accumulation of OSCM within a blocked tube leading to a chronic inflammatory reaction, or anaphylaxis if the OSCM enters blood vessels or lymphatics. There were no trials assessing tubal flushing with WSCM versus no treatment or WSCM versus OSCM. Further randomised controlled trials are needed to evaluate the potential therapeutic effects of tubal flushing with water-soluble media. There was no evidence of difference in the rates of adverse events between any of these interventions.

WSCM allows better imaging of the tubal mucosal folds and ampullary rugae (internal tube architecture) compared to OSCM. OSCM has a high viscosity which leads to slow filling of the tubes; often, this requires a late film after 24 hours. However, sometimes, this 'late' film can offer additional information, such as adhesions after slow peritoneal spillage. It is slower to resorb and remains in the pelvic cavity for longer. OSCM may be associated with less pain probably because there is less irritation of the peritoneum. WSCM is cheaper than OSCM.

2.2 Laparoscopy and Dye

The laparoscopy and dye test is regarded as the 'gold standard' for assessing tubal patency. Historically, laparoscopy and dye was the first line screening evaluation for women with subfertility. However, HSG or hysterosalpingo-contrast-sonography (HyCoSy), when available is a less invasive procedure. At present, it is still considered the most accurate diagnostic test available for assessing tubal related infertility. It enables the operator to directly visualise the abdominal cavity and pelvic structures, including the external appearance of the Fallopian tubes and the fimbrial ends. In addition, pelvic pathologies such as endometriosis which may contribute to infertility may be diagnosed and treated. Through insertion of a cannula into the cervix (traditionally a Spackman), diluted methylene blue is instilled into the uterine cavity and the Fallopian tubes.

It is common that dye does not pass through an apparently normal tube due to the preferential flow of blue dye to the opposite tube. To overcome this problem, application of a gentle pressure using a laparoscopic forceps over the tube with the preferential flow of dye (Figure 8.3), allows for the redirection of blue dye to the other tube, and avoids the erroneous diagnosis of 'blockage' of an apparently normal Fallopian tube.

It is also important to ensure that an adequate seal is obtained at the level of the Spackman cannula and the cervix. A significant amount of methylene blue can flow back into the vagina if there is an inadequate seal over the cervix; with insufficient dye passing up the uterine cavity into the Fallopian tubes, patency cannot be shown. In this scenario, reapplication of the instruments to secure a better seal or the use of two tenaculae, one over the anterior and the other over the posterior lip of the cervix may ensure sufficient seal. However, in the event that the latter is not possible, the insertion of a Foley catheter into the uterine cavity, with the pulling back of the inflated balloon onto the internal cervical os, will ensure a better seal. Methylene blue can then be injected through the catheter without the problem of excessive backflow of dye into the vagina.

There are, however, serious though rare complications associated with laparoscopy including injury to the bladder, bowel and blood vessels. The risk of a laparotomy as a result of a severe complication is 1.4 to 3.1 per 1000 cases. This risk is increased in patients with previous abdominal or pelvic surgery, previous pelvic inflammatory disease or obesity. A prospective study reported a complication rate of 5.7 per 1000 cases, with the most commonly observed being haemorrhage from the epigastric vessels and injury to the bowel [5].

2.3 Hysterosalpingo-Contrast-Sonography (HyCoSy)

HyCoSy assesses tubal patency and the uterine cavity by transvaginal ultrasonography (TVUS) and the concomitant instillation of an echogenic contrast medium into the uterine cavity via a catheter inserted through the cervical os. An echogenic contrast medium is required in HyCoSy as there is no tissue–fluid interface in normal tubes. Fallopian tubes may only be visualised when there is a hydrosalpinx or free fluid in the pelvis outlining the tubes, or fluid is introduced in the tubal lumen or the pelvis. The cheap and cost-effective option is the use of saline mixed with air, which produces a contrast fluid due to the presence of air bubbles. However, these air bubbles stand for a short period, making tubal assessment practically more difficult. Ex-Foam can be used as an alternative to saline solution and remains stable for several minutes. The foam is created by diluting gel (containing glycerol and hydroxyethyl cellulose)

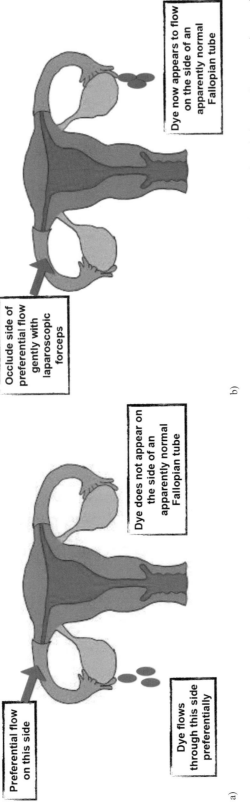

Fig. 8.3a and 8.3b Laparoscopy and dye. Occlusion of the side of the Fallopian tube with preferential flow will facilitate methylene blue to pass through the opposite apparently normal Fallopian tube.

purified in water, and little air bubbles are formed by pushing the gel through small openings in syringes or tubes. HyCoSy is usually done in the mid proliferative phase (day 6–10 of a 28-day cycle) of the menstrual cycle, after menstruation stops but before ovulation, to reduce the risk of disrupting an early pregnancy.

HyCoSy has high diagnostic accuracy in the assessment of the uterine cavity and allows for concomitant assessment of ovarian morphology; TVUS is a common imaging technique for the diagnosis of ovarian cysts. There is a good statistical concordance with HSG and laparoscopy with dye [6]. The agreement of HyCoSy compared with standard X-ray HSG was 94%, the sensitivity 50% and specificity 97% [7].

This examination has been shown to be safe and well tolerated with shorter examination times and fewer side effects compared to HSG. It avoids the risk of radiation, whilst providing the same information as HSG. It is relatively low cost. The procedure has no major complications; the most common complications include nausea and vomiting and abdominal pain. The risk of pelvic infection and associated peritonitis is about 1%. Failure to perform or complete the procedure is documented in approximately 7% cases [8].

HyCoSy is not a widely available investigation. There is a steep learning curve for professionals training to perform the procedure. As with HSG, there is also an issue with record keeping; unless the images are recorded in real time, they cannot be easily kept for retrospective review.

The National Institute for Health and Care Excellence (NICE) recommends HyCoSy as a primary investigation for tubal assessment for low-risk women without a history suggestive of tubal damage [9]. It is an effective alternative to HSG when the expertise is available. Women with comorbidities such as inflammatory disease, previous ectopic pregnancies or endometriosis, should be offered laparoscopy and dye in order for tubal and other pelvic structures to be assessed at the same time.

2.4 Fertiloscopy or Transvaginal Hydrolaparoscopy

Fertiloscopy is a relatively new development. One prospective multicentre study ('FLY study') compared the two endoscopic techniques of laparoscopy and fertiloscopy in routine evaluation of the pelvis in infertile women; they showed that both have similar sensitivity and negative predictive values, and concluded that fertiloscopy may be considered an alternative to diagnostic laparoscopy in the routine assessment of women without clinical or ultrasound evidence of pelvic disease [10].

Fertiloscopy (Figure 8.4) is done under either general or local anaesthetic and involves introducing 100–200 mls of saline via a Veress needle into

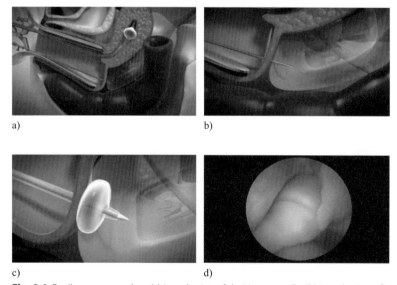

a)

b)

c)

d)

Fig. 8.4 Fertiloscopy procedure. (a) Introduction of the Veress needle, (b) introduction of 100–200 mls of saline into the posterior fornix of vagina through pouch of Douglas, (c) insertion of trocar for mini-laparoscope, and (d) insertion of mini-laparoscope for visualisation of posterior uterus, ovaries and Fallopian tubes.

posterior fornix of the vagina and through the pouch of Douglas. This is followed by the insertion of a trocar through which a mini-laparoscope (less than 3 mm) is inserted. This allows visualisation of the posterior pelvis, including the posterior aspect of the uterus, ovaries and the Fallopian tubes. Methylene blue can be injected into the uterine cavity for tubal patency to be assessed. If tubal pathology is found, falloposcopy can be performed at the same time. It is also possible to perform small interventions such as adhesiolysis, ovarian drilling and coagulation of endometriosis spots at the same time.

Fertiloscopy is minimally invasive, substantially harmless and well accepted by patients. It is easily performed, even in obese patients. It permits a very 'physiological approach' as it does not require mobilisation of the tubes and ovaries for the examination. The procedure is quick, lasting 10–15 minutes and is easy to learn. The development of surgical capabilities may in the future reduce the number of laparoscopies for conditions such as mild endometriosis.

Although studies have shown that there is good correlation between fertiloscopy and laparoscopy, fertiloscopy is still not widely practised. Firstly, there is concern that it is associated with rectal and uterine injuries (although studies seem to show that this is not the case [11]). Secondly, it is contraindicated in cases where there is evident pelvic pathology, requiring laparoscopy; these include pelvic masses occupying the pouch of Douglas (including posterior myomas, ovarian cysts and women with fixed uterine retroflexion). One of the limitations of fertiloscopy is the inability to visualise the anterior aspect of the uterus and uteri-vesical fold. There is low operative capacity and currently, fertiloscopy is only considered as a diagnostic procedure.

2.5 Falloposcopy or Salpingoscopy

Falloposcopy is mainly used as a research tool and is a highly specialised procedure that allows direct vision of the inside of the Fallopian tube. There are suggestions that falloposcopy may be a more discriminatory test of tubal pathology, as one study has shown that women with normal Fallopian tubes at falloposcopy have higher rates of spontaneous pregnancy (27.6%) compared to those with mild or severe endotubal lesions (11.5% to 0%) [12].

Falloposcopy involves cannulation of the Fallopian tubes, via the cervix and uterus with ultrasound or hysteroscopic guidance. There are two main types of falloposcope: coaxial and linear everting catheter. In the coaxial technique, the uterotubal ostium is identified and a guidewire is introduced into the Fallopian tube until the fimbrial end or an obstruction is reached. A fibreoptic endoscope, usually no more than 5 mm in width, then replaces the guidewire. There is constant irrigation and distension of the tubes as the fibreoptic endoscopy is slowly withdrawn; this allows visualisation of the Fallopian tube mucosa in a retrograde fashion. The linear everting catheter technique is a different kind of falloposcopy which does not require a guidewire.

Substantial training and investment is required for this highly technical procedure. It is used as a research tool, as there are still significant technical difficulties, such as cannulation difficulties and problems with visualisation. Complications include pinhole tubal perforations and tubal wall dissection. One study examining the technical aspects of this procedure revealed that only 57% of patients received a complete evaluation by the test [13].

2.6 Chlamydia Testing

Chlamydia immunoglobulin G antibodies are thought to persist for many years and so have been assessed as markers of previous *Chlamydia trachomatis* infection. Chlamydia antibody testing has been shown to be a non-invasive and cost-effective method of screening for potential past chlamydia infection and for tubal factor subfertility. A meta-analysis of 23 studies, showed that the discriminative capacity of the chlamydia antibody detected using enzyme linked immunosorbent assay (ELISA), micro-immunofluorescence or immunofluorescence in the assessment of tubal pathology was comparable to that of HSG in the diagnosis of tubal occlusion [14]. In addition, there was a positive correlation between the level of antibody titre and the degree of tubal damage. An elevated antibody level is significantly associated with poor live birth rates, but not pregnancy rates. Micro-immunofluorescence has been shown to be superior in the assessment of tubal pathology and therefore should be used as the first choice test [15].

Chlamydia antibody testing (CAT) is a low-risk screening modality, with minimal inconvenience to the patient, and should be considered an initial infertility investigation, prior to laparoscopy. It can be performed at any time during the menstrual cycle.

While a negative CAT can be reassuring, a positive test warrants further assessment using invasive diagnostic procedures such as laparoscopy. For CAT negative patients with subfertility, they should have further investigation with, for example, HyCoSy if available. CAT however, does have limitations; it is unable to identify women with non-infectious cases of tubal factor infertility (e.g. endometriosis, previous pelvis surgeries), antibody titres may decline over time, and false positives are possible.

For detection of current infection of chlamydia, samples can be taken from the cervix or urethra for culture. An alternative for urethral/cervical cultures is nucleic acid amplification tests (NAATs) that can be performed on urinary samples or self-administered vulvo-vaginal swab. The three types of commercially available NAATs are polymerase chain reaction (PCR), transcription-mediated amplification and strand displacement amplification. Cook et al. conducted a systematic review which showed that all three NAATs had greater than 95% specificity for chlamydia and gonorrhoea infections in urine, cervical and urethral samples. Urine samples were comparable in sensitivity to cervical or urethral samples [16].

Chlamydia screening has a favourable cost-effectiveness; the risk of pelvic inflammatory disease (PID) after lower genital tract chlamydia is in the range up to 30%. The risks of developing tubal infertility after PID are 10–20%. A cost-effectiveness model estimated a risk of tubal infertility in up to 4.6% of the women with a positive antibody screen [17].

3 Conclusion

Half a millennium on, tubal assessment essentially entails the assessment of tubal patency. It must, however, be appreciated that a patent tube does not equate to a functional tube and that 'routine' tubal testing is not always necessary. The clinician must, in planning for the investigations of a subfertile couple, be able to individualise their care. A change of paradigm in tubal assessment will be when diagnostic tools are available to facilitate the assessment of tubal damage, patency and last but not least, tubal function.

References

1. Swart P, Mol BW, van der Veen F, van Beurden M, Redekop WK, et al. (1995) The accuracy of hysterosalpingography in the diagnosis of tubal pathology: a meta-analysis. *Fertil Steril* 64: 486–491.

2. Sulak PJ, Letterie GS, Coddington CC, Hayslip CC, Woodward JE, et al. (1987) Histology of proximal tubal occlusion. *Fertil Steril* 48: 437–440.

3. Collins J (1988) Diagnostic assessment of the infertile female partner. *Curr Probl Obstet Gynecol Fertil*: 6–42.

4. Mohiyiddeen L, Hardiman A, Fitzgerald C, Hughes E, Mol BW, et al. (2015) Tubal flushing for subfertility. *Cochrane Database Syst Rev* Issue 5. Art. No.: CD003718.

5. Jansen FW, Kapiteyn K, Trimbos-Kemper T, Hermans J, Trimbos JB (1997) Complications of laparoscopy: a prospective multicentre observational study. *Br J Obstet Gynaecol* 104: 595–600.

6. Dijkman AB, Mol BW, van der Veen F, Bossuyt PM, Hogerzeil HV (2000) Can hysterosalpingocontrast-sonography replace hysterosalpingography in the assessment of tubal subfertility? *Eur J Radiol* 35: 44–48.

7. Spalding H, Martikainen H, Tekay A, Jouppila P (1999) Transvaginal salpingosonography for assessing tubal patency in women previously treated for pelvic inflammatory disease and benign ovarian tumors. *Ultrasound Obstet Gynecol* 14: 205–209.

8. de Kroon CD, de Bock GH, Dieben SW, Jansen FW (2003) Saline contrast hysterosonography in abnormal uterine bleeding: a systematic review and meta-analysis. *BJOG* 110: 938–947.

9. National Institute for Health and Care Excellence. Fertility: Assessment and treatment for people with fertility problems. NICE Clinical Guideline CG156. Published February 2013. www.nice.org.uk/guidance/cg156/resources/fertility-problems-assessment-and-treatment-pdf-35109634660549

10. Watrelot A, Nisolle M, Chelli H, Hocke C, Rongieres C, et al. (2003) Is laparoscopy still the gold standard in infertility assessment? A comparison of fertiloscopy versus laparoscopy in infertility. Results of an international multicentre prospective trial: the 'FLY' (Fertiloscopy-LaparoscopY) study. *Hum Reprod* 18: 834–839.

11. Gordts S, Watrelot A, Campo R, Brosens I (2001) Risk and outcome of bowel injury during transvaginal pelvic endoscopy. *Fertil Steril* 76: 1238–1241.

12. Dechaud H, Daures JP, Hedon B (1998) Prospective evaluation of falloposcopy. *Hum Reprod* 13: 1815–1818.

13. Rimbach S, Bastert G, Wallwiener D (2001) Technical results of falloposcopy for infertility diagnosis in a large multicentre study. *Hum Reprod* 16: 925–930.

14. Mol BW, Dijkman B, Wertheim P, Lijmer J, van der Veen F, et al. (1997) The accuracy of serum chlamydial antibodies in the diagnosis of tubal pathology: a meta-analysis. *Fertil Steril* 67: 1031–1037.

15. Broeze KA, Opmeer BC, Coppus SF, Van Geloven N, Alves MF, et al. (2011) Chlamydia antibody testing and diagnosing tubal pathology in subfertile women: an individual patient data meta-analysis. *Hum Reprod Update* 17: 301–310.

16. Cook RL, Hutchison SL, Ostergaard L, Braithwaite RS, Ness RB (2005) Systematic review: noninvasive testing for Chlamydia trachomatis and Neisseria gonorrhoeae. *Ann Intern Med* 142: 914–925.

17. Land JA, Van Bergen JE, Morre SA, Postma MJ (2010) Epidemiology of Chlamydia trachomatis infection in women and the cost-effectiveness of screening. *Hum Reprod Update* 16: 189–204.

Endometriosis
Diagnosis and Treatment Strategies to Improve Fertility

Ertan Saridogan

1 Endometriosis and Infertility Association

The association between endometriosis and infertility is controversial, as endometriosis can be present in both fertile and infertile women. A review of the published studies showed that the prevalence of endometriosis was 4% in women with proven fertility undergoing laparoscopic sterilisation, whilst this figure was 13.5% in infertile population[1]. Furthermore, this review demonstrated that endometriosis tends to be more advanced in infertile women, compared to women with proven fertility. A recent epidemiological study showed that endometriosis was associated with an age-adjusted two-fold increased risk of subsequent infertility, but only in women under the age of 35 years[2].

2 Causes of Infertility in Endometriosis

Advanced endometriosis (American Society of Reproductive Medicine, ASRM Stage III and IV disease) causes significant distortion to the pelvic anatomy (Figure 9.1). Periovariotubal adhesions affect tubal mobility and the ability of the tubes to capture the released oocyte. Ovarian endometriomas may not prevent ovulation, but may change the anatomical relationship between the fallopian tubes and ovaries, with resultant failure of ovum capture. Distal tubal obstruction and hydrosalpinx formation may prevent gamete/embryo transport. Coital frequency may be reduced due to endometriosis related pain (Box 9.1).

It is however unclear why early stage (ASRM Stage I and II) endometriosis causes infertility, when the pelvic anatomy is not usually affected (Figure 9.2). There are a number of publications which indicate possible mechanisms for endometriosis associated infertility, even in early stages (Box 9.2). Endometriotic implants secrete a number of proinflammatory substances such as prostaglandin E2, interleukins

and tumour necrosis factor-α which may all have toxic effects on gametes, embryo and tubal function [3]. Peritoneal fluid in women with endometriosis has an inhibitory effect on tubal ciliary activity and this may potentially compromise gamete and embryo transport[4]. Some researchers demonstrated presence of an ovum capture inhibitor in the peritoneal fluid of women with endometriosis. This substance was found to prevent the ability of fimbria to capture the cumulus–oocyte complex in vitro and was not found in the peritoneal fluid of women without endometriosis[5]. Others suggested that subtle changes of the fimbrial end such as fimbrial agglutination, blunting or phimosis are more frequently found in women with early endometriosis compared to women without endometriosis[6].

Endometriosis may also affect sperm–endosalpinx interaction; sperm may be more likely to bind to the tubal epithelium in women with endometriosis compared to controls, an effect which appears to have been reversed by the use of gonadotrophin releasing hormone analogues[7].

3 Diagnosis

Tools for the diagnosis of endometriosis in infertile women are history, clinical examination, ultrasound assessment of the pelvis and laparoscopy. Evidence for the predictive value of symptoms in diagnosing endometriosis is relatively weak. However, it is thought that presence of dysmenorrhoea, dyspareunia, non-cyclical pelvic pain and fatigue together with a history of infertility should raise the possibility of endometriosis[8]. Clinical examination may also give some clue in detecting endometriosis in infertile women, although the evidence for the value of this approach is again weak. It may be possible to feel ovarian endometriomas and rectovaginal nodules during bimanual examination. A normal examination does not however rule out possibility of endometriosis.

A.

B.

C.

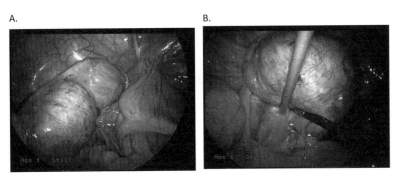

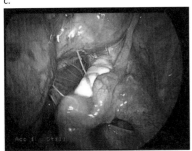

Fig. 9.1 Pelvic structures in severe endometriosis. A. Significantly distorted pelvic anatomy in the presence of a large left ovarian endometrioma B. Large left ovarian endometrioma and left hydrosalpinx C. Significant perituboovarian adhesions

Box 9.1 Possible causes of infertility in advanced endometriosis

- Significant mechanical distortion to pelvic anatomy
- Tubal damage
  - Distal tubal obstruction
  - Hydrosalpinx with or without distal tubal obstruction
- Perituboovarian adhesions affecting tubal motility and limiting access of fimbriae to ovarian surface
- Ovarian endometriomas causing anatomical distortion and disturbing tuboovarian relationship
- Reduced coital frequency due to pain

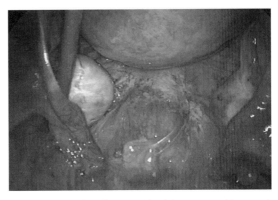

Fig. 9.2 Relatively well preserved pelvic anatomy with normal Fallopian tubes in early endometriosis

The contribution of transvaginal pelvic ultrasound (TVUS) examination to the diagnosis of endometriosis has increased significantly in recent years. TVUS is not only very reliable in detecting ovarian endometriomas [9] but in experienced hands is also very useful in identifying deep endometriotic nodules[10]. Typical ultrasound characteristics of endometriomas are ground glass echogenicity, one to four compartments and absence of papillary structures with significant blood flow[11]. There are also indirect TVUS findings that may indicate the possibility of pelvic endometriosis such as reduced mobility of ovaries and obliteration of the pouch of Douglas. The use of TVUS in screening for possible endometriosis may help in identifying women who may benefit from surgical confirmation and treatment. TVUS is also beneficial in detecting hydrosalpinges which may need to be treated prior to assisted reproduction treatment.

Box 9.2 Possible causes of infertility in early endometriosis

- Increased concentrations of proinflammatory substances (prostaglandin E2, interleukins and tumour necrosis factor-α) in the peritoneal fluid and their possible toxic effect on gametes and embryo
- Inhibition of tubal ciliary activity
- Presence of a possible ovum capture inhibitor
- Subtle fimbrial changes
- Adhesions between the ovaries and ovarian fossae
- Increased sperm binding to tubal epithelium

Laparoscopy remains the gold standard for the diagnosis of endometriosis, however its use has recently become more selective in line with improvements in the success of assisted reproductive technology (ART) and better understanding of the impact of surgery on ovarian reserve. Laparoscopy is more commonly used when improvements in spontaneous pregnancy are anticipated following surgical therapy, particularly in younger women with good ovarian reserve.

4 Management of Endometriosis Associated Subfertility

4.1 Medical Treatment

It is now well established that hormonal treatments do not have any benefit in treating endometriosis associated infertility[12]. In fact, most hormonal treatment options have contraceptive effects and are only likely to cause a delay in spontaneous or treatment associated conceptions. In addition, they are associated with significant side effects.

4.2 Surgery

Surgical treatment of endometriosis aims to eliminate endometriotic lesions, divide adhesions and restore pelvic anatomy as much as possible. This may in turn, in theory, improve chances of spontaneous pregnancy by addressing the possible causative factors which are outlined in Boxes 9.1 and 9.2. Elimination of endometriotic lesions may be carried out by excising them, such as removal of ovarian cysts, superficial peritoneal or deep endometriotic lesions, or destroying them such as coagulation of superficial ovarian or peritoneal lesions or the inner surface of an ovarian endometrioma using diathermy, laser or plasma energy. Earlier studies included outcomes from both laparoscopic and open approaches, however with the advance and widespread availability of laparoscopic surgery, this has become the norm in most centres.

Possible benefit of surgery in early endometriosis was evaluated in three randomised controlled trials (RCT) which were included in a Cochrane review[13]. This review showed that laparoscopic surgery was associated with an almost two-fold increase in live birth or ongoing pregnancy rates, compared with diagnostic laparoscopy only.

The evidence for benefit of surgery in advanced endometriosis is weaker, as there are no RCTs confirming a definite advantage. However, there are a number of retrospective case series indicating a probable benefit of surgery in improving spontaneous pregnancy rates. In fact a long-term cohort study suggests that cumulative spontaneous pregnancy rates are very similar after surgical treatment in all stages of endometriosis[14]. A review of retrospective studies on surgical treatment of ovarian endometriomas (which usually indicate stage III or IV disease) showed pregnancy rates varying between 30 and 70%[15]. This wide range in success rates may be due to differences in patient populations, including presence or absence of history of infertility, duration of infertility and level of experience of the clinician.

A meta-analysis of two RCTs comparing excision of cyst capsule and bipolar electrocoagulation of ovarian endometriomas larger than 3 cm showed considerably high pregnancy rates after excision, with an OR of 5.21 (95% CI 2.04–13.29) for spontaneous conceptions rates for excisional surgery compared to electrocoagulation[16]. Excisional surgery has the additional advantages of lower risk of cyst recurrence or recurrence of pain symptoms.

Potential disadvantages of surgical treatment are surgical complications and a reduction in ovarian reserve after treatment of ovarian endometriomas. Surgical complications are uncommon, especially for early disease, but the risk increases with more advanced disease. Surgical treatment of deep endometriosis affecting the bowel can be challenging and its impact on infertility outcome is not well established. In fact, a non-randomised study comparing the fertility outcome after surgery for rectovaginal endometriosis showed similar pregnancy rates compared to expectant management after 24 months[17].

Inevitably, surgical removal or coagulation of endometriomas may result in loss or destruction of some normal ovarian tissue. In fact, there is now significant data that suggest reduction in anti-Mullerian hormone levels (AMH) after surgery. In addition, the ovaries that have undergone surgery for endometriomas do not show the same level of response to ovarian stimulation compared to the contralateral ovary. It is however unclear whether this impact is due to the presence of the original endometrioma itself or due to surgery as antral follicle count in the affected ovary tends to be lower both before and after surgery, compared to the contralateral ovary[18].

Due to the potential impact of surgery on ovarian reserve, a decision for surgery to aid fertility needs to be carefully considered in women who have had previous surgery, in those with reduced ovarian reserve and those with bilateral endometriomas[19].

Postsurgical hormonal therapy is prescribed by some clinicians, usually in the form of gonadotrophin releasing hormone analogues (GnRHa). However, evidence from RCTs and a meta-analysis suggest that this practice does not offer any benefit in improving spontaneous pregnancy rates[20].

4.3 Intrauterine Insemination

Intrauterine insemination (IUI) is less frequently used in the United Kingdom since the publication of 2013 Guidelines of National Institute for Health and Clinical Excellence (NICE) on fertility[21]. NICE guidelines advised against routine use of IUI for couples who are having regular sexual intercourse. However, this treatment is still regularly used outside the United Kingdom as there is some, although old and low quality, evidence which supports use of IUI with controlled ovarian stimulation in couples with stage I and II endometriosis and infertility[22]. There is also evidence that stimulated IUI is more effective than unstimulated IUI in couples with endometriosis associated infertility[23]. Stimulated IUI may be used after surgical treatment of early endometriosis instead of expectant management[8]. Disadvantages of stimulated IUI include multiple pregnancies and relatively low success rates.

4.4 Assisted Reproductive Technology

ART refers to treatments which include handling of gametes or embryo for the purpose of establishing a pregnancy. Hence in vitro fertilisation and embryo transfer (IVF-ET) and intracytoplasmic sperm injection come under this category. ART is now an established treatment in endometriosis associated subfertility when tubal function is compromised, when there is concomitant male factor infertility or when other treatment approaches have failed[8]. There is an ongoing debate as to whether ART is less successful in women with endometriosis compared to controls without endometriosis. There are a number of systematic reviews and meta-analyses which indicate that this might be the case[24, 25]. However, large national databases such as the Human Fertilisation and Embryology database do not show a significant difference in success rates in women with endometriosis compared to other diagnostic categories.

Presence of endometriomas can sometimes create difficulties in gaining access to ovarian follicles during egg collection procedures. In addition, some clinicians believe endometriomas may affect oocyte quality. Hence clinicians may be tempted to perform surgery to remove endometriomas prior to IVF. There is, however, significant evidence that surgery for endometriomas prior to IVF does not improve success rates[26]. In fact, evidence from at least one RCT suggests that ovarian stimulation takes longer, requires a higher dosage of gonadotrophins and leads to lower oestradiol and fewer oocytes without improving the pregnancy rates after surgery compared to controls[27]. Hence, surgery should only be considered in these women for the treatment of pain or to improve ovarian accessibility. Similarly, surgery for deep endometriosis is not thought to be beneficial to improve ART outcome and should only be considered in the context of treatment of pain[8].

There is some data to support the practice of extended (3–6 months) GnRHa down-regulation in women with endometriosis, prior to IVF treatment. Data from three small RCTs show significantly higher clinical pregnancy rates with extended GnRHa use (OR 4.28, 95% CI 2.00–9.15)[28]. Potential disadvantages of this approach might be difficult ovarian stimulation after prolonged down-regulation and its additional cost.

Increased oestrogen levels during ovarian stimulation for ART may, in theory, increase the risk of recurrent endometriosis. However, published cumulative recurrence rates do not seem to increase following ART[29,30]. Hence, women can be encouraged to undergo IVF when clinically indicated, without expecting a significant increase in their risk of recurrent endometriosis.

5 Conclusion

Endometriosis is a well-known cause of infertility, although the mechanisms of reduced fecundity in early endometriosis are not clearly understood. Surgery and medically assisted reproduction (IUI and ART) are two effective forms of treatment for endometriosis associated subfertility. Surgery may represent first line treatment in young women with good ovarian reserve and otherwise unexplained infertility, as it is known to increase spontaneous pregnancy rates significantly. This seems to be applicable to endometriosis in all stages, as long as the tubal function is not compromised and it is possible to restore

the pelvic anatomy to near normal status at surgery. Excisional treatment of endometriomas appears to offer higher spontaneous pregnancy rates compared to drainage and electrocoagulation. Surgery for ovarian endometriomas may however reduce ovarian reserve, and should be considered carefully in older women, in women with reduced ovarian reserve or history of previous endometrioma surgery, when the tubal function is compromised or when there is concomitant male factor. ART may be a better choice in these circumstances. Success rates of ART may be somewhat lower in women with endometriosis compared to other diagnostic categories; however, this is disputed on the basis of data from large national databases. ART does not appear to increase the risk of recurrent endometriosis; hence, women should be encouraged to consider ART when clinically indicated without the fear of recurrence.

References

(1) d'Hooghe TM, Debrock S, Hill JA, Meuleman C. Endometriosis and subfertility: is the relationship resolved? *Semin Reprod Med* 2003 May;21(2):243–54.

(2) Prescott J, Farland LV, Tobias DK, Gaskins AJ, Spiegelman D, Chavarro JE, et al. A prospective cohort study of endometriosis and subsequent risk of infertility. *Hum Reprod* 2016 31(7):1475–82.

(3) Giudice LC. Clinical practice: Endometriosis. *N Engl J Med* 2010 Jun 24; 362(25):2389–98.

(4) Lyons RA, Djahanbakhch O, Saridogan E, Naftalin AA, Mahmood T, Weekes A, et al. Peritoneal fluid, endometriosis, and ciliary beat frequency in the human fallopian tube. *Lancet* 2002 Oct 19;360(9341):1221–2.

(5) Suginami H, Yano K. An ovum capture inhibitor (OCI) in endometriosis peritoneal fluid: an OCI-related membrane responsible for fimbrial failure of ovum capture. *Fertil Steril* 1988 Oct;50(4):648–53.

(6) Abuzeid MI, Mitwally MF, Ahmed AI, Formentini E, Ashraf M, Abuzeid OM, et al. The

prevalence of fimbrial pathology in patients with early stages of endometriosis. *J Minim Invasive Gynecol* 2007 Jan;14(1):49–53.

(7) Reeve L, Lashen H, Pacey AA. Endometriosis affects sperm-endosalpingeal interactions. *Hum Reprod* 2005 Feb;20(2):448–51.

(8) Dunselman GA, Vermeulen N, Becker C, Calhaz-Jorge C, D'Hooghe T, De BB, et al. ESHRE guideline: management of women with endometriosis. *Hum Reprod* 2014 Mar;29(3):400–12.

(9) Moore J, Copley S, Morris J, Lindsell D, Golding S, Kennedy S. A systematic review of the accuracy of ultrasound in the diagnosis of endometriosis. *Ultrasound Obstet Gynecol* 2002 Dec;20(6):630–4.

(10) Hudelist G, Ballard K, English J, Wright J, Banerjee S, Mastoroudes H, et al. Transvaginal sonography vs. clinical examination in the preoperative diagnosis of deep infiltrating endometriosis. *Ultrasound Obstet Gynecol* 2011 Apr;37(4):480–7.

(11) Van HC, Van CB, Guerriero S, Savelli L, Paladini D, Lissoni AA, et al. Endometriomas: their

ultrasound characteristics. *Ultrasound Obstet Gynecol* 2010 Jun;35(6):730–40.

(12) Hughes E, Brown J, Collins JJ, Farquhar C, Fedorkow DM, Vandekerckhove P. Ovulation suppression for endometriosis. *Cochrane Database Syst Rev* 2007; Issue 3. Art. No.: CD000155. DOI: 10.1002/14651858.CD000155.pub2.

(13) Duffy JMN, Arambage K, Correa FJS, Olive D, Farquhar C, Garry R, Barlow DH, Jacobson TZ. Laparoscopic surgery for endometriosis. *Cochrane Database Syst Rev* 2014, Issue 4. Art. No.: CD011031.

(14) Vercellini P, Fedele L, Aimi G, De GO, Consonni D, Crosignani PG. Reproductive performance, pain recurrence and disease relapse after conservative surgical treatment for endometriosis: the predictive value of the current classification system. *Hum Reprod* 2006 Oct;21(10):2679–85.

(15) Vercellini P, Somigliana E, Vigano P, Abbiati A, Barbara G, Crosignani PG. Surgery for endometriosis-associated infertility: a pragmatic approach.

Hum Reprod 2009 Feb; 24(2):254–69.

(16) Hart RJ, Hickey M, Maouris P, Buckett W. Excisional surgery versus ablative surgery for ovarian endometriomata. *Cochrane Database Syst Rev* 2008;Issue 2. Art. No.: CD004992.

(17) Vercellini P, Pietropaolo G, De GO, Daguati R, Pasin R, Crosignani PG. Reproductive performance in infertile women with rectovaginal endometriosis: is surgery worthwhile? *Am J Obstet Gynecol* 2006 Nov; 195(5):1303–10.

(18) Muzii L, Di TC, Di FM, Marchetti C, Perniola G, Panici PB. The effect of surgery for endometrioma on ovarian reserve evaluated by antral follicle count: a systematic review and meta-analysis. *Hum Reprod* 2014 Oct 10;29(10):2190–8.

(19) Garcia-Velasco JA, Somigliana E. Management of endometriomas in women requiring IVF: to touch or not to touch. *Hum Reprod* 2009 Mar;24(3):496–501.

(20) Yap C, Furness S, Farquhar C. Pre and post operative medical therapy for endometriosis surgery. *Cochrane Database Syst Rev* 2004; Issue 3. Art. No.: CD003678. DOI:

10.1002/14651858.CD003678. pub2.

(21) National Institute for Health and Clinical Excellence. Fertility; assessment and treatment for people with fertility problems. RCOG; 2013.

(22) Tummon IS, Asher LJ, Martin JS, Tulandi T. Randomized controlled trial of superovulation and insemination for infertility associated with minimal or mild endometriosis. *Fertil Steril* 1997 Jul;68(1):8–12.

(23) Nulsen JC, Walsh S, Dumez S, Metzger DA. A randomized and longitudinal study of human menopausal gonadotropin with intrauterine insemination in the treatment of infertility. *Obstet Gynecol* 1993 Nov;82(5):780–6.

(24) Hamdan M, Omar SZ, Dunselman G, Cheong Y. Influence of endometriosis on assisted reproductive technology outcomes: a systematic review and meta-analysis. *Obstet Gynecol* 2015 Jan;125(1):79–88.

(25) Harb HM, Gallos ID, Chu J, Harb M, Coomarasamy A. The effect of endometriosis on in vitro fertilisation outcome: a systematic review and meta-analysis. *BJOG* 2013 Oct;120(11):1308–20.

(26) Hamdan M, Dunselman G, Li TC, Cheong Y. The impact of endometrioma on IVF/ICSI outcomes: a systematic review and meta-analysis. *Hum Reprod Update* 2015 Nov;21(6):809–25.

(27) Demirol A, Guven S, Baykal C, Gurgan T. Effect of endometrioma cystectomy on IVF outcome: a prospective randomized study. *Reprod Biomed Online* 2006 May;12(5):639–43.

(28) Sallam HN, Garcia-Velasco JA, Dias S, Arici A. Long-term pituitary down-regulation before in vitro fertilization (IVF) for women with endometriosis. *Cochrane Database Syst Rev* 2006; Issue 1. Art. No.: CD004635. DOI: 10.1002/14651858.CD004635. pub2.

(29) Benaglia L, Somigliana E, Vercellini P, Benedetti F, Iemmello R, Vighi V, et al. The impact of IVF procedures on endometriosis recurrence. *Eur J Obstet Gynecol Reprod Biol* 2010 Jan;148(1):49–52.

(30) d'Hooghe TM, Denys B, Spiessens C, Meuleman C, Debrock S. Is the endometriosis recurrence rate increased after ovarian hyperstimulation? *Fertil Steril* 2006 Aug;86(2):283–90.

Chapter 10

Congenital Uterine Abnormalities

Kanna Jayaprakasan

1 Introduction

A structurally normal and functionally competent uterus is essential for the process of reproduction including sperm transport, embryo implantation, fetal development and growth, and the process of labour and birth. Any uterine abnormalities including congenital anomalies may adversely influence some of these uterine functions, precluding a successful pregnancy. Congenital uterine anomalies are deviations from normal anatomy resulting from embryological maldevelopment of the Mullerian ducts and are not uncommon. While most of these anomalies are asymptomatic and are associated with normal reproductive outcome, some may be associated with adverse reproductive outcomes.

2 Development of Normal Uterus and Anomalies

Normal development of the female reproductive tract involves a series of complex processes characterized by the differentiation, migration, fusion and subsequent canalization of the Mullerian duct system (Figure 10.1). Uterine anomalies result when these processes are interrupted [1, 2]. The primordial germ cells that develop at around the fourth week of life among the endodermal cells in the dorsal wall of the yolksac migrate to the primitive gonads. The primitive gonads appear on the gonadal ridge medial to mesonephros, and subsequently Wolffian and Mullerian ducts develop. By the seventh week, sex determining region-Y (SRY) antigen in male fetus differentiate the primitive gonad into testis, which secretes anti-Mullerian hormone (AMH) and testosterone, which allows Mullerian duct to regress and Wolffian duct to develop into male internal genitalia. Absence of the SRY gene in female embryos allows the gonads to develop into ovaries. The subsequent lack of AMH causes regression of the Wolffian ducts and allows the Mullerian ducts to

develop into fallopian tubes, the uterus and upper vagina, while the lack of androgens permits differentiation of the indifferent external genitalia into the labia majora, labia minora and the clitoris. The lower tip of the fused Mullerian ducts makes contact with the urogenital sinus, causing proliferation of the endodermal sinovaginal bulbs, which form the vaginal plate. This then canalizes to form the vagina with the upper portion derived from Mullerian duct and lower portion from the sinovaginal bulbs. Mullerian development occurs separately from gonadal development, and women with Mullerian anomalies usually have normal ovaries and ovarian hormone production. By contrast, Mullerian development occurs in close association with the development of the urinary tract, and renal anomalies are occasionally identified in those with Mullerian anomalies.

There are three phases of Mullerian duct development (Table 10.1)

1. Organogenesis – developmental defect leads to agenesis or aplasia – Mayer Rokitansky Kuster Hauser (MRKH) Syndrome if bilateral agenesis and Unicornuate uterus if unilateral agenesis.
2. Fusion
   a. **Horizontal fusion** (lower segments of paired Mullerian duct fuse to form uterus, cervix and upper vagina). Varying degrees of fusion defect causes bicornuate uterus and didelphys.
   b. **Vertical fusion** (between the descending Mullerian duct and ascending sinovaginal bulbs to form vaginal canal). Fusion defects cause an imperforate hymen or a transverse vaginal septum
3. Septal resorption of the horizontally fused Mullerian ducts – failure of resorption leads to septate uterus.

While certain types of congenital malformation are the result of a clear disturbance in one stage of

Table 10.1 Phases of Mullerian duct development and defects

Phases of Mullerian duct development	Defect	Anomaly
Organogenesis: Development of Mullerian duct	Failure to develop bilaterally	Aplasia/ agenesis (MRKH syndrome)
	Failure to develop unilaterally	Unicornuate uterus
Fusion or Unification: between paired Mullerian ducts between fused Mullerian duct and urogenital sinus (sinovaginal bulbs)	Horizontal fusion defect	Bicornuate uterus Uterus didelphys
	Vertical fusion defect	Transverse vaginal septum Imperforate hymen
Septal resorption or canalization	Defect in resorption or canalization	Septate uterus Arcuate

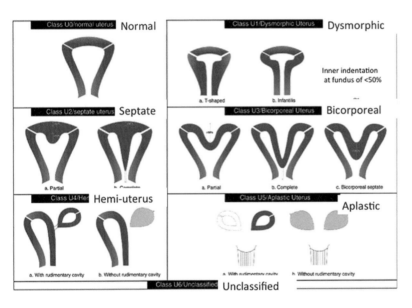

Fig. 10.1 Congenital malformations of the female genital tract

embryologic development, others are the result of disturbances in more than one stage of normal formation. The combination of malformations, which occur at different stages of development, seems to be the reason for the extremely wide anatomical variations and the large observed number of combinations of congenital malformation of the female genital tract (Figure 10.1).

3 Classification of Uterine Anomalies

While different classification systems have been proposed for Mullerian anomalies, the classification described by the American Society of Reproductive Medicine (ASRM; formerly known as the American Fertility Society [AFS]) remains the most widely used [3]. This classification is based on the extent of failure of Mullerian development and divides anomalies into groups with similar clinical manifestations, management requirements and prognosis. However, this classification is not without limitations; for example, it does not include combined or complex anomalies (obstructive-like cervical or vaginal aplasias), which are often incorrectly identified, and inaccurately reported. There has been criticism on arcuate uterus being included as separate class as well.

The European Society of Human Reproduction and Embryology (ESHRE) and the European Society for Gynaecological Endoscopy (ESGE), recognizing the clinical significance of female genital anomalies, have established a common working group under the name CONUTA (CONgenital UTerine Anomalies), with the goal of developing a new updated classification system [4]. The ESHRE/ESGE classification system is based on anatomy. Anomalies are classified into the following main classes, expressing uterine anatomical deviations deriving from the same embryological origin: U0, normal uterus; U1, dysmorphic uterus; U2, septate uterus; U3, bicorporeal uterus; U4, hemi-uterus; U5, aplastic uterus; U6, for still unclassified cases. Main classes have been divided into subclasses expressing anatomical varieties with clinical significance. Cervical and vaginal anomalies are classified independently into subclasses having clinical significance. Embryological origin has been adopted as the secondary basic characteristic in the design of the main classes. Cervical and vaginal anomalies are classified in independent coexistent subclasses according to increasing severity of the anatomical deviation (C0 to C4 and V0 to V4); the less severe variants are placed in the beginning, the more deformed types at the end, with C0 being normal cervix and C4 being cervical aplasia and with V0 being normal vagina and V4 being vaginal aplasia. Arcuate uterus is considered as a normal variant and is not included in this classification. While it seems that the new system fulfils the needs and expectations of a large group of experts in the field, the practical usefulness of this classification system is yet to be tested.

4 Prevalence

The reported population prevalence rates in individual studies have varied between 0.06% and 38% and the observed wide variation is possibly due to the assessment of different study populations and the use of different diagnostic techniques [5]. The lack of universally agreed-upon standardized classification systems and invasive nature of the gold standard diagnostic tests (combined laparoscopy and hysteroscopy) has made difficult to assess the true population prevalence of congenital uterine anomalies in the past. The advent of 3D ultrasound with its ability to define both internal and external contours of the uterus has made the diagnosis of uterine anomalies easier and less invasive. Recently two well-conducted systematic reviews have evaluated the prevalence of uterine

anomalies, categorizing the diagnostic tests used into optimal and suboptimal tests [5, 6].

Chan et al. (2011) evaluated the prevalence of congenital uterine anomalies in the unselected population and in women with a history of infertility, including those undergoing in vitro fertilization (IVF) treatment, miscarriage, infertility and recurrent miscarriage combined, and preterm delivery [5]. In their review they classified investigations, as proposed by Saravelos et. al. (2008), into optimal tests that are capable of accurately identifying and classifying congenital uterine anomalies (3D transvaginal ultrasound, laparoscopy or laparotomy with hysteroscopy or hysterosalpingogram [HSG], magnetic resonance imaging [MRI] and saline sono-hysterography) and suboptimal tests that can identify and differentiate most but not all anomalies (2D transvaginal ultrasound, hysteroscopy, HSG and clinical assessment at the time of Caesarean section). In an overall pooled sample of more than 89,000 women from 94 studies, the authors reported prevalence of different types of uterine anomalies in various population subtypes depending on whether they were subjected to optimal or suboptimal tests (Table 10.2). Overall, 5.5% (95% confidence interval [CI], 3.5–8.5) of the unselected population were shown to have a uterine anomaly diagnosed by an optimal test. The prevalence was not increased in women with infertility (8.0%; 95% CI, 5.3–12.0, P = 0.239) when compared with the unselected population. Women with a history of miscarriage (13.3%; 95% CI, 8.9–20; P = 0.011) and miscarriage in association with infertility (24.5%; 95% CI, 18.3–32.8; P = 0.001) were all shown to have significantly higher rates of uterine anomalies than the unselected population. The prevalence of congenital uterine anomalies diagnosed by optimal tests in women with two or more miscarriages (10.9%; 95% CI, 3.6–33.3) was not significantly different (P = 0.572) from those with three or more miscarriages (15.4%; 95% CI, 10.3–23). The prevalence of all uterine anomalies in various populations diagnosed by suboptimal tests was found to be consistent with those diagnosed by optimal tests (Table 10.2). The observed higher rate of major congenital uterine anomalies in the high-risk groups, with the exception of isolated subfertility, suggests a causal role in poor reproductive outcome.

Subgroup analyses showed that the specific anomalies, which were increased in the high-risk populations of miscarriage, are mainly canalization or

Table 10.2 The prevalence of uterine anomalies in different study populations stratified by the accuracy of the diagnostic test used to classify uterine anomalies

Population	Diagnostic test	Prevalence of all anomalies % (95% CI)	Arcuate % (95% CI)	Canalization defects % (95% CI)	Unification Defects			Others % (95% CI)
					Bicornuate % (95% CI)	Unicornuate % (95% CI)	Didelphys % (95% CI)	
Unselected	Optimal	5.5 (3.5–8.5)	3.9 (2.1–7.1)	2.3 (1.8–2.9)	0.4 (0.2–0.6)	0.1 (0.1–0.3)	0.3 (0.1–0.6)	0.1 (0–2.2)
	Suboptimal	4.6 (2.3–9.1)	2.2 (0.9–5.2)	0.2 (0–0.9)	0.2 (0–0.7)	0.2 (0.1–0.5)	0.1 (0.1–0.2)	2.5 (1.6–3.7)
Infertility	Optimal	8.0 (5.3–12.0)	1.8 (0.8–4.1)	3.0 (1.3–6.7)	1.1 (0.6–2.0)*	0.5 (0.3–0.8)*	0.3 (0.2–0.5)	0.9 (0.4–1.8)
	Suboptimal	6.1 (3.9–9.5)	5.8 (3.4–10.1)	2.7 (1.5–4.6)*	0.8 (0.5–1.4)	0.8 (0.5–1.2)	0.4 (0.2–0.9)	1.0 (0.4–2.4)
Miscarriage	Optimal	13.3 (8.9–20)*	2.9 (0.9–9.6)	5.3 (1.7–16.8)*	2.1 (1.4–3)*	0.5 (0.3–1.1)*	0.6 (0.3–1.4)	0.9 (0.1–12.6)
	Suboptimal	15.8 (11.9–20.9)*	8.9 (6.4–12.4)*	4.3 (2.3–8.2)*	2.8 (1.6–5)*	0.5 (0.3–0.9)	0.6 (0.2–1.6)	4.5 (2–9.8)*
Mixed infertility & recurrent miscarriage	Optimal	24.5 (18.3–32.8)*	6.6 (2.8–15.7)	15.4 (12.5–19)*	4.7 (2.9–7.6)*	3.1 (2–4.7)*	2.1 (1.4–3.2)*	0.3 (0–2.3)
	Suboptimal	31.8 (20.7–48.8)	No study found	None diagnosed	None diagnosed	4.5 (1.5–14.1)	None diagnosed	27.3 (17.2–43.3)*

resorption defects, namely subseptate or septate uteri, and unification or fusion defects. Of note, based on studies employing optimal tests, the most commonly diagnosed uterine anomaly in the unselected or general population was the arcuate uterus. The arcuate uterus is, however, no more prevalent in any of the high-risk groups studied than in the unselected population. The canalization defect was the most common anomaly in all of the high-risk groups (Table 10.2).

5 Diagnosis

While most uterine anomalies are asymptomatic and detected incidentally, accurate diagnosis and correct classification is important for appropriate counselling of women about their potential prognosis and risks associated with reproduction and for planning any intervention with a view to improve the reproductive outcome. Accurate evaluation of the internal and external contours of the uterus is the key in making a diagnosis and correctly classifying a uterine anomaly. Considering this, the gold standard test is the combination of laparoscopy and hysteroscopy as you can directly visualize both the external and internal

uterine contours. However, imaging modalities such as ultrasonography, HSG, sonohysterogram and MRI are less invasive modes of screening and classifying various uterine anomalies [5]. HSG is an excellent method of evaluating the uterine cavity but definitive diagnosis requires evaluation of the external uterine contour, which is poorly defined by HSG. While conventional transvaginal ultrasound and HSG are good in screening for uterine anomalies, 3D ultrasound and MRI could correctly classify the type of anomaly [7, 8].

Conventional transvaginal ultrasound is minimally invasive and a less expensive way of assessing uterine morphology and ruling out uterine anomalies [9]. Timing the ultrasound study in the second half of menstrual cycle (secretory phase) provides more accurate visualization of the endometrium and is therefore more appropriate for evaluating the uterus for congenital anomalies. Visualization of double endometrial complex on a transverse plane is indicative of a uterine anomaly (Figure 10.2B), which could be a bicornuate, septate, subseptate or arcuate uterus. Systematic scanning through longitudinal plane of uterus may reveal a uterine complex which then

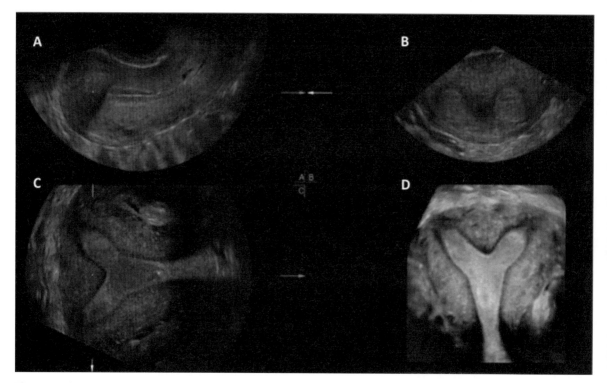

Fig. 10.2 Ultrasound assessment of uterine anomaly. A and B conventional longitudinal and transverse view of uterine anomaly. C and D 3D resolution of the same.

disappears while moving to the opposite side, followed by appearance of a second uterine complex suggesting that the uterus may be bicornuate. The transverse plane provides more information and widely placed double endometrial echoes especially at the upper portion of uterus towards fundus and an indentation at the fundus on an oblique plane (if obtainable) are typical of a bicornuate uterus. However, 3D ultrasound through its unique feature of providing the coronal plane of uterus (Figure 10.2C) facilitates simultaneous visualization of both external (serosal surface) and internal (endometrial) contours of the uterine fundus and can correctly classify the uterine anomaly into bicornuate, septate or subseptate or arcuate uterus [10]. Uterus didelphys, although rarer, also shows two endometrial complexes in the transverse plane of conventional 2D scan whilst 3D ultrasound and the clinical demonstration of two cervices confirm the diagnosis. Two uterine horns may be symmetrical or asymmetrical and two separate vaginas may be seen on speculum examination. In cases of unicornuate uterus, a normal-looking long axis of the uterus is seen on one side in the pelvis with no or a rudimentary uterine shadow on the other side. A rudimentary or severely hypoplastic uterine horn is seen as isoechoic pear-shaped structure with or without a central thin echogenic endometrial line. On the transverse plane, at the level of the fundus, a beak-like projection from the endometrial shadow (cornua) is seen on one side. 3D

ultrasound, again, is confirmatory, demonstrating a banana-shaped uterine cavity and single interstitial portion of fallopian tube in the coronal plane. Saline infusion sonography has been suggested as a method for diagnosing rudimentary horns as saline can be clearly seen in the unicornuate uterus, with no passage into the rudimentary horn.

3D transvaginal ultrasound is now considered the gold standard tool for the assessment of uterine anomalies as it is less invasive and can correctly classify the types of uterine anomalies. Although the method for diagnosis is agreed-upon, set international ultrasound criteria have yet to be agreed upon. However, criteria for the classification of uterine anomalies based on 3D ultrasound have been well described in the literature [10](Table 10.3). The morphology of the uterus is best examined in the coronal plane, using the interstitial portions of the fallopian tubes as reference points. Three measurements should be taken – W, the width of the uterine cavity which is measured as the distance between the internal tubal ostia; F, the septum length or fundal indentation which is measured as the distance from the midpoint of a line joining the tubal ostia and the tip of the fundal indentation or septum; and C, the length of the unaffected cavity from the tip of the septum or fundal indentation to the internal os, and then the diagnosis made with the diagnostic criteria as shown in Table 10.3. The degree of distortion of the cavity can be

Table 10.3 Classification of uterine anomalies based on 3D ultrasound

Uterine morphology	Internal contour	External contour
Normal (Figure 10.4A)	Straight or convex	Uniformly convex or with indentation < 10 mm
Arcuate (Figure 10.4B)	Concave fundal indentation with central point of indentation at obtuse angle (> 90°)	Uniformly convex or with indentation < 10 mm
Subseptate (Figure 10.4C)	Presence of septum, which does not extend to cervix, with central point of septum at an acute angle (< 90°)	Uniformly convex or with indentation < 10 mm
Septate (Figure 10.4D)	Presence of uterine septum that completely divides cavity from fundus to cervix	Uniformly convex or with indentation < 10 mm
Unicornuate (Figure 10.4E)	Single well-formed uterine cavity with a single interstitial portion of Fallopian tube and concave fundal contour	Fundal indentation > 10 mm dividing the two cornua if rudimentary horn present
Bicornuate (Figure 10.4F)	Two well-formed uterine cornua	Fundal indentation > 10 mm dividing the two cornua
T-shaped	T-shaped uterine cavity	

calculated by F/ (F+C) (Figure 10.3). Good inter- and intra-observer reproducibility for these measurements has been reported.

Congenital uterine anomalies may be associated with congenital renal anomalies because of closely related embryogenesis and therefore an abdominal scan is recommended in all women diagnosed to have uterine anomalies. MRI, due to its ability to demonstrate both external and internal contours of the uterus, is sensitive and specific for diagnosing nearly all uterine anomalies. MRI is helpful in delineating the endometrium and detecting uterine horns as well as in defining aberrant gonadal location or renal anatomy and is less invasive compared to laparo-hysteroscopy. While MRI is not routinely recommended in all women suspected to have a uterine anomaly, it proves useful for those patients with suspected complex anomalies and for those at higher risk for associated anomalies.

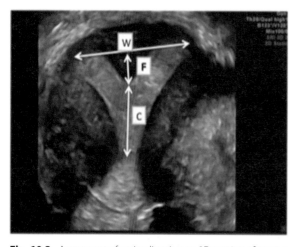

Fig. 10.3 Assessment of cavity distortion on 3D scaning of uterine anomaly.

6 Clinical Implications

Congenital uterine anomalies are often diagnosed incidentally during the work up for common gynae-cologic complaints such as subfertility, recurrent pregnancy loss or menstrual disorders [8]. Mullerian anomalies associated with obstruction, such as uni-cornuate uterus with a rudimentary horn; uterine

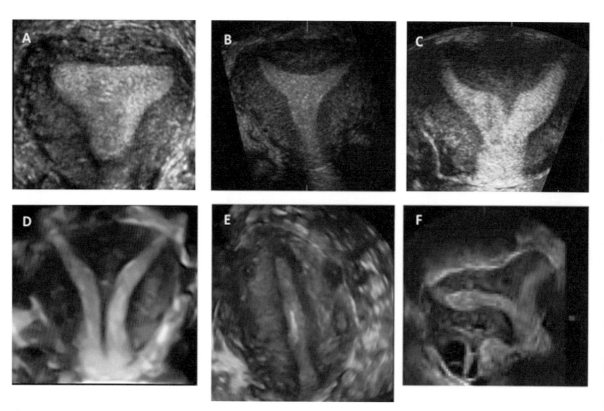

Fig. 10.4 3D appearance of uterine morphology of different anomalies - see classification; Table 10.3

didelphys with obstructed hemivagina; or vaginal or cervical agenesis or anomalies often present with pelvic pain secondary to haematometra, haematocolpos or endometriosis. Such pain may be either cyclic or non-cyclic, and located in the pelvis or vagina, depending on the level of obstruction. Patients with haematometra or haematocolpos may present with a painful mass on bimanual examination. Patients with agenesis such as MRKH syndrome or segmental hypoplasia often present with primary amenorrhoea. For conditions associated with longitudinal vaginal septa, such as uterine didelphys, patients may report dyspareunia or bleeding despite use of a single tampon [11, 12].

Uterine anomalies have been implicated as a potential cause of infertility, recurrent pregnancy loss, preterm delivery and fetal malpresentation. The various types of uterine anomaly are individually associated with varying degrees of adverse outcomes, with greater effects being evident in women with more significant defects. A systematic review incorporating 3,805 patients has reported the impact of congenital uterine anomalies on reproductive outcome by including only studies that have appropriate control groups and that considered the effect of the subtypes of uterine anomaly [13]. Women with canalization defects, such as septate and subseptate uteri, appear to have the poorest reproductive performance with a reduced conception rate and increased risk of first-trimester miscarriage, preterm birth and fetal malpresentation at delivery. When compared with women with subseptate uteri, women with septate uteri have poorer outcomes throughout the course of pregnancy (Table 10.4). The association between various uterine anomalies and adverse reproductive outcome has been detailed in Table 10.4.

While the association between canalization defects and suboptimal reproductive performance appears to be evident, the exact aetiology and pathophysiological processes underlying infertility and pregnancy loss remain uncertain. Various hypotheses have been put forward such as endometrium overlying the septum being abnormal and thus a poor site for implantation, disorderly and decreased blood supply insufficient to support placentation and embryo growth, more frequent or uncoordinated

Table 10.4 Impact of various uterine anomalies on reproductive outcome

Anomaly		Conception rate	First trimester miscarriage	Second trimester miscarriage	Preterm labour	Malpresentation at birth
Arcuate		1.03 (0.94 to 1.12)	1.35 (0.81 to 2.26)	2.39 (1.33 to 4.27)**	1.53 (0.70 to 3.34)	2.53 (1.54 to 4.18)***
Canalization defects	Subseptate	0.80 (0.57 to 1.11)	2.94 (1.90 to 4.54)***	1.86 (0.56 to 6.22)	2.01 (1.16 to 3.51)*	5.29 (1.89 to 14.86)**
	Septate	0.93 (0.75 to 1.17)	2.37 (1.64 to 3.43)***	3.74 (1.57 to 8.91)**	2.30 (1.46 to 3.62)***	6.15 (3.96 to 9.53)***
	All	**0.86 (0.77 to 0.96)***	**2.89 (2.02 to 4.14)***	**2.22 (0.74 to 6.65)**	**2.14 (1.48 to 4.47)***	**6.24 (4.05 to 9.62)***
Unification defects	Bicornuate	0.86 (0.61 to 1.21)	3.40 (1.18 to 9.16)*	2.32 (1.05 to 5.15)*	2.55 (1.57 to 4.17)***	5.38 (3.15 to 9.19)***
	Didelphys	0.9 (0.79 to 1.04)	1.10 (0.21 to 5.66)	1.39 (0.44 to 4.41)	3.58 (2.00 to 6.40)***	3.70 (2.04 to 6.70)***
	Unicornuate	0.74 (0.39 to 1.41)	2.15 (1.03 to 4.47)*	2.22 (0.53 to 9.19)	3.47 (1.94 to 6.22)***	2.74 (1.30 to 5.77)**
	All	**0.87 (0.68 to 1.11)**	**2.56 (0.89 to 7.38)**	**1.94 (0.92 to 4.09)**	**2.97 (2.08 to 4.23)***	**3.87 (2.42 to 6.18)***

* P < 0.05, ** P < 0.01, ***P < 0.001

uterine contractions or a reduced uterine capacity causing miscarriage and preterm birth. Both conditions may also explain the increased incidence of fetal malpresentation, although this may simply reflect the anatomical distortion.

Unification defects, such as the bicornuate, unicornuate and didelphic uterus, do not appear to reduce fertility but are associated with increased risk of adverse outcome during pregnancy (Table 10.4). The risks are, however, dependent on the type of anomaly. Women with bicornuate and unicornuate uteri have an increased risk of miscarriage, preterm birth and fetal malpresentation while women with uterus didelphys seem to have an increased risk of preterm labour and malpresentation. These findings are consistent with those of previous studies. The arcuate uterus, a minor uterine defect considered a normal variant rather than a uterine anomaly by many, was specifically associated with an increase in pregnancy loss during the second trimester. Women with arcuate uteri also are at an increased risk of experiencing fetal malpresentation.

7 Management of Congenital Uterine Anomalies

Management of congenital uterine abnormalities aims to treat pain and anatomical distortion associated with obstructed abnormalities and to improve reproductive outcome and ultimately increase live birth rates. Treatment of patients with obstructive Mullerian anomalies and agenesis need appropriate correction of anatomical defects to relieve the symptoms and to improve the quality of life. They also need psychosocial counselling to address the functional and emotional effects of genital anomalies [12]. Future fertility options should be addressed with adolescents and their parents or guardians. While unicornuate uterus as such does not warrant surgical intervention, functioning rudimentary uterine horns frequently associated with unicornuate uterus need surgical removal to prevent the risk of haematometra or pregnancy occurring in the horn, although the presence of associated renal tract anomalies needs to be ruled out prior to any surgery.

While there is evidence of a strong association between unification (fusion) defects and canalization (resorption) defects and adverse reproductive outcome, the effectiveness of treating such nonobstructed uterine anomalies surgically to improve the reproductive outcome, especially if they are incidentally diagnosed, is still debated. Traditionally, abdominal metroplasty was performed to unify or restore the shape of the uterus. However, surgery is associated with a number of complications and risks, including prolonged hospital stay, long recovery period, post-operative intraperitoneal adhesions and uterine rupture during subsequent pregnancy. It is still the only surgical treatment available for women with unification defects such as bicornuate or didelphic uteri. However, surgical intervention for unification defects is not generally considered in the absence of significant adverse reproductive history. Evidence on improving the reproductive outcome following abdominal metroplasty in unification defect in women with past history of repeated pregnancy loss or preterm deliveries is limited. Data from only one controlled study of 21 patients with 13 managed conservatively and 8 managed with abdominal metroplasty did not show an improved obstetric outcome [14].

Hysteroscopic metroplasty or trans-cervical resection or division of the uterine septum has become the established treatment of choice for septate uterus [12]. It has largely replaced abdominal metroplasty as treatment for septate uterus as it is a relatively quick and simple surgical procedure that can be performed on a day case basis. Hysteroscopic metroplasty has more advantages over the abdominal approach as it has lower morbidity, fewer adhesions and shorter hospital stay and possibly reduced risks during pregnancy and labour such as uterine rupture. A variety of instruments can be used for the resection of a septum such as micro-scissors, a bipolar electrosurgical needle or a resectope with an operating loop. Transabdominal ultrasound or laparoscopic guidance is utilized intraoperatively to monitor the procedure with a view to reducing the risk of uterine perforation and to ensure adequacy of the procedure. It is a good practice to measure the septal length preoperatively using 3D ultrasound or other imaging modalities so that it may help the surgeon on appropriate planning of the septal resection to ensure its safety and efficacy. Preoperative endometrial suppression is not routinely done but may improve visualization and operative precision. If used, endometrial suppression with a single dose of gonadotrophin-releasing hormone (GnRH) agonist 3–4 weeks prior to the procedure is adequate. When suppression is not used, the procedure is preferably performed in the early follicular phase. Incision of the septum may be undertaken with any standard hysteroscopic scissors, bipolar electrode or resectoscope. The length of the uterine septum may vary from a small septum of 1 cm to a full septum extending from the fundus to the internal cervical os. The presence of a residual septum 0.5–1.0 cm in length does not adversely influence outcome [12]. Moving the hysteroscope from side to side and visualization of both ostia on a panoramic view from the level of internal os verifies completion of resection. Endometrial re-epithelialization of the cut surface can occur centripetally by the proliferation of endometrial tissue and centrifugally from the base of the remaining glands to the margin of the incision. Re-evaluation by hysteroscopy or HSG or saline infusion sonography at two months post-operatively is done to evaluate for adhesion formation and for any residual septum. Postponement of pregnancy attempts for two months after surgery is recommended although definite evidence for such approach is lacking. While there is no evidence of benefit of using intrauterine devices or an intrauterine balloon to reduce the risk of adhesions, some clinicians routinely use this. Post-operative hormone treatment, especially if preoperative GnRH agonist given, is frequently used to enhance endometrial proliferation and to reduce adhesion formation. Conjugated oestrogen at 2.5–5 mg per day or oestradiol 2 mg daily may be used for 5 to 6 weeks and 10–20 mg of medroxyprogesterone acetate is added during the final 10 days.

The effectiveness and possible complications of hysteroscopic metroplasty have never been tested in a randomised controlled trial. Various self-controlled studies and studies with cases and contemporaneous controls in women with no history of surgery have reported significant improvements in pregnancy outcome in terms of reduced miscarriage rates and increased live birth rates [15–17]. A recent systematic review and meta-analysis of controlled studies have reported a decreased probability of spontaneous first and second trimester miscarriage in women treated with hysteroscopic removal of septum compared to women who were not treated (RR 0.37, 95% CI, 0.25 to 0.55; heterogeneity I2 = 0%; six datasets). On the other hand, conception rates (RR 1.14, 95% CI, 0.79 to 1.65; heterogeneity I2 = 80%; four datasets) and preterm delivery rates (RR 0.66, 95% CI, 0.29 to 1.49; heterogeneity I2 = 0%; six datasets) were similar between the hysteroscopic resection and control groups. Although observational studies have found a benefit in removing the septum in women with a history of subfertility and miscarriage, a Cochrane review of the evidence for hysteroscopic metroplasty in women with recurrent miscarriage and a septate uterus in 2011, found no evidence to recommend it as routine practice [18]. They have recommended hysteroscopic metroplasty should not be practised unless as part of a randomised controlled trial. A multicentre randomised controlled trial in women having recurrent miscarriage is currently underway in Netherlands.

The National Institute for Health and Care Excellence (NICE) have recently produced guidance on hysteroscopic metroplasty of a uterine septum for recurrent miscarriage and for primary infertility [19, 20]. While evidence on the safety of hysteroscopic metroplasty of a uterine septum for recurrent miscarriage includes some serious but rare complications, evidence on efficacy is adequate to support the use of this procedure provided that normal arrangements are in place for clinical governance, consent and audit. A multidisciplinary team including specialists in reproductive medicine, uterine imaging and hysteroscopic surgery should undertake patient selection and treatment. In the guideline for management of septum in primary infertility patients, NICE recommends that current evidence on efficacy is inadequate in quantity and quality and therefore this procedure should only be used with special arrangements for clinical governance, consent and audit or research.

8 Conclusion

Uterine anomalies are commonly seen in women presenting with a history of reproductive problems. While 2D ultrasound and HSG are adequate for screening for uterine anomalies, 3D ultrasound, MRI and combined laparoscopy and hysteroscopy can correctly classify the type of uterine anomaly due to their ability to show both external and internal contours of the uterus. However, MRI and combined laparoscopy and hysteroscopy are reserved for diagnosing complex Mullerian anomalies.

While uterine anomalies are associated with adverse reproductive outcomes such as miscarriage, preterm labour and malpresentation in labour, high quality evidence on the efficacy and safety of surgical treatment to improve the reproductive outcome is lacking. However, controlled studies have indicated that hysteroscopic septal resection reduces miscarriage rates and increases live birth rates. Based on the evidence from the controlled studies, NICE has recommended that the evidence on efficacy of hysteroscopic metroplasty of a uterine septum for recurrent miscarriage is adequate to support the use of this procedure provided that normal arrangements are in place for clinical governance, consent and audit.

References

1. Lin, P.C., et al., *Female genital anomalies affecting reproduction. Fertil Steril*, 2002. **78**(5): p. 899–915.

2. W, S.T., *Langman's Medical Embryology*, 12th Edition. 2012: p. 243 – 259.

3. AFS, *The American Fertility Society classifications of adnexal adhesions, distal tubal occlusion, tubal occlusion secondary to tubal ligation, tubal pregnancies, mullerian anomalies and intrauterine adhesions. Fertil Steril*, 1988. **49**(6): p. 944–55.

4. Grimbizis, G.F., et al., *The ESHRE/ESGE consensus on the classification of female genital tract congenital anomalies. Hum Reprod*, 2013. **28**(8): p. 2032–44.

5. Chan, Y.Y., et al., *The prevalence of congenital uterine anomalies in unselected and high-risk populations: a systematic review. Hum Reprod Update*, 2011. **17**(6): p. 761–71.

6. Saravelos, S.H., K.A. Cocksedge, and T.C. Li, *Prevalence and diagnosis of congenital uterine anomalies in women with reproductive failure: a critical appraisal. Hum Reprod Update*, 2008. **14**(5): p. 415–29.

7. Marcal, L., et al., *Mullerian duct anomalies: MR imaging. Abdom Imaging*, 2011. **36**(6): p. 756–64.

8. Jayaprakasan, K., et al., *Prevalence of uterine anomalies and their impact on early pregnancy in women conceiving after assisted reproduction treatment. Ultrasound Obstet Gynecol*, 2011. **37**(6): p. 727–32.

9. Puscheck, E.E. and L. Cohen, *Congenital malformations of the uterus: the role of ultrasound. Semin Reprod Med*, 2008. **26**(3): p. 223–31.

10. Salim, R., et al., *Reproducibility of three-dimensional ultrasound diagnosis of congenital uterine anomalies. Ultrasound Obstet Gynecol*, 2003. **21**(6): p. 578–82.

11. Reichman, D.E. and M.R. Laufer, *Congenital uterine anomalies affecting reproduction. Best Pract Res Clin Obstet Gynaecol*, 2010. **24**(2): p. 193–208.

12. Letterie, G.S., *Management of congenital uterine abnormalities. Reprod Biomed Online*, 2011. **23**(1): p. 40–52.

13. Chan, Y.Y., et al., *Reproductive outcomes in women with congenital uterine anomalies: a systematic review. Ultrasound Obstet Gynecol*, 2011. **38**(4): p. 371–82.

14. Maneschi, F., et al., *Reproductive performance in women with bicornuate uterus. Acta Eur Fertil*, 1993. **24**(3): p. 117–20.

15. Valle, R.F. and G.E. Ekpo, *Hysteroscopic metroplasty for the septate uterus: review and meta-analysis. J Minim Invasive Gynecol*, 2013. **20**(1): p. 22–42.

16. Homer, H.A., T.C. Li, and I.D. Cooke, *The septate uterus: a review of management and reproductive outcome. Fertil Steril*, 2000. **73**(1): p. 1–14.

17. Venetis, C.A., et al., *Clinical implications of congenital uterine anomalies: a meta-analysis of comparative studies. Reprod Biomed Online*, 2014. **29**(6): p. 665–83.

18. Kowalik, C.R., et al., *Metroplasty versus expectant management for women with recurrent miscarriage and a septate uterus. Cochrane Database Syst Rev*, 2011. Issue 6. Art. No.: CD008576.

19. NICE, *Hysteroscopic metroplasty of a uterine septum for recurrent miscarriage*. nice.org.uk/guidance/ipg510, 2014.

20. NICE, *Hysteroscopic metroplasty of a uterine septum for primary infertility*. guidance.nice.org.uk/ipg509, 2015.

Fibroids and Fertility

Yakoub Khalaf

Sesh K. Sunkara

1 Introduction

Uterine fibroids are the most common pelvic tumours, occurring in 30% of women over the age of 30 years. Their incidence increases with age, and they are more common in certain ethnic populations. The frequency of fibroids reported in literature varies widely due to differences in diagnostic tests used, populations studied and study design. The largest study to date, prospectively followed up 95,061 female nurses in America aged between 25 and 44 years with questionnaires every two years, to determine the incidence of fibroids among premenopausal women by age and race [1]. The diagnosis of fibroids was self reported and confirmed for a sample of cases. The crude incidence rate in this study was 12.8 per 1,000 woman years. The standardised rates were much higher in black women than in white women, 30.6 and 8.9 per 1,000 woman years respectively. Even after adjusting for variables such as body mass index, infertility and contraception, the rates among black women were significantly higher than those amongst white women (RR 3.25; 95% CI 2.71–3.88). Another large American survey included 1,364 women aged between 35 and 49 years who were randomly selected from an urban health plan. All recruited women underwent transvaginal ultrasonography. The cumulative incidence of fibroids at 50 years of age was 70 and >80% for whites and African Americans respectively. The prevalence of fibroids is lower in Europe, although still remarkable from the healthcare point of view. An Italian cohort study documented an incidence of ultrasonographically detectable fibroids of 21% in a series of 341 unselected women residing in an urban zone aged between 30 and 60 years [2]. A Swedish study recruiting 335 unselected subjects from an urban district and who accepted to undergo transvaginal ultrasonography showed a prevalence of 3% in women aged between 25 and 32 years and 8% in those aged between 33 and 40 years [3].

2 Classification of Fibroids

Numerous classifications of fibroids can be found in the literature. They are traditionally classified according to their anatomical location and divided into submucous, intramural or subserous. Submucous fibroids are those that distort the uterine cavity and are further divided into three subtypes: pedunculated (type 0); sessile with less than 50% intramural extension of the fibroid (type I); and sessile with 50% or greater intramural extension (type II). The FIGO classification describes eight fibroid locations (0–7; 0 = pedunculated intracavitary, 1 = submucosal with <50% intramural, 2 = submucosal with ≥50% intramural, 3 = 100% intramural and contact with endometrium, 4 = intramural, 5 = subserosal with ≥50% intramural, 6 = subserosal with <50% intramural, 7 = pedunculated subserosal) as well as other forms which include cervical and parasitic fibroids [4].

3 Clinical Presentation of Uterine Fibroids

Symptoms associated with the presence of uterine fibroids include heavy and prolonged periods, pelvic pressure (from large fibroids), pain (resulting from torsion of a pedunculated fibroid or degeneration), urinary symptoms and constipation resulting from pressure by anterior and posterior fibroids. Whether they cause infertility is the subject of considerable speculation. Although most women with fibroids are fertile, fibroids may interfere with fertility secondary to anatomical distortion and alterations to the uterine environment [5]. For those women afflicted with fibroids, the risk of miscarriage [6] and pregnancy complications such as pain are also increased.

4 Do Fibroids Impair Fertility?

A decreased risk of fibroids in parous women when compared with nulliparous women has been repeatedly reported. The observation that parity is associated with a reduction in the risk of fibroids could be interpreted in two ways. Parity may be a protective factor or, alternatively, fertility may be partly compromised in women with fibroids. Studies investigating the association between fibroids and history of infertility may be of help in clarifying this issue, but unfortunately evidence on this regard is scarce. Overall, the question therefore remains about causality of the association. Does pregnancy protect from fibroid development or, conversely, do fibroids affect fertility?

5 How Could Fibroids Impair Fertility?

Whilst fibroids are associated with infertility in 5–10% of cases, they are estimated to be the sole cause of infertility in 2–3% of cases [7]. Fibroids can impair fertility through several possible mechanisms such as: anatomic distortion of the uterine cavity and subsequent alterations to endometrial function, functional changes such as increased uterine peristalsis and impairment of the endometrial and myometrial blood supply and changes to the local hormone milieu and paracrine molecular changes induced by fibroids, which could impair gamete transport [5,8]. The effect of fibroids on fertility is dictated largely by the location and size of the fibroid.

6 Effect of Fibroids on Embryo Implantation

The advent of assisted reproductive techniques (ART) and, in particular, of in vitro fertilisation (IVF) treatment has offered a useful tool to elucidate the relationship between fibroids and fertility. Results from IVF treatment provide precious information on the impact of uterine fibroids on embryo implantation.

There have been meta-analyses that have aimed to assess the impact of fibroids in IVF cycles. A meta-analysis of studies investigating the influence of fibroids located at different sites in IVF cycles showed that myomas negatively affect pregnancy rates [8]. Although based on a small number of studies, submucous fibroids appeared to strongly interfere with the chance of pregnancy: OR (95% CI) for conception and delivery being 0.3 (0.1–0.7) and 0.3 (0.1–0.8) respectively. The impact of intramural fibroids was less dramatic although still statistically significant: OR (95% CI) for conception and delivery being 0.8 (0.6–0.9) and 0.7 (0.5–0.8) respectively. In a follow-

up study, intramural fibroids were shown to have an adverse effect on live birth rate after three consecutive cycles of IVF treatment [9]. In general, these effects appeared to be more relevant when considering the delivery rate compared to the clinical pregnancy rate. Conversely, subserosal fibroids did not seem to affect pregnancy rates.

A systematic review evaluated the effects on fertility by location of fibroids [10]. The results demonstrated that women with submucous fibroids, compared with infertile women without fibroids, demonstrated a significantly lower clinical pregnancy rate (RR 0.36; 95% CI 0.17–0.73), implantation rate (RR 0.28; 95% CI 0.12–0.64) and ongoing pregnancy/ live birth rate (RR 0.31; 95% CI 0.11–0.85) and a significantly higher miscarriage rate (RR 1.67; 95% CI 1.37–2.05). Women with intramural fibroids also had a significantly lower clinical pregnancy rate, implantation rate and ongoing pregnancy/ live birth rate and a significantly higher miscarriage rate. When women with subserous fibroids were compared with women without fibroids, no difference was observed for any outcome measure.

There is controversy on the impact of intramural fibroids that do not distort the uterine cavity on IVF treatment outcome. The first prospective observational study reported an adverse effect of such fibroids on outcome of IVF [11]. This was further addressed in a comprehensive systematic review that looked at 19 observational studies comprising a total of 6,087 IVF cycles. Meta-analysis of these studies showed a significant decrease in live birth (RR 0.79; 95% CI 0.70–0.88) and clinical pregnancy rates (RR 0.85; 95% CI 0.77–0.94) in women with non-cavity distorting intramural fibroids compared to those without fibroids, following IVF treatment [12]. However, there is currently lack of evidence from randomised controlled trials whether any intervention in this group of women would improve the outcome of IVF treatment and restore live birth rates to the levels expected in women without fibroids.

7 Fibroids and Miscarriage

An early review comprising reports on women with symptomatic, palpable fibroids published from 1957 to 1980 identified a reduction in miscarriage from 41% to 19%, in a cohort of women with symptomatic fibroids who underwent myomectomy [7]. A small, uncontrolled series of 19 asymptomatic women who conceived with fibroids reported a reduction in miscarriage post myomectomy compared to the pre-myomectomy rate (24% vs 60%) [13].

A study involving 143 women with ultrasonographically identified fibroids in the first trimester reported a nearly two-fold increase in miscarriage rate, when compared to 715 age-matched controls without fibroids (14% vs 7.6%, $P < 0.5$) [6]. Although the fibroid size was not associated with the spontaneous loss rate, the presence of multiple fibroids was a significant predictor of spontaneous loss and among the 88 patients with only a single fibroid, there was no increased risk of miscarriage compared with controls. A meta-analysis of controlled studies of intramural fibroids and IVF outcome which reported on miscarriage showed a miscarriage rate of 22% in women with intramural fibroids compared with 15.4% in the control group [14]. Data are currently unavailable to evaluate the risk of miscarriage in women with submucosal fibroids. Another observational study reported miscarriages in 5 of 9 (53%) pregnant women with submucosal fibroids and 9 out of 21 women (43%) who underwent prior myomectomy [15].

8 Fertility after Myomectomy

Before the advent of less invasive options, hysterectomy was the standard treatment for women troubled with fibroid-associated symptoms. This option is understandably unacceptable for women wishing to conserve their fertility. Myomectomy which involves the removal of the fibroid with conservation of the uterus is the alternative surgical treatment option for women wishing to conceive. The procedure may be performed abdominally, laparoscopically or hysteroscopically. Several reviews of literature on pregnancy rates following myomectomy have been published. One of the early reviews focussing on studies published between 1933 and 1980 by Buttram and Reiter [7] reported a 40% pregnancy rate following abdominal myomectomy (480 out of 1,202 cases). This rate was 54% when patients with other causes of infertility were excluded. Another review by Vercellini et al [16] confirmed this rate of success following myomectomy. They reported a post-surgical pregnancy rate of 57% across prospective studies. When including women with unexplained infertility, this rate was 61%. The advent of endoscopic surgery did not seem to modify this result. In a review by Donnez and Jadoul [5] the pregnancy rate among women undergoing hysteroscopic and laparoscopic myomectomy was reported as 45% and 49% respectively. These findings have further been confirmed by more recent and larger studies.

9 IVF Outcome after Myomectomy

Whilst there is a consistent body of literature on the adverse influence of fibroids on pregnancy outcome, the impact of myomectomy has been less extensively investigated. An early study investigating the effect of myomectomy on 27 women with submucosal fibroids found that the delivery rate was not significantly different in women who underwent myomectomy compared to women without fibroids (37% and 22% respectively, $P = 0.13$) [17]. Surrey et al [18] reported a pregnancy rate of 62% and 68% respectively in women operated for submucous fibroids and controls without fibroids following IVF treatment. From these studies we can infer that although the overall evidence is scarce, previous myomectomy did not seem to negatively affect the pregnancy rate following IVF treatment.

A prospective comparative study has provided further evidence on the effectiveness of myomectomy prior to IVF treatment. Women with intramural and/or subserosal fibroids with at least one lesion >5 cm were allocated to myomectomy or no surgery based on their decision. They reported a live birth rate of 25% and 12% respectively in women who did and did not undergo surgery prior to IVF treatment [19].

10 Non Surgical Treatments for Fibroids

Several non-surgical approaches for the treatment of fibroids have emerged over the last few decades, with medical therapies as well as radiological interventions being proposed. The medical therapies traditionally used are gonadotrophin releasing hormone (GnRH) analogues and, more recently, selective progesterone receptor modulators (SPRM), e.g. ulipristal acetate (UPA). Radiological interventions include uterine artery embolisation (UAE) and the use of magnetic resonance-guided high-intensity focused ultrasound (MRgFUS).

GnRH agonists, the mainstay of medical therapy for fibroids, work by creating a hypogonadotrophic hypogonadal state and produce a significant reduction in uterine size. Their use in the context of infertility treatment remains questionable since ovulation is generally inhibited during treatment and the fibroids usually resume their pretreatment dimension within a few months after stopping treatment. Selective progesterone receptor modulators are thought to stimulate apoptosis and inhibit cell proliferation in fibroids. Ulipristal acetate is approved in the European Union as a preoperative treatment for moderate to severe symptoms associated with uterine fibroids and for intermittent treatment of fibroid symptoms in women of reproductive age. However, treatment beyond four courses of three months of therapy has not been formally studied, and it is noted in the assessment report for this product that unnecessary interventions for assessment of endometrial normality may be a consequence [20].

Significant adverse effects of UAE on endometrium and fertility have been described. Routine hysteroscopic examination after UAE showed intracavitary abnormal findings including intrauterine adhesions, protruding myomas, myometrial fistula and necrotic tissue in approximately 60% of women [21]. A follow-up study involving 61 women after UAE found a low monthly fecundability rate of 0.1% (95% CI 0–0.3%). This study found no reduction in ovarian reserve after UAE, and it concluded that UAE might have an adverse effect on fertility and should not be routinely offered to women desiring childbearing [22]. In a retrospective analysis of pregnancy outcomes following UAE, 33 (58.9%) out of 56 pregnancies had successful outcomes; out of these, six (18.2%) were premature, seventeen (30.4%) were miscarriages, three were terminations, two were stillbirths and one was an ectopic pregnancy. Of the 33 deliveries, 24 (72.7%)

were delivered by caesarean section. There were 13 elective sections and the indication for nine was fibroids. There were six cases of postpartum haemorrhage (18.2%). The study concluded that there was a significant increase in delivery by caesarean section and an increase in preterm delivery, postpartum haemorrhage, miscarriage and lower pregnancy rates following UAE compared to the general obstetric population [23]. Data regarding pregnancy outcome with MRgFUS is scanty as most women who wish to conserve fertility have been excluded from these treatments due to safety concerns. Recently, uterine leiomyomas have become an attractive target for gene therapy. Gene therapy is the introduction of genetic material into patients' cells to achieve a therapeutic benefit. Gene therapy strategies include: mutation compensation of dysregulated genes; replacement of defective tumour-suppressor genes; inactivation of oncogenes; introduction of suicide genes; immunogenic therapy and anti-angiogenesis based approaches. Preclinical studies of gene therapy have shown promising results in uterine leiomyomas and researchers are of the view that this approach is not far from becoming a medical reality [24].

11 Conclusion

Given the evidence of the impact of fibroids on fertility based on the location, size and number, clinicians should pursue a comprehensive and personalised approach, taking into account the pros and cons of myomectomy in terms of alleviating fibroid symptoms, improving fertility outcomes and balancing against potential surgical risks.

References

1. Marshall LM, Spiegelman D, Barbieri RL, Goldman MB, Manson JE, Colditz GA, et al. Variation in the incidence of uterine leiomyoma among premenopausal women by age and race. *Obstet Gynecol* 1997;90:967–973.

2. Marino JL, Eskanazi B, Warner M, Samuels S, Vercellini P, Gavoni N, Olive D. Uterine leiomyoma and menstrual cycle characteristics in a population based cohort study. *Hum Reprod* 2004;19:2350–2355.

3. Borgfeldt C, Andolf E. Transvaginal ultrasonographic findings in the uterus and the endometrium: low prevalence of leiomyoma in a random sample of women age 25–40 years. *Acta Obstet Gynecol Scand* 2000;79:202–207.

4. Munro GM, Critchley HO, Broder MS, Fraser IS for the FIGO Working Group on Menstrual Disorders. FIGO classification system (PALM-COEIN) for causes of abnormal uterine bleeding in nongravid women of reproductive age. *Int J Gynecol Obstet* 2011;113:3–13.

5. Donnez J, Jadoul P. What are the implications of myomas on fertility? A need for a debate? *Hum Reprod* 2002;17:1424–1430.

6. Benson CB, Chow JS, Chang-Lee W et al. Outcome of pregnancies in women with uterine leiomyomas identified by sonography in the first trimester. *J Clin Ultrasound* 2001; 29: 261–264.

7. Buttram VC Jr, Reiter RC. Uterine leiomyomata: etiology,

symptomatology, and management. *Fertil Steril* 1981;36:433–445.

8. Somigliana E, Vercellini P, Dagauti R, Pasin R, De Giorgi O, Crosignani PG. Fibroids and female reproduction: a critical analysis of evidence. *Hum Reprod Update* 2007;13:465–476.

9. Khalaf Y, Ross C, El-Toukhy T, Hart R, Seed P, Braude P. The effect of small intramural uterine fibroids on the cumulative outcome of assisted conception. *Hum Reprod.* 2006 Oct;21:2640–2644.

10. Pritts EA, Parker WH, Olive DL. Fibroids and Infertility: an updated systematic review of evidence. *Fertil Steril* 2009;91:1215–1223.

11. Hart R, Khalaf Y, Yeong CT, Seed P, Taylor A, Braude P. A prospective controlled study of the effect of intramural uterine fibroids on the outcome of assisted conception. *Hum Reprod.* 2001;16:2411–2417.

12. Sunkara SK, Khairy M, El-Toukhy T, Khalaf Y, Coomarasamy A. The effect of intramural fibroids without uterine cavity involvement on the outcome of IVF treatment: a systematic review and meta-analysis. *Hum Repro* 2010;25:418–429.

13. Li TC, Mortimer R, Cooke ID. Myomectomy: a retrospective study to examine reproductive performance before and after surgery. *Hum Reprod.* 1999;14:1735–1740.

14. Klatsky PC, Tran ND, Caughey AB, Fujimoto VY. Fibroids and reproductive outcomes: a systematic literature review from conception to delivery. *Am J Obstet Gynecol.* 2008;198:357–366.

15. Casini ML, Rossi F, Agostini R, Unfer V. Effects of the position of fibroids on fertility. *Gynecol Endocrinol.* 2006;22:106–109.

16. Vercellini P, Maddalena S, De Giorgi O, Aimi G, Crosignani PG. Abdominal myomectomy for infertility: a comprehensive review. *Hum Reprod.* 1998;13:873–879.

17. Narayan R and Goswamy RK. Treatment of submucous fibroids and outcome of assisted conception. *J Am Assoc Gynecol Laparosc* 1994; 1:307–311.

18. Surrey ES, Minjarez D, Stevens J and Schoolcraft WB. Effects of myomectomy on the outcome of assisted reproductive technologies. *Fetil Steril* 2005; 83:1473–1479.

19. Bulletti C, DE Ziegler D, Levi Setti P, Cicinelli E, Polli V and Stefanetti M. Myomas, pregnancy outcome, and in vitro fertilisation. *Ann N Y Acad Sci* 2004;1034:84–92.

20. Donnez J, Vázquez F, Tomaszewski J, Nouri K, Bouchard P, Fauser BC, Barlow DH, Palacios S, Donnez O, Bestel E, Osterloh I, Loumaye E; PEARL III and PEARL III Extension Study Group. Long-term treatment of uterine fibroids with ulipristal acetate. *Fertil Steril.* 2014;101:1565–1573.

21. Mara M, Horak P, Kubinova K, Dundr P, Belsan T, Kuzel D. Hysteroscopy after uterine fibroid embolization: evaluation of intrauterine findings in 127 patients. *J Obstet Gynaecol Res.* 2012;38:823–831.

22. Torre A, Paillusson B, Fain V, Labauge P, Pelage JP, Fauconnier A. Uterine artery embolization for severe symptomatic fibroids: effects on fertility and symptoms. *Hum Reprod* 2014;29:490–501.

23. Walker WJ, McDowell SJ Pregnancy after uterine artery embolization for leiomyomata: a series of 56 completed pregnancies. *Am J Obstet Gynecol.* 2006;195:1266–1271.

24. Markowski DN, Holzmann C, Bullerdiek J. Genetic alterations in uterine fibroids - a new direction for pharmacological intervention? *Expert Opin Ther Targets.* 2015;19:1485–1494.

Tubal Factor Infertility and Tubal Surgery

Mostafa Metwally
Tulay Karasu

1 Introduction

Tubal factor infertility is a common cause for infertility worldwide. Prior to the introduction of in vitro fertilisation (IVF), tubal surgery was the mainstay of fertility treatment in women with tubal disorders. However, in the era of assisted reproductive technology the use of tubal surgery has gradually declined. This chapter investigates tubal factor infertility and the current role of tubal surgery in the age of assisted reproductive technology. In conclusion, tubal surgery remains an important option that can supplement and in some cases substitute IVF treatment.

Diseased fallopian tubes are an important cause for infertility worldwide and are responsible for 30% to 35% of female infertility [1]. Tubal disease can involve the proximal, midtubal, distal or entire fallopian tube and vary in severity. Pelvic inflammatory disease is the most common cause of tubal disease, representing more than 50% of cases, and may affect the fallopian tube at multiple sites [2]. Other causes for tubal damage are ectopic pregnancy and sterilisation.

Prior to the introduction of IVF, tubal surgery was the mainstay of fertility treatment in women with tubal disorders. The introduction of IVF in 1978 witnessed a gradual decline in the use of tubal surgery leading many to believe that tubal surgery is now an obsolete art, a common misconception held by many. Indeed an editorial in *Fertility and Sterility* some years ago was titled 'Infertility surgery is dead, only the obituary remains' [3]. However, in this chapter it is argued that tubal surgery remains an integral part of fertility treatment. In many cases tubal surgery is an essential adjuvant treatment to IVF aimed at increasing the success rates of assisted reproductive procedures. In many other cases tubal surgery, in well-trained hands can, in fact, be a substitute for IVF treatment, yielding similar results. This chapter investigates tubal factor infertility and the current role of tubal surgery in the age of assisted reproductive technologies.

2 Proximal Tubal Blockage

Proximal tubal blockage demonstrated at hysterosalpingogram by failure of the dye to enter the fallopian tubes is not an uncommon finding and is diagnosed in about 10–25% of cases of tubal infertility [4]. Bilateral proximal tubal occlusion is found in about 3% of cases of proximal tubal disease and the condition is unilateral in about 2% of cases [5].

When this clinical situation is presented, a decision needs to be made as to whether to proceed directly with IVF treatment or to investigate further. The decision depends on many variables, taking into consideration the patient's wishes and values. For example in the presence of an additional fertility problem such as severe male factor or in the case of advanced maternal age, the decision may be made to proceed directly with IVF. However, in many cases the decision is made to investigate further and therefore proceed with laparoscopic assessment of the fallopian tubes.

2.1 Causes of Proximal Tubal Blockage

The causes of proximal tubal blockage include the following:

1. **Tubal spasm**

    This is one of the commonest causes of proximal tubal blockage diagnosed particularly at the time of hysterosalpingogram, where considerable pain can lead to tubal spasm and a false diagnosis of tubal occlusion. These women should proceed to have laparoscopic inspection under a general anaesthetic and with the pain no longer a confounding factor, often these tubes are found to easily fill with dye.

2. **Mucous plug**

    This is a common cause of proximal tubal blockage. The presence of a small amount of mucous or endometrial debris can lead to a temporary occlusion of the proximal fallopian tube. Injection of dye under laparoscopic guidance often relieves the problem. In these cases, if necessary, tubal cannulation is quite successful at dislodging the obstructing mucous plug.

3. **Preferential tubal flow**

This is often the case during hysterosalpingogram or even during laparoscopy when the dye will pass preferentially through one fallopian tube rather than the other. This can be excluded by gently blocking the proximal end of the patent tube using an atraumatic instrument followed by injection of the dye. The dye can then be seen to flow freely through the contralateral fallopian tube previously thought to be obstructed.

4. **True proximal tubal occlusion**

This may be as a result of a number of tubal and pelvic pathologies, such as endometriosis and pelvic inflammatory disease. Chronic inflammation and nodular thickening of the proximal tube is sometimes seen at laparoscopy and is known as salpingitis isthmica nodosa. This is a particular pathology that surgeons should look for, as its presence is a poor prognostic factor for attempted tubal surgery.

5. **Intrauterine pathology**

Proximal tubal obstruction may occasionally be caused by the presence of endometrial pathology such as intrauterine adhesions or an endometrial polyp, which overlies the tubal ostium. Hysterosalpingogram may give rise to suspicion by showing an irregular endometrial cavity as is often the case in Asherman's syndrome, or the presence of a filling defect as in the presence of a polyp. Performing combined hysteroscopic and laparoscopic examination will diagnose and often allow treatment of the cause.

2.2 Diagnosis of Proximal Tubal Disease

1- **Hysterosalpingogram**

This is the usual initial screening test performed in the absence of high risk factors for tubal disease as recommended by the NICE guidelines [6]. Hysterosalpingogram correlates with laparoscopic findings in about 75% of cases, with a false positive rate of 6–25% and a false negative of 8–24% [7]. Although a good test for excluding proximal tubal disease, failure of the

dye to pass into the fallopian tubes is often a result of a false positive test due to, as indicated above, a mucous plug, tubal spasm or preferential flow. The presence of proximal tubal blockage on hysterosalpingogram is an indication for further assessment of the tube using laparoscopy.

2- **Laparoscopy and chromotubation**

Diagnostic laparoscopy will allow a detailed examination of the fallopian tube. False positive diagnoses, as a result of preferential flow, mucous plug or tubal spasm are easily excluded during laparoscopic assessment. Combined laparoscopic and hysteroscopic assessment will also allow exclusion of intrauterine factors which may be obstructing the tubal ostium. If true proximal tubal obstruction is diagnosed then laparoscopic assessment of the remainder of the tube as well as assessment of other relevant pelvic pathologies is essential to determine the feasibility of surgical correction. The presence of bipolar tubal disease (proximal and distal blockage), the presence of salpingitis isthmica nodosa or significant pelvic pathology such as grade IV endometriosis would be a contraindication for proximal tubal cannulation and may be an indication to proceed with IVF treatment.

3- **Hysterosalpingocontrastsonography**

Although a recent meta-analysis showed that hysterosalpingocontrastsonography (HyCoSy) was comparable to hysterosalpingogram for diagnosis of proximal tubal disease, the study noted that there was no differentiation between proximal versus distal tubal disease in individual reports [7]. It remains, however, that in well-trained hands, hysterosalpingosonography can be a useful diagnostic tool for diagnosing proximal tubal disease with a potential advantage of avoiding exposure to radiation.

4- **Fluoroscopic guided salpingography**

Proximal tubal cannulation can also be performed under fluoroscopic control and several studies have reported encouraging results [7,4]. In addition, fluoroscopic balloon tuboplasty can be performed [8]. However, hysteroscopic tubal cannulation does offer several advantages over performing the procedure under only fluoroscopic control as a full evaluation of the endometrial cavity can be performed. This allows the option to deal with any adhesions or endometrial polyps.

Furthermore, performing the procedure only under fluoroscopic control does lead to the potential of missing significant pathologies such as bipolar tubal disease, which would be achieved using a combined hysteroscopic and laparoscopic approach.

2.3 Treatment of Proximal Tubal Obstruction by Hysteroscopic Tubal Cannulation

A 5 mm saline hysteroscopy is performed allowing inspection of the uterine cavity. This also allows exclusion of any intrauterine adhesions or endometrial polyps. A dedicated tubal catheter is then passed through the hysteroscope into the tubal ostium. In our Unit the Cook Novy® catheter is used. This has an outer sheath that curves towards the cornu and hence facilitates placement of the inner catheter and guide wire that are used to cannulate the tube. The procedure should be performed under laparoscopic guidance to avoid undue trauma and perforation of the fallopian tube (occurring in rare cases). The catheter should only be introduced a few millimetres through the tubal ostium. This usually results in the treatment of the blockage. Dye can then be injected (selective salpingography) and free flow of the dye can be observed laparoscopically. The process of hysteroscopic tubal cannulation is a simple procedure with a short learning curve, requires only basic diagnostic hysteroscopic skills and when successful can be highly rewarding to both the patient and the surgeon.

2.3.1 Success Rate of Laparoscopic Guided Hysteroscopic Tubal Catheterisation

In a recent study it was found that tubal cannulation could lead to a significant improvement in pregnancy rates, resulting in a cumulative pregnancy rate of approximately 43% over a two-year period [9]. The procedure was successful in tubal cannulation in up to 62% of patients. This study also found a clinically significant higher pregnancy rate in those who required only unilateral cannulation. Other studies have also shown similar encouraging results with one study reporting a recanalisation success rate of about 26% and a pregnancy rate approaching 28% [10] and a second study reporting a recanalisation success rate of 67% and pregnancy rate of 55% [11].These success rates are extremely encouraging and approach or

sometimes even exceed the results expected after IVF treatment. This emphasises the importance that the reproductive surgeon considers the option of hysteroscopic tubal cannulation in women with proximal tubal obstruction.

2.3.2 Complications of Tubal Hysteroscopic/Fluoroscopic Tubal Cannulation

The main complication is the potential risk for perforation of the fallopian tube. Again, this is where laparoscopic guidance offers a clear advantage where the assistant can help during the process of hysteroscopic cannulation by gently straightening the fallopian tube therefore minimising the risk of the guide wire perforating the tube. Furthermore, the guide wire should never be advanced beyond the few millimetres required to unblock the proximal part of the fallopian tube. In the presence of a longer segment of obstruction, hysteroscopic cannulation is not a suitable technique. Other options would include either proceeding with IVF or microsurgical tubocornual anastomosis.

2.4 Microsurgical Tubal Anastomosis/Cornual Reimplantation

In the presence of significant proximal tubal blockage where tubal cannulation has either been unsuccessful or is deemed to have a low success rate such as in women with salpingitis isthmica nodosa or fibrosis and obstruction affecting a long segment, then microsurgical reanastomosis is a valid option. The surgeon first excises the occluded portion of fallopian tube, taking extreme care not to extend the dissection into the broad ligament where troublesome bleeding may occur. After identification of the patent proximal and distal portions of the fallopian tube, 7/0 or 8/0 of a monofilament delayed absorbable sutures can be used to reinsert the tube into the uterine cornua or reanastomose the two ends of the tube. This is best achieved using the operative microscope for correct placement of the sutures. The fallopian tube is approximated in two layers, seromuscular and serosal while avoiding the tubal lumen. A tubal stent of Prolene 0 or 1 suture can be used at the time to facilitate correct approximation of the tubal lumen. The procedure should, of course, be carried out using microsurgical principles to minimise trauma and ensure a moist, relatively blood-free operating field with minimal tissue handling and the use of anti-adhesion agents at the end of the procedure. With adequate training and careful patient selection, intrauterine pregnancy rate following tubal anastomosis can be extremely encouraging reaching between 38 and 68% [12].

2.5 Distal Tubal Disease

Distal tubal disease is one of the most significant tubal disorders faced by the reproductive medicine specialist as it can have a serious impact on the results of the fertility treatment, in particular, assisted conception treatment. Distal tubal disease can vary from partial to complete occlusion of the distal end of the fallopian tube. This may be associated with a wide spectrum of damage to the remainder of the fallopian tube and can be combined with proximal tubal disease (bipolar disease).

Distal tubal disease is commonly caused by pelvic inflammatory disease as a result of chlamydial infection. Women with at least one previous attack of chlamydia have a 30% increased risk of pelvic inflammatory disease, ectopic pregnancy and tubal factor infertility over their lifetime [13]. Other causes of distal tubal disease include pelvic adhesions as a result of previous pelvic surgery, endometriosis and inflamed pelvic organs such as appendicitis. Distal tubal disease can result in complete occlusion and distension of the fallopian tube with fluid leading to a hydrosalpinx.

2.6 Effect of Hydrosalpinges on the Results of Assisted Conception

The negative effect of hydrosalpinges and the significant improvement in pregnancy rates after treatment has been clearly demonstrated in many studies including a Cochrane meta-analysis which has shown that treatment of a hydrosalpinx by salpingectomy, salpingostomy or occlusion can result in almost doubling the chance of conceiving [14].

Hydrosalpinges can impair pregnancy chances by several mechanisms including embryo toxicity, decreasing endometrial receptivity or mechanical flushing of the embryos from the uterine cavity [[15,16,17]. Hydrosalpingeal fluid has an effect on cytokines and integrins essential for successful implantation. Studies have shown that leukaemia inhibitory factor (LIF) expression is reduced in the mid-luteal endometrium of women with a hydrosalpinx and improved following salpingectomy or salpingostomy [18,19]. Furthermore, alteration of HOXA10 and HOXA11 expression has been associated with decreased implantation in women with a hydrosalpinx. HOX genes are essential for endometrial development and receptivity [20].

Another study demonstrated impaired endometrial and ovarian blood flow in women with hydrosalpinges, which may have an effect on endometrial receptivity and oocyte quality [21].

The effect is so significant that the suspicion of a hydrosalpinx during fertility investigations should almost always be investigated further to either confirm or refute the diagnosis. In this context it is important to remember that ultrasound is not an accurate method for diagnosing hydrosalpinges and furthermore hydrosalpinges can be intermittent and therefore may not always be seen on ultrasound scan. Therefore, if a hydrosalpinx is suspected then a laparoscopy should always be considered.

2.7 The Diagnosis of Distal Tubal Disease

Similar to proximal tubal disease, laparoscopy is the gold standard for diagnosis of distal tubal disease and is usually the first line of investigation in women with significant risk factors such as previous chlamydial infection [6]. This offers the opportunity to both diagnose and treat at the same time. It is imperative at laparoscopy that a full assessment of the degree of tubal damage is performed. The presence of a hydrosalpinx is significant regardless of whether it is partial or complete, unilateral or bilateral. The thickness of the wall, the presence of peri-tubal adhesions and intraluminal adhesions should be assessed and the presence of bipolar disease should be excluded. A proper assessment of the extent of tubal damage by an experienced surgeon is fundamental to planning future management and deciding whether to undertake surgical correction or proceed directly with IVF after removal of the hydrosalpinx.

A hydrosalpinx may also be seen when a hysterosalpingogram has been performed. This should usually be followed by a laparoscopy to evaluate further and decide the best approach for treatment (salpingectomy, salpingostomy or occlusion).

Some studies have advocated the use of chlamydial antibody testing as a screening method for tubal disease. However, evidence for the efficacy of this approach remains controversial; while some studies have shown a strong correlation between tubal factor and fertility and anti-chlamydial antibody testing [22], others have shown doubtful value [23]. Similarly centres that perform HyCoSy may identify possible hydrosalpinges but again the opportunity to fully assess the fallopian tube and its suitability for restorative surgery versus excisional treatment is lost except by performing a laparoscopy.

2.8 Treatment of Hydrosalpinges in Women Seeking Fertility

There are only a few conditions in reproductive medicine, which are supported with such strong evidence for the necessity of treatment as a hydrosalpinx is. The question remains whether every hydrosalpinx should be treated and the best approach to treatment, whether excisional (salpingectomy), reparative (salpingostomy) or occlusion. As a general rule, treatment is indicated in all women with a hydrosalpinx wishing to conceive either naturally or with assisted conception treatment as treatment can result in a significant improvement in pregnancy rate. Exceptions might be where there is a significant risk in undertaking open or laparoscopic surgery, for example, where there has been extensive prior surgery.

2.8.1 Salpingectomy

Salpingectomy is the usual approach for women with hydrosalpinges and is a simple procedure that can be performed by most gynaecological surgeons. However, the reproductive surgeon needs to be aware of the possible implications of salpingectomy on future assisted conception treatment.

Since the ovary receives its blood supply both from the ovarian and uterine vessels running along the mesosalpinx, removal of the fallopian tube may, in theory, result in a compromise of ovarian function and deterioration of the ovarian reserve. However, several recent studies have been reassuring regarding the absence of an immediate effect of salpingectomy on ovarian reserve, although a long-term effect cannot be excluded [24,25]. Nevertheless, the reproductive surgeon should always be careful to minimise any trauma to the ovarian blood supply during a salpingectomy. Therefore, the incision should be kept as close to the fallopian tube and as far away from the ovary as possible.

2.8.2 Salpingostomy

This is a less commonly performed surgical procedure and requires particular expertise and therefore should not be undertaken except by surgeons who have had particular training in this area. The key to successful salpingostomy is good selection of patients who may benefit from this procedure. With experience and proper case selection, the success rates are extremely encouraging with one study showing a cumulative pregnancy rate of 40% over 36 months after salpingostomy [26]. The key to good case selection is being able to effectively identify the severity of tubal disease. One of the most important factors is the assessment of the tubal lumen. In tubes where the mucosal folds have been preserved and there are no significant intraluminal adhesions, success rates are significantly better. In women where there is significant destruction of the tubal lumen, salpingostomy should not be undertaken. One particular study has demonstrated that the success rates of salpingostomy are directly correlated to the stage of tubal disease, where women with mild stage 1 disease had success rates of around 39% while those with more severe stage 3–4 disease had a success rate of as low as 8% [27].

The presence of bipolar disease or other concomitant causes of infertility such as significant male factor would be a contraindication to salpingostomy and an indication to proceed with salpingectomy followed by IVF.

2.8.2.1 Technique of Salpingostomy

After careful evaluation of tubal condition and confirming its provisional suitability for salpingostomy (small hydrosalpinx with thin wall, no associated proximal tubal disease, no significant intraluminal adhesions), the first step is to restore the anatomical relationship between the fimbrial end of the fallopian tube and the ovary. Often the fimbrial end is buried inside adhesions and should be carefully dissected and exposed. Adhesions between the fallopian tube and ovary should also be carefully treated to restore the normal anatomical relationship between the two structures.

The surgeon next proceeds to carefully open the distal end of the fallopian tube. This is usually facilitated by prior injection of methylene blue dye to help identify the site of the occluded ostium and hence the site where the incision should be made. It is best to avoid electrosurgical dissection so as to minimise thermal damage to the fallopian tube.

After incising the ostium and carefully stretching the opening, the surgeon should then proceed with examination and assessment of the tubal mucosa. This is by far the most important step from the prognostic point of view. This can be done by eversion of the fallopian tube and visually inspecting the mucosa. The presence of pink, intact mucosal folds with minimal adhesions is reassuring. However, a more accurate technique is by performing a salpingoscopy. This is achieved using a 3–5 mm hysteroscope, which can be introduced through any of the laparoscopic ports. The hysteroscope is carefully inserted into the opening of the fallopian tube. Saline infusion is started and the fallopian tube is distended. The hysteroscope is then advanced gradually into the fallopian tube and this allows an adequate inspection of the mucosa and assessment of intraluminal adhesions. If salpingostomy is shown to be feasible then the surgeon should evert the mucosa. This is achieved using a pair of atraumatic forceps to grasp the mucosa and carefully evert it to form a cuff taking care not to tear the tube. To prevent reocclusion 3–4 fine monofilament sutures such as PDS 3/0 are inserted at 6, 12, 3 and 9 o'clock positions to fix the mucosa to the outside surface of the fallopian tube. It is occasional practice that surgeons may use bipolar or monopolar energy to fuse the everted edge of the tube to the serosal surface. However, this may result in thermal damage of the tube and is not advised.

2.9 Cost Effectiveness of Surgical Treatment of Hydrosalpinges

One study demonstrated that the cost per live birth in 51 patients undergoing a salpingectomy was €22,823, significantly less than those who did not undergo the treatment (n=44), €29,517 [28].

Salpingostomy can also be a viable alternative to women who may choose not to proceed with IVF as their first choice of treatment. In many countries including the United Kingdom, there is limitation on IVF funding, and in many cases IVF is neither a valid nor affordable treatment. Furthermore, patients may have cultural or personal objections to IVF treatment or simply prefer to try a natural approach in the first instance. It is important to note that following a salpingostomy, a hydrosalpinx may recur. Therefore, if conception has not occurred after a significant period of time and the couple decide to proceed with IVF then reocclusion and recurrence of the hydrosalpinx should be confirmed, in which case a salpingectomy is usually performed. Furthermore, the patient should be informed about the risk of an ectopic pregnancy following salpingostomy.

2.9.1 Occlusion of the Fallopian Tube

This can be performed either laparoscopically, similar to tubal sterilisation, with the application of a Filshie clip or hysteroscopically by insertion of one of the hysteroscopic tubal sterilisation devices (Essure has been withdrawn from UK market). Tubal occlusion has been demonstrated to be effective in improving clinical pregnancy rate [14]. However, it does leave behind a diseased fallopian tube, which has the potential of future infection with the formation of a pyosalpinx and pelvic abscess.

Tubal occlusion is best suited in women where salpingectomy or salpingostomy is difficult to perform such as in the presence of significant pelvic adhesions. The safety of the hysteroscopic occlusion techniques on any ensuing pregnancy however is still a matter for debate although reports so far have been reassuring [29–33].

A recent systematic review and meta-analysis evaluated the use of ESSURE® in women with hydrosalpinx prior to embryo transfer. They confirmed higher clinical pregnancy rates in women treated with ESSURE® when compared to women without any intervention. However, the miscarriage rate was higher when compared to women with other interventions [34]. Hysteroscopic tubal occlusion should therefore only be considered if a laparoscopic procedure is difficult to be performed and ESSURE itself has been removed from the UK and other markets.

Current evidence however does not support ultrasound aspiration of the hydrosalpinx to improve pregnancy rates [14]. Furthermore, aspiration of the fallopian tube at the time of egg collection may merely be followed by reaccumulation by the time of embryo transfer. Finally, aspiration may lead to the risk of infection and development of pelvic abscess. Therefore, aspiration is not an advisable approach for women with hydrosalpinges.

3 Conclusion

In conclusion, tubal surgery is by no means obsolete and remains an important option that can supplement and in some cases substitute assisted conception treatment. Many cases of proximal tubal disease can easily be treated using proximal tubal cannulation and microsurgical anastomosis. The presence of a hydrosalpinx almost always necessitates surgical intervention in women wishing to conceive either naturally from a contralateral normal fallopian tube or through assisted conception. The usually performed technique is salpingectomy with care not to damage the ovarian blood supply. However, with adequate experience salpingostomy may salvage the tube, avoid damage to the ovarian blood supply and provide the patient with a viable alternative to IVF treatment. Where neither salpingostomy nor salpingectomy can be performed because of technical difficulties, tubal occlusion should be considered, mainly through the laparoscopic route.

References

1. Kawwass, J. F., Crawford, S., Kissin, D. M., Session, D. R., Boulet, S. & Jamieson, D. J. 2013. Tubal factor infertility and perinatal risk after assisted reproductive technology. *Obstet Gynecol*, 121, 1263–71.

2. Honore, G. M., Holden, A. E. & Schenken, R. S. 1999. Pathophysiology and management of proximal tubal blockage. *Fertil Steril*, 71, 785–95.

3. Feinberg, E. C., Levens, E. D. & Decherney, A. H. 2008. Infertility surgery is dead: only the obituary remains? *Fertil Steril*, 89, 232–6.

4. Cobellis, L., Argano, F., Castaldi, M. A., Acone, G., Mele, D., Signoriello, G. & Colacurci, N. 2012. Selective salpingography: preliminary experience of an office operative option for proximal tubal recanalization. *Eur J Obstet Gynecol Reprod Biol*, 163, 62–6.

5. Wadin, K., Lonnemark, M., Rasmussen, C. & Magnusson, A. 1994. Frequency of proximal tubal obstruction in patients undergoing infertility evaluation. *Acta Radiol*, 35, 357–60.

6. NICE 2016. Fertility problems: assessment and treatment.

7. Knuttinen, M. G., Jajko, R. & Scoccia, B. 2014. Fluoroscopic tubal recanalization in tubal factor related infertility. *Semin Intervent Radiol*, 31, 269–71.

8. Osada, H., Kiyoshi Fujii, T., Tsunoda, I., Tsubata, K., Satoh, K. & Palter, S. F. 2000. Outpatient evaluation and treatment of tubal obstruction with selective salpingography and balloon tuboplasty. *Fertil Steril*, 73, 1032–6.

9. Hou, H. Y., Chen, Y. Q., Li, T. C., Hu, C. X., Chen, X. & Yang, Z. H. 2014. Outcome of laparoscopy-guided hysteroscopic tubal catheterization for infertility due to proximal tubal obstruction. *J Minim Invasive Gynecol*, 21, 272–8.

10. Mekaru, K., Yagi, C., Asato, K., Masamoto, H., Sakumoto, K. & Aoki, Y. 2011. Hysteroscopic tubal catheterization under laparoscopy for proximal tubal obstruction. *Arch Gynecol Obstet*, 284, 1573–6.

11. Chung, J. P., Haines, C. J. & Kong, G. W. 2012. Long-term reproductive outcome after hysteroscopic proximal tubal cannulation – an outcome analysis. *Aust N Z J Obstet Gynaecol*, 52, 470–5.

12. Dubuisson, J. B., Chapron, C., Ansquer, Y. & Vacher-Lavenu, M. C. 1997. Proximal tubal occlusion: is there an alternative to microsurgery? *Hum Reprod*, 12, 692–8.

13. Davies, B., Turner, K. M., Frolund, M., Ward, H., May, M. T., Rasmussen, S., Benfield, T., Westh, H. & Danish Chlamydia Study, G. 2016. Risk of reproductive complications following chlamydia testing: a population-based retrospective cohort study in Denmark. *Lancet Infect Dis*, 16, 1057–64.

14. Johnson, N., Van Voorst, S., Sowter, M. C., Strandell, A. & Mol, B. W. 2010. Surgical treatment for tubal disease in women due to undergo in vitro fertilisation. *Cochrane Database Syst Rev*, Issue 1. Art. No.: CD002125. DOI: 10.1002/14651858.CD002125.pub3.

15. Strandell, A., Waldenstrom, U., Nilsson, L. & Hamberger, L. 1994. Hydrosalpinx reduces in-vitro fertilization/embryo transfer pregnancy rates. *Hum Reprod*, 9, 861–3.

16. Strandell, A. & Lindhard, A. 2002. Why does hydrosalpinx reduce fertility? The importance of hydrosalpinx fluid. *Hum Reprod*, 17, 1141–5.

17. Mukherjee, T., Copperman, A. B., Mccaffrey, C., Cook, C. A., Bustillo, M. & Obasaju, M. F. 1996. Hydrosalpinx fluid has embryotoxic effects on murine embryogenesis: a case for prophylactic salpingectomy. *Fertil Steril*, 66, 851–3.

18. Seli, E., Kayisli, U. A., Cakmak, H., Bukulmez, O., Bildirici, I., Guzeloglu-Kayisli, O. & Arici, A. 2005. Removal of hydrosalpinges increases endometrial leukaemia inhibitory factor (LIF) expression at the time of the implantation window. *Hum Reprod*, 20, 3012–7.

19. Zhong, Y., Li, J., Wu, H., Ying, Y., Liu, Y., Zhou, C., Xu, Y., Shen, X. & Qi, Q. 2012. Effect of surgical intervention on the expression of leukemia inhibitory factor and L-selectin ligand in the endometrium of hydrosalpinx patients during the implantation window. *Exp Ther Med*, 4, 1027–1031.

20. Du, H. & Taylor, H. S. 2016. The role of hox genes in female reproductive tract development, adult function, and fertility. *Cold Spring Harb Perspect Med*, 6, a023002.

21. El-Mazny, A., Ramadan, W., Kamel, A. & Gad-Allah, S. 2016. Effect of hydrosalpinx on uterine and ovarian hemodynamics in women with tubal factor infertility. *Eur J Obstet Gynecol Reprod Biol*, 199, 55–9.

22. Surana, A., Rastogi, V. & Nirwan, P. S. 2012. Association of the serum anti-chlamydial antibodies with tubal infertility. *J Clin Diagn Res*, 6, 1692–4.

23. Singh, S., Bhandari, S., Agarwal, P., Chittawar, P. & Thakur, R. 2016. Chlamydia antibody testing helps in identifying females with possible tubal factor infertility. *Int J Reprod Biomed (Yazd)*, 14, 187–92.

24. Demir, B., Bozdag, G., Sengul, O., Kahyaoglu, I., Mumusoglu, S. & Zengin, D. 2016. The impact of unilateral salpingectomy on antral follicle count and ovarian response in ICSI cycles: comparison of contralateral side. *Gynecol Endocrinol*, 1–4.

25. Qin, F., Du, D. F. & Li, X. L. 2016. The effect of salpingectomy on ovarian reserve and ovarian function. *Obstet Gynecol Surv*, 71, 369–76.

26. Singhal, V., Li, T. C. & Cooke, I. D. 1991. An analysis of factors influencing the outcome of 232 consecutive tubal microsurgery cases. *Br J Obstet Gynaecol*, 98, 628–36.

27. Winston, R. M. & Margara, R. A. 1991. Microsurgical salpingostomy is not an obsolete procedure. *Br J Obstet Gynaecol*, 98, 637–42.

28. Strandell, A., Lindhard, A. & Eckerlund, I. 2005. Cost–effectiveness analysis of salpingectomy prior to IVF, based on a randomized controlled trial. *Hum Reprod*, 20, 3284–92.

29. Legendre, G., Moulin, J., Vialard, J., Ziegler, D. D., Fanchin, R., Pouly, J. L., Watrelot, A., Belaisch Allart, J., Massin, N. & Fernandez, H. 2014. Proximal occlusion of hydrosalpinges by Essure((R)) before assisted reproduction techniques: a French survey. *Eur J Obstet Gynecol Reprod Biol*, 181, 300–4.

30. Ozgur, K., Bulut, H., Berkkanoglu, M., Coetzee, K. & Kaya, G. 2014. ICSI pregnancy outcomes following hysteroscopic placement of Essure devices for hydrosalpinx in laparoscopic contraindicated patients. *Reprod Biomed Online*, 29, 113–8.

31. Arora, P., Arora, R. S. & Cahill, D. 2014. Essure((R)) for management of hydrosalpinx prior to in vitro fertilisation – a systematic review and pooled analysis. *BJOG*, 121, 527–36.

32. Veersema, S., Mijatovic, V., Dreyer, K., Schouten, H., Schoot, D., Emanuel, M. H., Hompes, P. & Brolmann, H. 2014. Outcomes of pregnancies in women with hysteroscopically placed micro-inserts in situ. *J Minim Invasive Gynecol*, 21, 492–7.

33. Cohen, S. B., Bouaziz, J., Schiff, E., Simon, A., Nadjary, M., Goldenberg, M., Orvieto, R. & Revel, A. 2016. In vitro fertilization outcomes after placement of essure microinserts in patients with hydrosalpinges who previously failed in vitro fertilization treatment: a multicenter study. *J Minim Invasive Gynecol*, 23, 939–43.

34. Barbosa, M. W., Sotiriadis, A., Papatheodorou, S. I., Mijatovic, V., Nastri, C. O. & Martins, W. P. 2016. High miscarriage rate in women submitted to Essure for hydrosalpinx before embryo transfer: a systematic review and meta-analysis. *Ultrasound Obstet Gynecol*, 48, 556–65.

Chapter 13

Fertility and the Hypogonadal Male

Andrew A. Dwyer
Richard Quinton

1 Developmental Physiology of the Male Reproductive Axis

1.1 Embryology and Developmental Physiology

The appearance of Leydig cells within the testes of a 46XY fetus from 7–10 weeks gestation marks the onset of testosterone (T) secretion stimulated by placental gonadotrophin (hCG). T diverts development from female default towards external male phenotype. The testes then begin their hormonally induced descent, while Sertoli cell–derived anti-mullerian hormone (AMH) induces regression of internal female reproductive organs.

In the third trimester, a diffuse network of approximately 2,000 specialised neurons in the mediobasal hypothalamus begins secreting coordinated pulses of gonadotrophin-releasing hormone (GnRH). GnRH secretion is the central neuroendocrine regulator of reproduction, stimulating pituitary gonadotrophs to secrete luteinising- (LH) and follicle-stimulating hormones (FSH) (Figure 13.1). Gonadotrophins spur T secretion, causing penile growth and completion of testicular descent (1). GnRH-stimulated gonadotrophin secretion is critical for testicular development, T production and, in postnatal life, spermatogenesis (2).

Around 80% of GnRH neurons originate within the embryonic olfactory placode, migrating during the first trimester to the hypothalamic arcuate nucleus along terminal-vomeronasal nerve fibres, with the rest having a neural crest origin (3). Developmental disorders disrupting the GnRH neural network result in congenital hypogonadotrophic hypogonadism (CHH), a rare condition characterised by absent or partial puberty and infertility (4).

1.2 Significance of Minipuberty in Boys

The hypothalamic-pituitary-gonadal (HPG) axis remains active for 4–6 months postnatally, when LH, FSH and T concentrations approach adult levels (5). This period of 'minipuberty' represents a key proliferative window for testicular germ cells and immature Sertoli cells although spermatogenesis is not initiated because Sertoli cells do not express the androgen receptor until the age of five (6).

Minipuberty is characteristically absent in congenital GnRH deficiency and combined pituitary hormone deficiency (CPHD) (Box 13.1), creating a brief diagnostic window-of-opportunity shortly after birth. For neonates with cryptorchidism ± micropenis, a single serum sample taken 4–8 weeks postnatally can pinpoint CHH more accurately than dynamic tests performed in later childhood or adolescence (4).

1.3 Puberty and Spermatogenesis

The HPG axis is quiescent during childhood, although subtle testicular development continues. Pubertal-onset is marked by sleep-entrained GnRH pulses, with nocturnal low-frequency GnRH pulses initially favouring FSH secretion over LH. The resulting rises in serum gonadotrophin and T levels progressively extend to the waking hours, culminating in reproductive maturity. Normal spermatogenesis requires the coordinated actions of both FSH and endogenously secreted T on testicular germs cells and seminiferous tubules (Box 13.2).

Broadly, LH stimulates interstitial Leydig cells to mature and secrete T. The resulting local micromolar concentrations of T exert a paracrine action on the seminiferous tubules to induce and maintain spermatogenesis in concert with FSH. T is also secreted into the testicular vein, whence it circulates at nanomolar concentrations to exert classic endocrine actions on body tissues. FSH is essential for development of the tubular compartment where spermatogenesis occurs, stimulating the proliferation of immature Sertoli cells, which secrete inhibin B and AMH and determine final seminiferous tubule length. With seminiferous tubules accounting for approximately 90% of testicular volume (TV), TV is thus a key indicator of fertility potential (6).

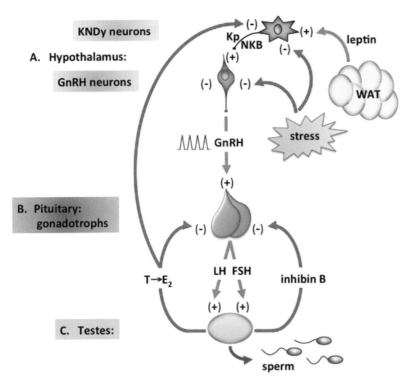

Fig. 13.1 Simplified schematic depicting the hypothalamic-pituitary-gonadal (HPG) axis and its modulation by homeostatic and environmental cues.
(A) Hypothalamic GnRH neurons (in blue) receive multiple inputs including stimulation from the KNDy neurons that receive permissive signals from leptin secreted by white adipose tissue. Both internal and external stressors in the form of glucocorticoids, prolactin, inflammatory cytokines and opiates can inhibit GnRH secretion, principally via inhibitory inputs to hypothalamic KNDy neurons.
(B) Pulsatile GnRH secretion into the hypophyseal portal circulation stimulates gonadotrophs in the anterior pituitary to release LH and FSH.
(C) The gonadotrophins circulate peripherally, stimulating the testes to produce hormones (T), regulatory peptides (inhibin B) and gametes (sperm). The HPG axis functions via feed-forward and feedback loops. T (particularly its aromatised form E_2) provides negative feedback on pituitary gonadotrophs and hypothalamic KNDy neurons. Inhibin B is a major regulator of FSH.
Stimulatory effects are depicted by (+) and green arrows and inhibitory effects by (-) and red arrows.
GnRH (gonadotrophin-releasing hormone); Kp (Kisspeptin); NKB (Neurokinin B); KNDy (Kp-NKB-dynorphin); WAT (white adipose tissue); LH (luteinising hormone); FSH (follicle stimulating hormone).

With the onset of puberty, rising intratesticular T ends the proliferative phase; Sertoli cells mature, sex cords lumenate to become tubules and spermatogenesis is initiated. Intratesticular T levels are around 30-times higher than serum concentrations, which is a paracrine requisite for spermatogenesis. Thus, FSH combined with hCG-induced T synthesis induces spermatogenesis in men with CHH, while FSH combined with exogenous T does not (7).

1.4 Disrupted GnRH Secretion/Action and Congenital Hypogonadotrophic Hypogonadism

Figure 13.1 illustrates physiological control of the adult male HPG axis, with the hypothalamus integrating internal-homeostatic and external-environmental signals to modulate secretion of GnRH and, consequently, gonadotrophin-mediated testicular function. The HPG axis is sexually dimorphic in three respects. First, the male axis lacks a sex steroid–mediated positive feedback pathway (via paraventricular kisspeptin neurons) on GnRH secretion. Second, obesity and corticosteroids both act to inhibit GnRH secretion, causing an HH-like biochemical picture, whereas in females they promote ovarian hyperandrogenism. Finally, the male axis appears more resistant to bioenergetic deficit that predisposes females to HH ('hypothalamic amenorrhoea').

Our understanding of these pathways has been greatly informed via clinical and genetic studies of patients with CHH, a rare disease affecting 1-in-

---

Box 13.1   Significance of absent minipuberty in CHH boys

- Healthy neonate males attain near adult levels of serum LH, FSH and T during minipuberty (4–8 weeks of life). Thus, male neonates exhibiting 'red flag' features prompting suspicion of CHH (*e.g.* cryptorchidism, micropenis, cleft lip/palate, hearing loss, absent erections on nappy-change, and/or family history of CHH) can be diagnosed by demonstrating low levels of LH, FSH and T.
- Minipuberty is critical for testicular development and descent, and testicular maldescent can have far reaching negative consequences on future fertility potential. The high prevalence of cryptorchidism exhibited by CHH boys underscores the crucial role of minipuberty in the final stages of testicular descent and in anchoring the testes securely within the scrotum. Sexual (penile) development occurs much earlier in fetal development; thus, hypospadias is not seen in CHH.
- Suppression of minipuberty in primates has been shown to impair subsequent testicular maturation at puberty.
- Even with gonadotrophin replacement or GnRH pump therapy, men with severe GnRH deficiency (lacking minipuberty) typically do not achieve normal testicular volumes and semen quality.

Box 13.2   Is testosterone good or bad for spermatogenesis?

- Whilst T secretion is essential for spermatogenesis, exogenous T treatment is noted as a cause of low sperm count in medical textbooks, websites and product inserts, which can cause confusion.
- Gonadotrophins are needed for spermatogenesis (FSH as well as LH to stimulate T secretion by the Leydig cells). T exerts central negative feedback, so when exogenous T treatment is started, endogenous LH and FSH are suppressed and, consequently, so is sperm production.
- This adverse effect only arises with T (or anabolic steroid) use under the following circumstances:
- In men who were eugonadal at baseline with intact spermatogenesis, *e.g.*
  - athletes or body-builders wishing to enhance their performance and/or appearance
  - normal men misdiagnosed with hypogonadism, *e.g.* following one-off non-fasting/post-prandial low serum T level, or as a result of a screening questionnaire without biochemical confirmation.
  - In hypogonadal men with partial gonadotrophin deficiency, *e.g.* pituitary tumour.
- In the above circumstances, a rise in serum T with exogenous therapy causes inhibition of pituitary gonadotrophin secretion and, consequently, a paradoxical *fall* in intratesticular T levels with consequent loss of (any residual) spermatogenesis.

4,000 men (4). The underlying gene defects comprise two broad clusters, namely (a) neuroendocrine regulation of GnRH secretion (resulting in a purely 'reproductive' phenotype) and (b) defective embryonic GnRH neuron migration/fate-specification, often associated with non-reproductive defects such as the absent sense of smell (anosmia) that defines Kallmann syndrome (KS) (8). HH is the only form of male infertility that is directly treatable with endocrine replacement therapy, without obligate use of assisted reproduction techniques (ART).

2 Differential Diagnosis, Classification and Fertility Prognosis of Male Hypogonadism

Male hypogonadism is typically associated with azoospermic infertility. The key distinction is between primary (hyp*er*gonadotrophic hypogonadism / primary testicular insufficiency) and secondary (hyp*o*gonadotrophic / central) hypogonadism (HH). (Box 13.3).

2.1 Hypergonadotrophic Hypogonadism

This is diagnosed biochemically with elevated gonadotrophins (LH and FSH) in the setting of low serum T levels and is progressive, irreversible and usually unresponsive to pharmacologic (hormonal) fertility treatment. Sperm-retrieval can be considered if identified early (*e.g.* adolescents with Klinefelter syndrome) (9) and prospective transwomen should consider sperm cryopreservation.

2.2 Hypogonadotrophic Hypogonadism (HH)

Beware of patients labelled as 'secondary hypogonadism' or 'HH' with inadequate characterisation; an identical biochemical profile (low T with low-normal, gonadotrophins) is also observed in eugonadal men

Box 13.3 Classification of male hypogonadism

- **Primary testicular insufficiency** = *Hyper*gonadotrophic hypogonadism = Intrinsic dysfunction of testis

    ↑ LH, ↑↑ FSH levels.

    Apart from acute castration, it is typically progressive with a post-pubertal onset.

    Spermatogenesis is typically lost before onset of overt hypogonadism/decline in T secretion.

    Common causes: Klinefelter syndrome (47XXY), age-related, post-orchitis, external beam radiation therapy, chemotherapy with alkylating agents and, increasingly, castration for gender reassignment.

    Fertility treatment: sperm/tissue storage, micro-testicular sperm extraction (mTESE) with intracytoplasmic sperm injection (ICSI), donor sperm.

- **Secondary / Central**: *Hypo*gonadotrophic hypogonadism = Deficient gonadotrophin stimulation

    ↓ LH and FSH levels, or 'inappropriately normal' or low serum T.

    Onset: Congenital forms present as pubertal failure; acquired forms (post-puberty) have variable presentations.

    Fertility: potentially restorable with gonadotrophin replacement (or pulsatile GnRH via pump unless there is primary hypopituitarism).

Box 13.4 Important causes and rule-outs of HH

I. Apparent / artefactual HH

- Physiological suppression of gonadotrophic axis due to chronic illness.
- Inappropriate timing of measurement: afternoon clinic, or postprandial venepuncture.
- Low level of sex hormone binding globulin (SHBG), such that calculated free testosterone men is normal range even with low total testosterone.
- Inaccurate measurement: low-quality T immunoassay.

II. Organic diseases causing HH

- Structural lesions of hypothamalus or pituitary gland.
- Gonadotroph failure secondary to iron overload, *e.g.* genetic haemochromatosis.
- GI malabsorption, *eg.* Coeliac disease, inflammatory bowel disease.

III. Functional / Reversible causes of HH

- HH secondary to opiate use/ abuse.
- HH secondary to post-anabolic steroid abuse
- HH secondary to hyperprolactinaemia (tumour- or drug-induced).
- Stress-induced HH related to high stress / low body mass index (BMI) / excessive exercise / and/or underlying eating disorder.
- HH secondary glucocorticoid excess: exogenous or endogenous.

under certain conditions (Box 13.3). The diagnosis of HH should be based on fasting venepuncture 8–10 am in an otherwise healthy (no systemic diseases), well-rested man (not during phase of night shift-work) (10) – also ideal for screening-out broader hypopituitarism and metabolic syndrome. In CHH, pituitary function is otherwise normal and other relevant conditions are excluded (4) (Box 13.4).

Further to correct interpretation of biochemistry, clinical features may frame the diagnosis within a defined medical syndrome, *e.g.* Kallmann's (CHH + anosmia); adult-onset HH with structural pituitary disease (*e.g.* visual field disturbance); functional/reversible HH secondary to opiate intake, or antipsychotic-induced hyperprolactinaemia (Box 13.4).

For a man started inappropriately on T following incorrect diagnosis of hypogonadism (*e.g.* as a result of 'screening questionnaire', afternoon non-fasted venepuncture, or in the context of chronic illness, stopping T will eventually permit reversion to previous fertility. Although clinical trial data are lacking, emerging data suggest possible benefits of oestrogen-antagonists (*e.g.* clomiphene citrate) and aromatase inhibitors (*e.g.* anastrazole) in improving sperm quality by boosting gonadotrophin secretion in men with functional HH, *e.g.* due to opiates, obesity or other chronic disease process. Organic HH is treatable with exogenous gonadotrophin therapy, although extended treatment periods (two years or longer) may be required for men with congenital disease (CHH). Whereas females achieve their lifetime supply of oocytes *in utero*, males require three distinct phases of testicular maturation to develop and sustain spermatogenesis, comprising the effects of placental hCG *in utero*, and of pituitary gonadotrophins during perinatal minipuberty and adolescent puberty.

2.3 CHH: Reproductive Phenotype, Genetic Basis and Relationship to Cryptorchidism

CHH is clinically and genetically heterogeneous and the degree of GnRH deficiency influences the clinical presentation. Males typically present in adolescence or early adulthood with impairment of puberty (4) and undeveloped testes, but the most severe cases exhibit neonatal cryptorchidism ± micropenis, or absent pubertal development (TV $\leq$ 4 mL) in adolescence. Around one-third have partial GnRH deficiency, evidenced by some spontaneous testicular development (TV > 4 mL) (4).

Most cases are sporadic, in keeping with impairment of fertility, although a third display familial inheritance, comprising autosomal dominant, autosomal recessive, X-linked recessive and oligogenic forms (8). Some 30 loci have been identified to date, with mutations acting alone or in synergy, but still only accounting for around 50% of cases. For the majority of CHH-associated genes, full disease penetrance probably occurs only with homozygous, hemizygous or compound heterozygous mutations (4). Clinical phenotypes may sign-post molecular defects: mirror movements (synkinesia) or renal agenesis suggest *KAL1*; clefting and skeletal defects, including dental agenesis, suggest *FGFR1, FGF8* or the FGF8 synexpression group, while deafness suggests *CHD7, IL17RD* or *SOX10* mutations. Notably, men with *KAL1* mutations (approximately 10% of male KS) respond least well to fertility treatment, even accounting for their higher prevalence of cryptorchidism (4).

Sons fathered by *KAL1* males are unaffected and daughters are carriers, but given the sometimes complex genetic architecture of CHH the potential for transmission to offspring is usually less predictable. Men usually welcome the opportunity to have a family despite the risk of transmission, being confident they could ensure their child was diagnosed promptly and treated at an appropriate age, but genetic counselling should be offered to couples pursuing fertility treatment (4).

Numerous studies have highlighted the high prevalence of cryptorchidism among CHH men with TV $\leq$ 4 mL (*i.e.* severe GnRH deficiency) (11). Cryptorchidism is a key adverse prognostic factor for fertility in CHH, especially if bilateral, but is not *per se* diagnostic of CHH as it affects 2–5% of full-term neonates and resolves spontaneously in approximately 75%, typically within the first six months of life (12, 13). However,

when testes remain undescended by one year, the impact on germ cell survival and long-term fertility can be dramatic, particularly with bilateral disease and higher-lying testes. Men with a history of bilateral cryptorchidism have lower serum inhibin B levels, smaller TV, lower sperm counts (14) and are six times more likely to be infertile compared to men with unilateral disease or normally descended testes (15).

Outcomes in boys who undergo orchidopexy later strongly favour earlier intervention and currently recommendations for timing is between 6 and 12 months of age (12, 13). However, for CHH infants lacking mini-puberty, combined gonadotrophin treatment to augment TV prior to orchidepexy would likely render surgery technically easier, or possibly even unnecessary, apart from having potential benefits on testicular and penile maturation (16).

3 Spermatogenesis Induction Protocols in Hypogonadotrophic Hypogonadism

HH men are typically azoospermic, but fall broadly into three prognostic categories in respect of predicted response to therapy. At the mildest end of the spectrum are men with adult-onset HH (*e.g.* secondary to pituitary adenoma), with the most unfavourable being those with severe CHH (or CPHD) and history of bilateral cryptorchidism. In between are the approximately one-third of CHH men with some spontaneous partial puberty at presentation (TV > 4 mL) (17).

Approaches to stimulate gonadal development and fertility include pulsatile GnRH therapy or subcutaneous gonadotrophins injections (4, 11). Although both approaches are equally effective in inducing spermatogenesis in the majority of CHH men (18), gonadotrophins are more readily available due to their obligate use in female superovulation protocols for ART and, importantly, are also effective in primary pituitary disease.

3.1 Predictors of Success for Fertility-Inducing Treatment in Men with CHH

Careful assessment of TV is key to estimating the pretreatment probability of successful spermatogenesis and of subsequent pregnancy (See Box 13.5) (4, 11, 17, 19). CHH men with absent pubertal development (baseline TV $\leq$ 4 mL) have impaired proliferation of immature Sertoli cells and germ cells – reflected

---

Box 13.5 Predicting the success of fertility treatments in HH

Positive predictors

- HH acquired post-pubertally (intact minipuberty)
- TV > 4mL, consistent with partial spontaneous puberty
- No history of testicular maldescent
- baseline serum inhibin B > 60 pg/mL
- Good spermatogenetic response in prior cycles

Negative predictors

- CHH, (absent minipuberty)
- TV ≤ 4mL, consistent with absent puberty
- History of bilateral cryptorchidism
    - thermal and/or surgical trauma-effects?
    - more severe neuroendocrine defect?
- Baseline serum inhibin B < 60 pg/mL
- *KAL1* mutation (X-linked Kallmann Syndrome)

---

biochemically in low serum inhibin B levels – and thus consistently poorer fertility outcomes (17). Optimal treatment for CHH during adolescence remains to be defined (*i.e.* gonadotrophins versus T) and prospective studies are needed, but exogenous androgen exposure is no longer believed to reduce the subsequent likelihood of attaining sperm thresholds for conception (18). However, high intratesticular T levels achieved during hCG-monotherapy can induce terminal differentiation of limited pre-proliferative Sertoli and germ cell populations.

3.2 Pulsatile GnRH Therapy

Although ineffective in pituitary disease, GnRH replacement is a logical approach for CHH men with GnRH deficiency. However, as continuous GnRH infusion causes pituitary de-sensitisation and suppression of gonadotrophin secretion (2), it must be administered as subcutaneous pulses every two hours via programmable micro-infusion device. Pulsatile GnRH successfully induces puberty and fertility, with approximately 75% of men developing spermatogenesis on long-term treatment (18). For pubertal induction, low-dose pulses are initiated with progressive upward titration, whereas studies targeting spermatogenesis as primary objective aimed to rapidly achieve gonadotrophin-stimulated serum T levels within the adult male range. Despite comparable outcomes to combined gonadotrophin therapy (18), GnRH use is limited in most countries by drug cost and availability, cost of micro-infusion device and ever-fewer clinicians experienced with its use.

3.3 Human Chorionic Gonadotrophin (hCG) Monotherapy

Serving as a long-acting LH-analogue, hCG given by subcutaneous self-injection 2–3 times per week,

---

Box 13.6 When to consider hCG monotherapy

Only consider hCG monotherapy in:

- Men with adult-onset HH (in whom other pituitary hormone replacement therapy, L-Thyroxine, hydrocortisone, *etc.* should first be optimised).
- CHH men without a history of cryptorchidism and baseline TV > 4 mL, reflecting some degree of endogenous gonadotrophin-induced testicular development.
- CHH men with the so-called fertile eunuch syndrome, characterised by enfeebled GnRH secretion that is sufficient to stimulate enough LH and FSH release to induce seminiferous tubule development, yet insufficient to stimulate serum T at levels needed for full virilisation. These men exhibit low-level spermatogenesis ('fertile') and, occasionally, may even achieve fertility without hCG.

---

typically gives an excellent serum T pharmacokinetic profile (11) Monotherapy with hCG is first-line therapy for spermatogenesis-induction in men with HH acquired post-puberty and typically induces testicular development, spermatogenesis and fertility within 3–9 months. If this is not achieved, remains suboptimal or conception has not occurred, FSH should be added to the regimen (Box 13.6).

However, hCG mono-therapy is only viable for CHH men at the mildest end of the spectrum (*i.e.* with partial to near-full testicular development). For men with TV ≤ 4 mL, less than half will develop any sperm in their ejaculate even with very prolonged treatment (11); 'normalisation' of semen quality by WHO criteria is almost never achieved (albeit that suboptimal sperm counts do not necessarily preclude fertility in CHH) (20).

Box 13.7   Take-home messages

- The neonatal minipuberty likely plays a key role in male fertility; its absence in CHH provides a unique diagnostic window-of-opportunity in postnatal life and also highlights a potential role for gonadotrophin therapy in improving outcomes for patients with testicular maldescent in childhood.
- Inform CHH men that fertility is possible; consider appropriate referrals to specialised centres while their partners are still young and refer for genetic counselling.
- Approximately 75–80% of CHH men can achieve spermatogenesis and low sperm counts do not preclude fertility/conception.
- Initial TV ≤ 4 mL, history of cryptorchidism, low inhibin B levels (<60 pg/mL) and *KAL1* gene mutations are key negative predictors of success in spermatogenesis induction.
- For men with CHH and TV ≤ 4 mL (with or without cryptorchidism) consider sequential gonadotrophin treatment with a two-month FSH pretreatment prior to starting FSH + hCG (or pulsatile GnRH) as this may enhance fertility outcome in these men.
- For men with CHH who have absent puberty there is no rationale for initiating hCG-only treatment; they require combined FSH + hCG therapy, typically lasting 18–24 months (or longer) to achieve fertility.
- During combined gonadotrophin therapy, adjust FSH dose to maintain serum levels 4–8 IU/L and titrate hCG dose based on trough levels to achieve normal adult serum T and E_2 levels; in some cases more than two years of combined treatment is necessary.
- ART can be helpful in a man with severely compromised sperm count and/or quality, or where there is an issue with his partner's fertility, including advancing age.
- Discuss sperm banking (cryopreservation) for long-term storage with patients who have developed sperm in their ejaculate.

3.4 Combined Gonadotrophin Therapy

Combined gonadotrophin therapy (hCG + FSH) is the mainstay of spermatogenesis induction in CHH men. FSH – recombinant (rFSH), highly purified urinary gonadotrophins (hMG) or long-acting analogue (*e.g.* cofollitropin-alpha) – is also given by subcutaneous self-injection; hMG also contains LH, but too little for significant Leydig cell stimulation (11).

The effectiveness of hCG + FSH at inducing fertility in CHH emerged in the mid-1980s. Over the next 30 years, a succession of larger clinical series reported outcomes – although subjects and drug-dosing schedules were highly variable. Median time to develop sperm in the ejaculate ranges from 9 to 12 months but men with prepubertal testes (i.e., TV ≤ 4 mL) are half as likely to develop sperm in the ejaculate compared to those men with larger testicular volume (summarised in (11). This is partly due to the fact that men with TV ≤ 4 mL were much more likely to have had cryptorchidism and maldescended testes restrict fertility outcomes. So, these men typically require longer treatment periods to achieve spermatogenesis – if at all.

Detailed analysis of a large cohort of 75 HH men (51 with CHH) receiving a standardised treatment regimen found that half the treatment programmes (58/116) resulted in pregnancy, of which only a few (7/58, 12%) required *in vitro* fertilisation (IVF) (19). Further, the median time to conception was 28 months, with median 7 months to developing sperm in the ejaculate. Interestingly, subgroup analysis of men who received multiple treatment programmes revealed that spermatogenesis was achieved two to three-fold faster in later programmes compared to the initial one. TV ≤ 4 mL is a key negative predictor as demonstrated in several studies using structured, combined gonadotrophin treatment regimens (summarised in (11)). Overall, 84% of participants developed sperm and 69% achieved a concentration ≥1.5 x 10^6/mL – compatible with spontaneous impregnation in CHH men, yet well below WHO criteria of normality (21). In 2014, a meta-analysis reported that combined gonadotrophin therapy induced spermatogenesis in 75% (CI: 69–81) of men with CHH, achieving a mean sperm concentration 5.9 x 10^6/mL (CI: 4.7–7.1), with better outcomes among men with baseline TV > 4 mL (18).

3.5 Implications of Historical Fixed-Dose 'hCG-first' Gonadotrophin Therapy Regimes

Despite exclud on of CHH men with a history of cryptorchidism, only three-quarters developed sperm with combined gonadotrophin regimes; the vast majority achieving maximal TV and sperm in the ejaculate within 12–18 months of treatment initiation

(4, 11). Four potential explanations are postulated for this 25% failure rate (even higher if cryptorchid men are included). First, absent minipuberty and the lack of critical hormonal stimulus during this window might be an insurmountable obstacle to fertility for some. Second, certain men might require an even longer period of continuous therapy to develop sperm. Third, these studies used fixed-dose FSH regimes (225–525 IU/week administered in 3–7 divided doses) rather than targeting a physiological serum FSH range (*e.g.* 4–8 IU/L). Finally, the traditional approach of starting with hCG and then adding FSH only after several weeks or months may be counterproductive.

The standard practice of initiating hCG-monotherapy for CHH men wanting fertility ironically entered into clinical practice with the introduction of highly purified hMG, recombinant-FSH (rFSH) and FSH-analogue molecules. In an effort to satisfy regulatory bodies that spermatogenesis was contingent upon introduction of the investigational FSH product, HH men who developed sperm during 3–6 months of hCG monotherapy were excluded from the active treatment phase. Notably, men who failed to normalise serum T levels on hCG were also typically excluded, with a view to eliminating men with underlying primary testicular defect who might confound the ultimate evaluation of drug effectiveness.

It can be difficult to normalise serum T levels with hCG-monotherapy in CHH men with TV $\leq$ 4mL, but this becomes much easier once FSH is added, possibly reflecting synergistic actions on Leydig cells. In 1998, Mark Vandeweghe presciently questioned the practice of deferring FSH therapy until after several months of hCG monotherapy, and advocated starting hCG and FSH simultaneously. Recently, data have raised the possibility that an initial phase of hCG monotherapy in men with severe CHH might actually compromise outcomes of subsequent combined hCG + FSH (or pulsatile GnRH).

3.6 FSH-First: A Sequential Approach to Spermatogenesis Induction in CHH

Men with the most severe GnRH deficiency (TV $\leq$ 4 mL) have the poorest outcomes for fertility-inducing treatment, with only about 68% (CI: 58–77) developing sperm on combined treatment (18). They also commonly have a history of bilateral cryptorchidism giving even worse outcomes. Given that 90% of TV is

determined by the seminiferous tubules, factors promoting tubule development (*i.e.* proliferation of immature Sertoli and germ cells) are critical for optimising spermatogenic capacity (22, 23). Therefore, a plausible approach to improve fertility in severely affected CHH men lies in recapitulating the gonadotrophin profile of early puberty by first providing unopposed FSH treatment, with the aim of proliferating immature Sertoli and germ cells prior to T-induced maturation (23).

Raivio first demonstrated the beneficial effects of rFSH on serum inhibin B and TV in three prepubertal HH boys (KS, CPHD and craniopharyngioma), reflecting FSH-induced Sertoli cell proliferation (24). In 2007, he reported the long-term follow-up of 14 prepubertal boys with diverse causes of gonadotrophin deficiency (including four CHH; two with history of cryptorchidism), all of whom had received variable rFSH regimens prior to pubertal-induction with hCG (25). Importantly, 3 of 4 with CHH developed sperm, suggesting that males with the most severe GnRH deficiency (TV $\leq$ 4 mL, cryptorchidism $\pm$ microphallus) might benefit from FSH-priming prior to hCG-induced maturation.

In 2013, an open-label randomised trial in CHH men with TV $\leq$ 4mL compared standard treatment (24 months pulsatile GnRH; n = 6) versus standard treatment *preceded* by four months of rFSH treatment (n = 7) (23). Men with a history of cryptorchidism or prior gonadotrophin therapy were excluded. During the four-month rFSH pretreatment phase, serum inhibin B levels normalised and TV (ascertained by ultrasound) doubled, whilst histologic studies revealed proliferation of Sertoli cells and spermatogonia, along with key cytoskeletal rearrangements. Crucially, 7/7 men receiving rFSH pretreatment developed sperm in their ejaculate compared to 4/6 in the GnRH-only group, with the pretreated group also trending towards higher maximal sperm counts.

Albeit a small sample, this sequential approach using pretreatment with FSH was 100% successful in inducing testicular growth and spermatogenesis in men with severe CHH and prepubertal testes, albeit underpowered for statistical significance. A larger prospective multicentre study, with approximately 28 subjects per treatment arm, is required – ideally also recruiting CHH men with a history of cryptorchidism, who are least responsive to gonadotrophin therapy.

4 Patient Monitoring during Spermatogenesis Induction

Careful clinical and biochemical monitoring and expert opinion from clinicians experienced in these specific fertility induction protocols are essential. Regular assessment of TV using a Prader orchidometer is important to evaluate growth, although as clinicians tend to slightly overestimate TV using this technique, calculated TV using sonography in three planes is more reliable and objective (26).

Patients should be informed of potential adverse effects. Gynaecomastia is seen in up to one-third of patients as a result of excess hCG-induced E_2-secretion (4, 11), with raised haematocrit being next most common. Both are avoidable by lowering the hCG dose; if necessary accepting slightly sub-normal serum T levels and, potentially, also lower patient-reported energy levels or libido. The half-life of hCG is approximately 36 hours so trough T and E_2 levels obtained prior to the subsequent injection are most informative.

Patients should be given proper instruction and be able to demonstrate aseptic self-injection technique, with therapeutic adherence assessed at each visit. Spermatogenesis can occur even in the setting of modest TV, so seminal fluid analysis should be performed (following 2–3 days of abstinence) once TV 5–8 mL is attained and repeated every 2–3 months thereafter.

4.1 hCG Dose Titration

Depending on locally available formulations, a typical hCG starting dose is around 3–5,000 IU per week, divided into at least two injections to ensure stable serum T levels. The dose may need adjusting to achieve the correct balance of serum T, haemoglobin, haematocrit and E_2, and to minimise risks of T-induced erythrocytosis or E_2-induced gynaecomastia. Serum levels should be checked every 4–6 weeks, with dose adjustments made until steady-state has been achieved. As the testes grow, it may be possible to slowly titrate-down the hCG dose while maintaining serum T levels. Steady-state weekly hCG doses range typically from 1,000 to 10,000 IU per week. Failure to achieve a serum T response to hCG treatment may result from poor adherence (27), or rarely, development of antibodies (4).

4.2 FSH (hMG/rFSH) Dose Titration

Typically FSH (hMG or rFSH) is given as a subcutaneous self-injection (75–150 IU) every other day (or three times per week) and adjusted to achieve serum FSH levels in the range of 4–8 IU/L. It may initially also be helpful to monitor serum inhibin B levels to gauge the Sertoli cells response to exogenous FSH. Given that CHH men have a limited Sertoli cell population and low intratesticular T levels, it is expected that baseline levels of inhibin B are low, so these levels could be used as a proxy for the proliferation of immature Sertoli cells during FSH treatment (4, 11, 23). In CHH men with severe GnRH deficiency, inhibin B levels typically plateau after two months of rFSH treatment (75 IU daily), suggesting this to be a sufficiently long pretreatment period with rFSH alone (23). Sharing laboratory results (i.e. increasing inhibin B levels) with patients can aid adherence early in treatment when subtle changes in TV may not yet be evident to them.

While no clear protocol has been established for men with a history of cryptorchidism, FSH pretreatment could be prolonged until inhibin B levels have plateaued. However, to avoid patients being hypogonadal for extended periods of time, it is plausible that exogenous T such as a transdermal gel – that would not raise intratesticular T levels – could be given to limit unfavourable symptoms of hypogonadism prior to the introduction of hCG.

4.3 Relationship between Testicular Volume and Spermatogenesis in CHH

Although seminal fluid analysis is the key outcome measure and should be repeated every 2–3 months, assessment of TV is a simple and key clinical indicator of response (28). Typically, TV of 8–10 mL is indicative of spermatogenesis, but men receiving fertility-inducing treatment who attain only limited testicular growth (*e.g.* TV 4–5mL) may still have sperm in their ejaculate (11). Indeed, CHH men with TV as small as 3 mL may have active spermatogenesis and, in rare cases, have been able to conceive naturally (23). The vast majority of CHH men will not achieve normal sperm counts as defined by the World Health Organization (i.e. >15 million/mL) (21), yet low sperm counts do not preclude fertility (20). Indeed, median sperm counts for conception range from 3 to 8 million/mL and median time to reach sperm is reported as 5 months (29). So, seminal fluid analysis can commence within a few months of starting treatment. However, those patients with smaller testes or who have a history of cryptorchidism can take 12–24 months to ejaculate sperm – even longer for men with a history of bilateral cryptorchidism (11, 30). Thus, when discussing fertility planning with patients, couples should be well-informed of the potential treatment period necessary to develop fertility (up to 24 months or longer), so that initiation of treatment can be planned accordingly (4, 11).

4.4 Role of Assisted Reproductive Technology (ART) in HH Men

Intracytoplasmic sperm injection (ICSI) was first used in CHH as an approach to shorten treatment duration (31) and it should be considered at an early stage where there is suspected dual-factor infertility or with an older female partner. However, in most cases, the rational approach is to defer ART until maximal testicular development has been achieved, evidenced by plateau in TV and sperm quality. The success rates of ICSI are high in HH, with fertilisation rates of 50–60% and pregnancy rates of ~30% per cycle (reviewed in (11)). If the ejaculate is consistently devoid of sperm then micro-testicular sperm extraction (TESE) may be effective. Reassuringly, detailed assessment of sperm quality in a group of CHH men undergoing combined gonadotrophin treatment revealed that CHH *per se* does not seem to impair DNA integrity, or increase the risk of chromosomal aberrations.

4.5 Securing the Benefits of Successful Spermatogenesis Induction

Treatment is typically continued after conception and into the second trimester, due to the possibility of early miscarriage. If the couple desires to conceive again quickly, hCG alone can be continued to maintain spermatogenesis, though sperm counts and TV tend to progressively diminish over time (32).

Although prior gonadotrophin treatment results in a two to three-fold shorter time to the appearance of first sperm on subsequent treatment cycles (29), the success of subsequent programmes cannot be guaranteed. Further in some countries (*e.g.* United Kingdom), entitlement to state-funded fertility treatments ceases with the birth of a child. Intrauterine insemination (IUI) with good-quality sperm is considerably cheaper than either ICSI or IVF. Even when sperm is of insufficient quality for IUI, IVF may still be more time- and cost-effective than restarting gonadotrophin therapy. Therefore, we encourage sperm cryopreservation prior to reverting back to T replacement.

5 Summary

Men with CHH have a hormonally treatable form of infertility. Existing data show that approximately 75–80% of these men are able to develop sperm in the ejaculate with appropriate combined gonadotrophin treatment, or GnRH pump. The effects of gonadotrophin therapy (*e.g.* testicular growth) may also ameliorate some of the psychosocial aspects of CHH and improve some health-related quality of life domains (33). This is not insignificant as many men struggle with psychosexual issues (34), increased depressive symptoms and impaired quality of life (27).

CHH covers a spectrum of GnRH deficiency and key factors affecting fertility outcomes include pre-treatment TV and whether or not there is a history of cryptorchidism. Men with some degree of spontaneous pubertal development and larger TV are at the milder end of the disease spectrum. These men are good responders and typically develop sperm within six months of starting treatment. In contrast, the most severe cases (*i.e.* TV $\leq$ 4 mL and/or history of bilateral cryptorchidism) have the poorest outcomes and should not be initiated on hCG-monotherapy. Although sequential protocols with FSH pretreatment offer better prospects for these men, a large multi-centre study is required to confirm the superiority of this novel approach.

Background Reading

Hamda A & Bouloux P-MG. 2013 Primary hypogonadism. In Oxford Endocrinology Library: *Testosterone Deficiency in Men*, TH Jones, Ed. Oxford University Press [ISBN 978-0-19-965167-2]; chapter 5: pp 35–44.

Balasubramanian R & Quinton R. 2013 Secondary hypogonadism. In Oxford Endocrinology Library: *Testosterone Deficiency in Men*, TH Jones, Ed. Oxford University Press [ISBN 978-0-19-965167-2]; chapter 5: pp 45–56.

Jones TH & Quinton R. 2013 Puberty & fertility. In Oxford Endocrinology Library: *Testosterone Deficiency in Men*, TH Jones, Ed. Oxford University Press [ISBN 978-0-19-965167-2]; chapter 5: pp 83–8.

Mitchell AL, Dwyer AA, Pitteloud N & Quinton R. Genetic basis and variable phenotypic expression of Kallmann syndrome: towards a unifying theory. *Trends in Endocrinology and Metabolism.* 2011; **22**: 249–58.

Anwalt BD. Approach to male infertility and induction of spermatogenesis. *Journal of Clinical Endocrinology and Metabolism.* 2013; 98: 3532–42.

Boehm U, Bouloux P-MG, Dattani M, *et al.* Expert consensus document: European consensus statement on congenital hypogonadotropic hypogonadism – pathogenesis, diagnosis and treatment. *Nature Reviews Endocrinology.* 2015; **11**: 547–64.

Dwyer AA, Raivio T & Pitteloud N. Gonadotrophin replacement for induction of fertility in hypogonadal men. *Best Practice & Research: Clinical Endocrinology & Metabolism.* 2015; 29: 91–103.

References

1. Hutson JM, Southwell BR, Li R, Lie G, Ismail K, Harisis G, et al. The regulation of testicular descent and the effects of cryptorchidism. *Endocrine Reviews.* 2013;34(5):725–52.

2. Belchetz PE, Plant TM, Nakai Y, Keogh EJ, Knobil E. Hypophysial responses to continuous and intermittent delivery of hypopthalamic gonadotropin-releasing hormone. *Science.* 1978;202(4368):631–3.

3. Casoni F, Malone SA, Belle M, Luzzati F, Collier F, Allet C, et al. Development of the neurons controlling fertility in humans: new insights from 3D imaging and transparent fetal brains. *Development.* 2016;143(21): 3969–81.

4. Boehm U, Bouloux PM, Dattani MT, de Roux N, Dode C, Dunkel L, et al. Expert consensus document: European Consensus Statement on congenital hypogonadotropic hypogonadism – pathogenesis, diagnosis and treatment. *Nature Reviews Endocrinology.* 2015;11(9):547–64.

5. Kuiri-Hanninen T, Sankilampi U, Dunkel L. Activation of the hypothalamic-pituitary-gonadal axis in infancy: minipuberty. *Hormone Research in Paediatrics.* 2014;82(2):73–80.

6. Rey RA, Musse M, Venara M, Chemes HE. Ontogeny of the androgen receptor expression in the fetal and postnatal testis: its relevance on Sertoli cell maturation and the onset of adult spermatogenesis. *Microscopy Research and Technique.* 2009;72 (11):787–95.

7. Schaison G, Young J, Pholsena M, Nahoul K, Couzinet B. Failure of combined follicle-stimulating hormone-testosterone administration to initiate and/or maintain spermatogenesis in men with hypogonadotropic hypogonadism. *The Journal of Clinical Endocrinology and Metabolism.* 1993;77(6):1545–9.

8. Mitchell AL, Dwyer A, Pitteloud N, Quinton R. Genetic basis and variable phenotypic expression of Kallmann syndrome: towards a unifying theory. *Trends in Endocrinology and Metabolism: TEM.* 2011;22(7):249–58.

9. Aksglaede L, Juul A. Testicular function and fertility in men with Klinefelter syndrome: a review. *European Journal of Endocrinology / European Federation of Endocrine Societies.* 2013;168(4):R67–76.

10. Bhasin S, Cunningham GR, Hayes FJ, Matsumoto AM, Snyder PJ, Swerdloff RS, et al. Testosterone therapy in men with androgen deficiency syndromes: an Endocrine Society clinical practice guideline. *The Journal of Clinical Endocrinology and Metabolism.* 2010;95(6):2536–59.

11. Dwyer AA, Raivio T, Pitteloud N. Gonadotrophin replacement for induction of fertility in hypogonadal men. *Best Practice & Research: Clinical Endocrinology & Metabolism.* 2015;29(1):91–103.

12. Chan E, Wayne C, Nasr A, Resource FfCAoPSE-B. Ideal timing of orchiopexy: a systematic review. *Pediatric Surgery International.* 2014;30(1):87–97.

13. Ritzen EM, Bergh A, Bjerknes R, Christiansen P, Cortes D, Haugen SE, et al. Nordic consensus on treatment of undescended testes. *Acta Paediatrica.* 2007;96(5): 638–43.

14. Trsinar B, Muravec UR. Fertility potential after unilateral and bilateral orchidopexy for cryptorchidism. *World Journal of Urology.* 2009;27(4):513–9.

15. Lee PA, O'Leary LA, Songer NJ, Coughlin MT, Bellinger MF, LaPorte RE. Paternity after bilateral cryptorchidism. A controlled study. *Archives of Pediatrics and Adolescent Medicine.* 1997;151(3):260–3.

16. Bouvattier C, Maione L, Bouligand J, Dode C, Guiochon-Mantel A, Young J. Neonatal gonadotropin therapy in male congenital hypogonadotropic hypogonadism. *Nature Reviews Endocrinology.* 2012;8(3):172–82.

17. Pitteloud N, Hayes FJ, Dwyer A, Boepple PA, Lee H, Crowley WF, Jr. Predictors of outcome of long-term GnRH therapy in men with idiopathic hypogonadotropic hypogonadism. *The Journal of Clinical Endocrinology and Metabolism.* 2002;87(9):4128–36.

18. Rastrelli G, Corona G, Mannucci E, Maggi M. Factors affecting spermatogenesis upon gonadotropin-replacement therapy: a meta-analytic study. *Andrology.* 2014;2(6):794–808.

19. Liu PY, Baker HW, Jayadev V, Zacharin M, Conway AJ, Handelsman DJ. Induction of spermatogenesis and fertility during gonadotropin treatment of gonadotropin-deficient infertile

men: predictors of fertility outcome. *The Journal of Clinical Endocrinology and Metabolism.* 2009;94(3):801–8.

20. Burris AS, Clark RV, Vantman DJ, Sherins RJ. A low sperm concentration does not preclude fertility in men with isolated hypogonadotropic hypogonadism after gonadotropin therapy. *Fertility and Sterility.* 1988;50(2):343–7.

21. Cooper TG, Noonan E, von Eckardstein S, Auger J, Baker HW, Behre HM, et al. World Health Organization reference values for human semen characteristics. *Human Reproduction Update.* 2010; 16(3):231–45.

22. Dwyer AA, Jayasena CN, Quinton R. Congenital hypogonadotropic hypogonadism: implications of absent mini-puberty. *Minerva Endocrinologica.* 2016;41(2):188–95.

23. Dwyer AA, Sykiotis GP, Hayes FJ, Boepple PA, Lee H, Loughlin KR, et al. Trial of recombinant follicle-stimulating hormone pretreatment for GnRH-induced fertility in patients with congenital hypogonadotropic hypogonadism. *The Journal of Clinical Endocrinology and Metabolism.* 2013;98(11):E1790–5.

24. Raivio T, Toppari J, Perheentupa A, McNeilly AS, Dunkel L. Treatment of prepubertal gonadotrophin-deficient boys with recombinant human follicle-stimulating hormone.

Lancet. 1997;350(9073): 263–4.

25. Raivio T, Wikstrom AM, Dunkel L. Treatment of gonadotropin-deficient boys with recombinant human FSH: long-term observation and outcome. *European Journal of Endocrinology / European Federation of Endocrine Societies.* 2007;156(1):105–11.

26. Behre HM, Nashan D, Nieschlag E. Objective measurement of testicular volume by ultrasonography: evaluation of the technique and comparison with orchidometer estimates. *International Journal of Andrology.* 1989;12(6):395–403.

27. Dwyer AA, Tiemensma J, Quinton R, Pitteloud N, Morin D. Adherence to treatment in men with hypogonadotrophic hypogonadism. *Clinical Endocrinology.* 2017;86(3):377–83.

28. Anawalt BD. Approach to male infertility and induction of spermatogenesis. *The Journal of Clinical Endocrinology and Metabolism.* 2013;98(9):3532–42.

29. Liu PY, Gebski VJ, Turner L, Conway AJ, Wishart SM, Handelsman DJ. Predicting pregnancy and spermatogenesis by survival analysis during gonadotrophin treatment of gonadotrophin-deficient infertile men. *Human Reproduction.* 2002;17(3):625–33.

30. Kirk JM, Savage MO, Grant DB, Bouloux PM, Besser GM. Gonadal

function and response to human chorionic and menopausal gonadotrophin therapy in male patients with idiopathic hypogonadotrophic hypogonadism. *Clinical Endocrinology.* 1994;41(1): 57–63.

31. Yong EL, Lee KO, Ng SC, Ratnam SS. Induction of spermatogenesis in isolated hypogonadotrophic hypogonadism with gonadotrophins and early intervention with intracytoplasmic sperm injection. *Human Reproduction.* 1997;12(6):1230–2.

32. Depenbusch M, von Eckardstein S, Simoni M, Nieschlag E. Maintenance of spermatogenesis in hypogonadotropic hypogonadal men with human chorionic gonadotropin alone. *European Journal of Endocrinology / European Federation of Endocrine Societies.* 2002;147(5):617–24.

33. Shiraishi K, Oka S, Matsuyama H. Assessment of quality of life during gonadotrophin treatment for male hypogonadotrophic hypogonadism. *Clinical Endocrinology.* 2014;81(2): 259–65.

34. Dwyer AA, Quinton R, Pitteloud N, Morin D. Psychosexual development in men with congenital hypogonadotropic hypogonadism on long-term treatment: a mixed methods study. *Sexual Medicine.* 2015;3(1):32–41.

Causes and Investigation of Ovarian Infertility

Adam H. Balen

1 Introduction

Conventional ovulation induction (OI) treatments are highly effective in achieving pregnancy when anovulation is the only factor in a couple's conception delay. Fertility declines with female age and lifestyle factors including smoking, alcohol intake and body weight negatively influence the success of treatment. Careful planning and monitoring of treatment is necessary to avoid complications such as multiple pregnancy and ovarian hyperstimulation syndrome (OHSS).

2 Aetiology

Ovulatory disorders are broadly classified by World Health Organization (WHO) as follows:

- Group I: hypothalamic pituitary failure (hypothalamic amenorrhoea or hypogonadotrophic hypogonadism)
- Group II: hypothalamic pituitary dysfunction (normogonadotrophic, predominately polycystic ovary syndrome).
- Group III: ovarian failure (hypergonadotrophic anovulation)

Table 14.1

Table 14.1 Gonadotrophin and oestradiol profiles in different clinical scenarios

Ovarian failure	↑ FSH	↑ LH	↓ Oestradiol
Hypothalamic or pituitary failure	↓ FSH	↓ ↓ LH	↓ Oestradiol
PCOS	n/↓ FSH	n/↑ LH	n/↑ Oestradiol
Mid-cycle, preovulatory	↑ FSH	↑↑ LH	↑ Oestradiol

3 History and Examination

Menstrual cycles are considered regular if they fall in the range of 23 to 35 days and have a month-to-month variation in cycle length of less than five days. It is estimated that at least 90–95% of normally menstruating women have ovulatory cycles. Women suspected of ovulatory dysfunction need careful assessment with appropriate investigations in order to be able to tailor treatment accordingly.

Measurement of height and weight should be performed in order to calculate the patient's body mass index (BMI). The normal range is 20–25 kg/m^2, and a value above or below this may suggest a diagnosis of weight-related amenorrhoea (which is a term usually applied to underweight women).

Signs of hyperandrogenism (acne, hirsutism, balding [alopecia]]) are suggestive of polcystic ovary syndrome (PCOS), although biochemical screening helps to differentiate other causes of androgen excess. It is important to distinguish between hyperandrogenism and virilization, which also occurs with high circulating androgen levels and causes deepening of the voice, breast atrophy, increase in muscle bulk and cliteromegaly. A rapid onset of hirsutism suggests the possibility of an androgen-secreting tumour of the ovary or adrenal gland. Hirsutism can be graded and given a 'Ferriman Gallwey Score' by assessing the amount of hair in different parts of the body (e.g. upper lip, chin, breasts, abdomen, arms, legs). It is useful to monitor the progress of hirsutism, or its response to treatment, by making serial records, either by using a chart or by taking photographs of affected areas of the body. It should be remembered, however, that not all hair on the body is necessarily responsive to hormone changes (for example the upper thighs). There may also be big ethnic variations in the expression of hirsutism, with women from South Asia and Mediterranean countries often having more pronounced problems, whereas those from the Far East may not have much in the way of bodily hair. Furthermore the degree of hirsutism does not correlate that well with the actual levels of circulating androgens.

Box 14.1 Endocrine normal ranges	
Follicle-stimulating hormone, FSH	1–10 IU/L (early follicular)
Luteinizing hormone, LH	1–10 IU/L (early follicular)
Prolactin	< 400 mIU/L
Thyroid-stimulating hormone, TSH	0.5–4.0 IU/L
Thyroxine (T4)	50–150 nmol/L
Free T4	9–22 pmol/L
Tri-iodothyronine (T3)	1.5–3.5 nmol/L
Free T3	4.3–8.6 pmol/L
Thyroid-binding globulin, TBG	7–17 mg/L
Testosterone (T)	0.5–3.5 nmol/L (ranges depend upon the assay being used)
Sex hormone-binding globulin, SHBG	16–120 nmol/L
Free androgen index [(T × 100) ÷ SHBG]	< 5
Dihydrotestosterone	0.3–1 nmol/L
Androstenedione	2–10 nmol/L
Dehydroepiandrosterone sulphate	3–10 μmol/L
Cortisol	
8 a.m.	140–700 nmol/L
Midnight	0–140 nmol/L
24-hour urinary	< 400 nmol/24 h
Oestradiol	250–500 pmol/L
Progesterone (mid-luteal)	> 25 nmol/L to indicate ovulation
17-hydroxyprogesterone	1–20 nmol/L
Anti-Mullerian hormone (AMH)	Values should be assessed with respect to age-related nomograms. Low levels indicate poor ovarian reserve, normal levels suggest normal fertility and high values are often seen in women with polycystic ovaries.

A measurement of total testosterone (T) is considered adequate for general screening (Box 14.1). It is unnecessary to measure other androgens unless total T is > 5 nmol/L (this will depend on the normal range of your local assay). Insulin may be elevated in overweight women and suppresses the production of sex hormone–binding globulin (SHBG) by the liver, resulting in a high free androgen index (FAI) in the presence of a normal total T. The measurement of SHBG is not required in routine practice but is a useful surrogate marker for insulin resistance (IR).

One should be aware of the possibility of Cushing's syndrome in women with stigmata of PCOS and obesity as it is a disease of insidious onset and dire consequences; additional clues are the presence of central obesity, moon face, plethoric complexion, buffalo hump, proximal myopathy, thin skin, bruising and abdominal striae (which alone are a common finding in obese individuals). Acanthosis nigricans (AN) is a sign of profound insulin resistance and is usually visible as hyperpigmented thickening of the skin folds of the axilla and neck; AN is associated with PCOS and obesity.

A testosterone concentration > 5 nmol/L should be investigated to exclude androgen-secreting tumours of the ovary or adrenal gland, Cushing's syndrome and late-onset congenital adrenal hyperplasia (CAH). Whereas CAH often presents at birth with ambiguous genitalia, partial 21-hydroxylase deficiency may present in later life, usually in the teenage years, with signs and symptoms similar to PCOS. In such cases, T may be elevated and the diagnosis confirmed by an elevated serum concentration of 17-hydroxyprogesterone (17-OHP); an abnormal ACTH-stimulation test may also be helpful (250 μg ACTH will cause an elevation of 17-OHP, usually between 65–470 nmol/L).

In cases of Cushing's syndrome, a 24-hour urinary-free cortisol will be elevated (> 700 nmol/24 hours). The normal serum concentration of cortisol is 140–700 nmol/L at 8 a.m. and less than 140 nmol/L at midnight. A low-dose dexamethasone suppression test (0.5 mg six-hourly for 48 hours) will cause a suppression of serum cortisol by 48 hours. A simpler screening test is an overnight suppression test, using a single midnight dose of dexamethasone 1 mg (2 mg if obese) and measuring the serum cortisol concentration at 8 a.m. when it should be less than 140 nmol/L. If Cushing's syndrome is confirmed, a high-dose dexamethasone suppression test (2 mg six-hourly for 48 hours) should suppress serum cortisol by 48 hours if there is a pituitary ACTH-secreting adenoma (Cushing's disease); failure of suppression suggests an adrenal tumour or ectopic secretion of ACTH; further tests and detailed imaging will then be required.

The measurement of other serum androgen levels can be helpful. Dehydroepiandrosterone sulphate (DHEAS) is primarily a product of the adrenal androgen pathway (normal range < 10 μmol/l). If the serum androgen concentrations are elevated, the possibility of an ovarian or adrenal tumour should be excluded by ultrasound or CT scans. The measurement of androstenedione can also be useful in some situations.

Amenorrhoiec women might have hyperprolactinaemia and galactorrhoea. It is important, however, not to examine the breasts before taking blood as the serum prolactin concentration may be falsely elevated as a result of physical examination. Stress may also cause minor elevation of prolactin. If there is suspicion of a pituitary tumour, the patient's visual fields should be checked, as bitemporal hemianopia secondary to pressure on the optic chiasm requires urgent attention.

Thyroid disease is common and the thyroid gland should be palpated and signs of hypothyroidism (dry thin hair, proximal myopathy, myotonia, slow-relaxing reflexes, mental slowness, bradycardia, etc.) or hyperthyroidism (goitre with bruit, tremor, weight loss, tachycardia, hyper-reflexia, exopthalmos, conjunctival oedema, ophthalmoplegia) elicited.

A baseline assessment of the endocrine status should include the measurement of serum prolactin and gonadotrophin concentrations and an assessment of thyroid function. Prolactin levels may be elevated in response to a number of conditions, including stress, a recent breast examination or even having a blood test. The elevation, however, is moderate and transient. A more permanent, but still moderate, elevation (greater than 700 mIU/L) is associated with hypothyroidism and is also a common finding in women with PCOS, where prolactin levels up to 2500 mIU/L have been reported. PCOS may also result in amenorrhoea, which can therefore create diagnostic and hence appropriate management difficulties, for those women with hyperprolactinaemia and polycystic ovaries. Amenorrhoea in women with PCOS is secondary to acyclical ovarian activity, yet oestrogen production by the ovaries continues and so the endometrium will be greater than 6 mm. A positive response to a progestogen challenge test (e.g. medroxyprogesterone acetate 10–20 mg [depending on body weight] daily for seven days), which induces a withdrawal bleed, will distinguish patients with PCOS-related hyperprolactinaemia from those with polycystic ovaries and unrelated hyperprolactinaemia, because the latter causes oestrogen deficiency and therefore failure to respond to the progestogen challenge because the endometrium is thin.

A serum prolactin concentration of greater than 1000 mIU/L warrants a repeat and then further investigation if still elevated. Computed tomography (CT) or magnetic resonance imaging (MRI) of the pituitary fossa may be used to exclude a hypothalamic tumour, a non-functioning pituitary tumour compressing the hypothalamus or a prolactinoma. Serum prolactin concentrations greater than 5000 mIU/L are usually associated with a macroprolactinoma, which by definition is greater than 1 cm in diameter.

Serum measurements of oestradiol are of limited value as they vary considerably, even in a patient with amenorrhoea. If the patient is well oestrogenized, the endometrium will be clearly seen on an ultrasound scan and should be shed on withdrawal of the progestogen.

Serum gonadotrophin measurements help to distinguish between cases of hypothalamic or pituitary failure and gonadal failure. Elevated gonadotrophin concentrations indicate a failure of negative feedback as a result of primary or premature ovarian insufficency (POI, formerly known as premature ovarian failure). A serum follicle-stimulating hormone (FSH) concentration of greater than 15 IU/L that is not associated with a preovulatory luteinizing hormone (LH) surge suggests impending ovarian failure. FSH levels of greater than 40 IU/L are suggestive of irreversible ovarian failure. The exact values vary according to individual assays, and so local reference levels should be checked. It is also important to assess serum gonadotrophin levels at baseline, that is, during the first three days of a menstrual period. In patients with oligo/amenorrhoea, it may be necessary to perform two or more random measurements, although combining an assessment of endocrinology with an ultrasound scan on the same day aids the diagnosis.

An elevated LH concentration, when associated with a raised FSH concentration, is indicative of ovarian failure. However, if LH is elevated alone (and is not attributable to the preovulatory LH surge), this suggests PCOS. This may be confirmed by a pelvic ultrasound scan. Rarely, an elevated LH in a phenotypic female may be due to androgen insensitivity syndrome (AIS), although this condition presents with primary amenorrhoea.

Inhibin B is thought to be the ovarian hormone which has the greatest influence on pituitary secretion of FSH. Previously, it was thought that serum concentrations of inhibin B might provide better quantification of ovarian reserve than serum FSH concentrations, however, the assay is no longer being used.

Anti-Mullerian hormone (AMH) is best known as a product of the testes during fetal development that suppresses the development of Mullerian structures. AMH is also produced by the preantral and antral follicles and appears to be a more stable predictor of the ovarian follicle pool as it does not fluctuate through the menstrual cycle. Indeed, it has been reported that higher AMH concentrations are associated with increased numbers of mature oocytes, embryos and clinical pregnancies during in vitro fertilization (IVF) treatment. Assays for AMH are now available for routine use and it is this hormone that currently offers the greatest promise for future assessment of ovarian reserve and function. The number of antral follicles in the ovary, as assessed by pelvic ultrasound, also correlates well with ovarian reserve and serum AMH levels. Indeed, it is the number of small antral follicles, 2–6 mm in diameter, that declines significantly with age while there is little change in the larger follicles of 7–10 mm, which is still below the size at which growing follicles have been recruited.

Failure at the level of the hypothalamus or pituitary is reflected by abnormally low levels of serum gonadotrophin concentrations, and gives rise to hypogonadotrophic hypogonadism. Kallmann's syndrome is the clinical finding of anosmia and/or colour blindness associated with hypogonadotrophic hypogonadism – usually a cause of primary amenorrhoea. CT or MRI should be performed if indicated.

Women with premature ovarian insufficiency (POI) (under the age of 40 years) may have a chromosomal abnormality (e.g. Turner syndrome [45X or 46XX/45X mosaic] or other sex chromosome mosaicisms). A number of genes have also been associated with familial POF, but have not been assessed in routine clinical practice. An autoantibody screen should also be undertaken in women with POI, although it can be difficult to detect antiovarian antibodies and many will have evidence of other autoantibodies (e.g. thyroid), which then indicates the need for further surveillance.

Measurement of bone mineral density (BMD) is indicated in amenorrhoeic women who are oestrogen-deficient. Measurements of density are made in the lumbar spine and femoral neck. The vertebral bone is more sensitive to oestrogen deficiency and vertebral fractures tend to occur in a younger age group (50–60 years) than fractures at the femoral neck (70+ years). However, it should be noted that crush fractures can spuriously increase the measured BMD. An X-ray of the dorsolumbar spine is therefore often complimentary, particularly in patients who have lost height.

Amenorrhoea may also have long-term metabolic and physical consequences. In women with PCOS and prolonged amenorrhoea, there is a risk of endometrial hyperplasia and adenocarcinoma. If on resumption of menstruation there is a history of persistent inter-menstrual bleeding, or on ultrasound there is a post-menstrual endometrial thickness of greater than 10 mm, an endometrial biopsy is indicated.

Serum cholesterol measurements are important because of the association of an increased risk of heart disease in women with POI. Women with PCOS, although not oestrogen-deficient, may have a subnormal high-density lipoprotein (HDL): total cholesterol ratio. This is as a consequence of the hypersecretion of insulin that occurs in many women with PCOS.

3.1 Glucose Tolerance

Women who are obese, and also many slim women with PCOS, may have insulin resistance and elevated serum concentrations of insulin (usually < 30 mIU/L fasting, although not measured in clinical practice). A 75 g oral glucose tolerance test (GTT) should be performed in women with PCOS and a BMI > 30 kg/m^2, with an assessment of the fasting and two-hour glucose concentration (Table 14.2). It has been suggested that South Asian women should have an assessment of glucose tolerance if their BMI is greater than 25 kg/m^2 because of the greater risk of insulin resistance at a lower BMI than seen in the white Caucasian population.

4 Polycystic Ovary Syndrome

The PCOS is a heterogeneous collection of signs and symptoms that, gathered together, form a spectrum of a disorder with a mild presentation in some but a severe disturbance of reproductive, endocrine and metabolic function in others. The pathophysiology of PCOS appears to be multifactorial and polygenic. The definition of the syndrome has been much debated. Key features include menstrual cycle disturbance, hyperandrogenism and obesity. There are many extraovarian aspects to the pathophysiology of PCOS, yet ovarian dysfunction is central. The joint ESHRE/ASRM (European Society for Human Reproduction and Embryology/American Society for Reproductive Medicine) consensus defined PCOS as requiring the presence of two out of the following three criteria:

1 oligo- and/or anovulation (that is oligomenorrhoea or amenorrhoea);

2 hyperandrogenism (clinical features and/or biochemical elevation of testosterone); and/or

3 polycystic ovaries assessed by ultrasound [1].

The consensus meeting that provided this definition was held in Rotterdam and so the ESHRE/ASRM criteria are often known as "the Rotterdam criteria" [1].

Other aetiologies of hyperandrogenism and menstrual cycle disturbance should be excluded by appropriate investigations, as described within this chapter. The morphology of the polycystic ovary (PCO) has been redefined as an ovary with 12 or more follicles measuring 2–9 mm in diameter and/or increased ovarian volume (> 10 cm^3) [2]. The use of higher resolution ultrasound than was available at the time of the Rotterdam meeting has led some to suggest that more follicles (19 or even 25) should define the polycystic ovary, but no consensus has been reached [3].

There is considerable heterogeneity of symptoms and signs among women with PCOS and for an individual these may change over time [1] (Box 14.2). PCOS may be familial, and various aspects of the syndrome may be differentially inherited. Polycystic ovaries can exist without clinical signs of the syndrome, which may then become expressed in certain circumstances. There are a number of factors that affect expression of PCOS; for example, a gain in weight is associated with a worsening of symptoms while weight loss may ameliorate the endocrine and metabolic profile and symptomatology.

Genetic studies have identified a link between PCOS and disordered insulin metabolism, and indicate that the syndrome may be the presentation of a complex genetic trait disorder. The features of obesity, hyperinsulinaemia and hyperandrogenaemia, which are commonly seen in PCOS, are also known to be factors that confer an increased risk of cardiovascular disease and non-insulin-dependent diabetes mellitus (Type 2 DM) [4]. There are studies indicating

Table 14.2 Definitions of glucose tolerance after a 75 g glucose tolerance test (GTT)

	Diabetes mellitus	Impaired glucose tolerance (IGT)	Impaired fasting glycaemia
Fasting glucose (mmol/L)	≥ 7.0	< 7.0	≥ 6.1 and < 7.0
2-hour glucose (mmol/L)	≥ 11.1	≥ 7.8 and ≤ 11.1	< 7.8

Box 14.2 Signs and symptoms of polycystic ovary syndrome.

Symptoms

Hyperandrogenism (acne, hirsutism, alopecia – *not* virilization)

Menstrual disturbance

Infertility

Obesity

Sometimes: asymptomatic, with polycystic ovaries on ultrasound scan

Serum endocrinology

↑ Fasting insulin (not routinely measured; insulin resistance or impaired glucose tolerance assessed by GTT)

↑ Androgens (testosterone and androstenedione)

↑ or normal luteinizing hormone (LH), normal follicle-stimulating hormone (FSH)

↓ Sex hormone binding globulin (SHBG), results in elevated 'free androgen index'

↑ Oestradiol, oestrone (neither measured routinely as very wide range of values)

↑ Prolactin

Possible late sequelae

Diabetes mellitus

Dyslipidaemia

Hypertension, cardiovascular disease

Endometrial carcinoma

that women with PCOS have an increased risk for these diseases, which pose long-term risks for health, and this evidence has prompted debate as to the need for screening women for PCOS [4].

Polycystic ovaries are commonly detected by ultrasound or other forms of pelvic imaging, with estimates of the prevalence in the general population being in the order of 20–33% [2]. Although the ultrasound criteria for the diagnosis of polycystic ovaries have not, until now, been universally agreed, the characteristic features are accepted as being an increase in the number of follicles and the amount of stroma compared with normal ovaries, resulting in

an increase in ovarian volume. The 'cysts' are not cysts in the sense that they do contain oocytes and indeed are follicles whose development has been arrested. The actual number of cysts may be of less relevance than the volume of ovarian stroma or of the ovary itself, which has been shown to closely correlate with serum testosterone concentrations.

4.1 Racial Differences in Expression of Polycystic Ovary Syndrome

Insulin resistance and hyperinsulinaemia are common antecedents of type 2 diabetes, with a high prevalence in South Asian people. Type 2 diabetes also has a familial basis, inherited as a complex genetic trait that interacts with environmental factors, chiefly nutrition, commencing during fetal life. We have found that South Asian people with anovulatory PCOS have greater insulin resistance and more severe symptoms of the syndrome than anovulatory white people with PCOS [4]. Furthermore, we have found that women from South Asia living in the United Kingdom appear to express symptoms at an earlier age than their white British counterparts [4].

4.2 Health Consequences of Polycystic Ovary Syndrome

Obesity and metabolic abnormalities are recognized risk factors for the development of ischaemic heart disease (IHD) in the general population, and these are also recognized features of PCOS. The question is whether women with PCOS are at an increased risk of IHD, and whether this will occur at an earlier age than for women with normal ovaries. The basis for the idea that women with PCOS are at a greater risk for cardiovascular disease is that these women are more insulin resistant than weight-matched controls and that the metabolic disturbances associated with insulin resistance are known to increase cardiovascular risk in other populations. Insulin resistance is defined as a diminution in the biological responses to a given level of insulin. In the presence of an adequate pancreatic reserve, normal circulating glucose levels are maintained at higher serum insulin concentrations. In the general population, cardiovascular risk factors include insulin resistance, obesity, glucose intolerance, hypertension and dyslipidaemia.

There have been a large number of studies demonstrating the presence of insulin resistance and

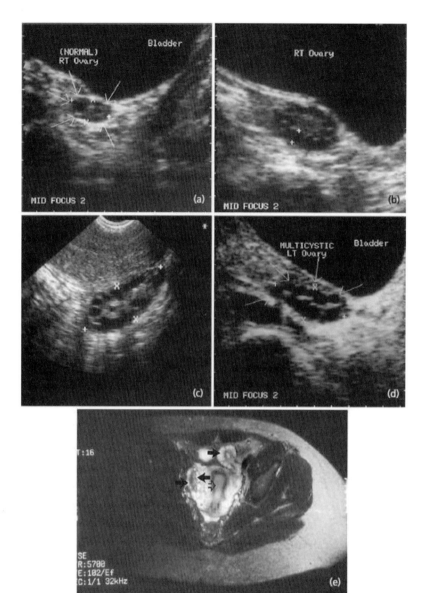

Fig. 14.1 (a) Transabdominal ultrasound scan of a normal ovary. (b) Transabdominal ultrasound scan of a polycystic ovary. (c) Transvaginal ultrasound scan of a polycystic ovary. (d) Transabdominal ultrasound scan of a multicystic ovary. (e) Magnetic resonance imaging (MRI) of a pelvis, demonstrating two polycystic ovaries (closed arrows) and a hyperplastic endometrium (open arrow). Reproduced from Balen AH. *Infertility in Practice*, 4th edn. London: Informa Healthcare, 2014, with permission.

corresponding hyperinsulinaemia in both obese and non-obese women with PCOS. Obese women with PCOS have consistently been shown to be more insulin resistant than weight-matched controls. It appears that obesity and PCOS have an additive effect on the degree and severity of the insulin resistance and subsequent hyperinsulinaemia in this group of women. The insulin resistance causes compensatory hypersecretion of insulin, particularly in response to glucose, so euglycaemia is usually maintained at the expense of hyperinsulinaemia. Insulin resistance is restricted to the extrasplanchnic actions

of insulin on glucose dispersal. The liver is not affected (hence the fall in SHBG and HDL), neither is the ovary (hence the menstrual problems and hypersecretion of androgens) nor the skin, hence the development of acanthosis nigricans. Women with PCOS who are oligomenorrhoeic are more likely to be insulin resistant than those with regular cycles, irrespective of their BMI, with the intermenstrual interval correlating with the degree of insulin resistance.

Women with PCOS have a greater truncal abdominal fat distribution as demonstrated by a higher waist:hip ratio. The central distribution of fat is independent of BMI and associated with higher plasma insulin and triglyceride concentrations and reduced HDL cholesterol concentrations. From a practical point of view, if the measurement of waist circumference is greater than 80 cm, there will be excess visceral fat and an increased risk of metabolic problems.

Thus, there is evidence that insulin resistance, central obesity and hyperandrogenaemia have an adverse effect on lipid metabolism, yet these are surrogate risk factors for cardiovascular disease. However, Wild et al. [6] reported the mortality rate in 1,028 women diagnosed as having PCOS between 1930 and 1979. All the women were older than 45 years and 770 women had been treated by wedge resection of the ovaries. A total of 786 women were traced; the mean age at diagnosis was 26.4 years and the average duration of follow-up was 30 years. There were 59 deaths, of which 15 were from circulatory disease. Of these 15 deaths, 13 were from ischaemic heart disease. There were six deaths from diabetes as an underlying or contributory cause compared with the expected 1.7 deaths. The standard mortality rate both overall and for cardiovascular disease was not higher in the women with PCOS than the national mortality rates in women, although the observed proportion of women with diabetes as a contributory or underlying factor leading to death was significantly higher than expected (odds ratio 3.6, 95% confidence interval [CI] 1.5–8.4). Thus, despite surrogate markers for cardiovascular disease, no increased rate of death from CVS disease could be demonstrated in this study [6,7].

4.3 Endometrial Cancer

Endometrial adenocarcinoma is the second most common female genital malignancy, but only 4% of cases occur in women aged under 40 years. The risk of developing endometrial cancer has been shown to be adversely influenced by a number of factors, including obesity, long-term use of unopposed oestrogens, nulliparity and infertility. Women with endometrial carcinoma have had fewer births than controls, and it has also been demonstrated that infertility *per se* increases the risk [7]. Hypertension and type 2 diabetes mellitus have long been linked to endometrial cancer – conditions that are now known also to be associated with PCOS. The true risk of endometrial carcinoma in women with clearly defined PCOS, however, is difficult to ascertain [7].

Endometrial hyperplasia may be a precursor to adenocarcinoma, although the rate of progression is difficult to predict. Although the degree of risk has not been clearly defined, it is generally accepted that for women with PCOS who experience amenorrhoea or oligomenorrhoea, the induction of artificial withdrawal bleeds to prevent endometrial hyperplasia is prudent management [7]. Indeed, we consider it important that women with PCOS shed their endometrium at least every three months.

For those with oligo-/amenorrhoea who do not wish to use cyclical hormone therapy, we recommend an ultrasound scan to measure endometrial thickness and morphology every 6–12 months (depending upon menstrual history). An endometrial thickness greater than 10 mm in an amenorrhoiec woman warrants an artificially induced bleed, which should be followed by a repeat ultrasound scan and endometrial biopsy if the endometrium has not been shed. Another option is to consider a progestogen-secreting intrauterine system, such as the Mirena® (Bayer Pharma, Newburg, UK).

Key References

1. Rotterdam ESHRE/ASRM-Sponsored PCOS Consensus Workshop Group. Revised 2003 consensus on diagnostic criteria and long-term health risks related to polycystic ovary syndrome. *Hum Reprod.*2004; 19, 41–47.

2. Balen AH, Laven JSE, Tan SL, Dewailly D. Ultrasound Assessment of the Polycystic Ovary: International Consensus Definitions. *Human Reproduction Update* 2003; 9: 505–514

3. Dewailly D, Lujan ME, Carmina E, Cedars MI, Laven J, Norman RJ, et al. Definition and significance of polycystic ovarian morphology: a task force report from the Androgen Excess and Polycystic Ovary Syndrome Society. *Hum Reprod Update* 2014;**20**: 334–352.

4. Wijeyeratne CN, Kumarapeli V, Seneviratne RdeA, Antonypillai CN, Seneviratne RdeA SR, Chaminda GJ, Yapa SC, Balen AH: Ethnic variations in the expression of polycystic ovary syndrome. *Current Management of Polycystic Ovary Syndrome.* Edited by AH Balen, S Franks and R Homburg. Proceedings of 59th RCOG Study Group, RCOG Press, London 2010; pp 25–46.

5. *Current Management of Polycystic Ovary Syndrome.* Edited by AH Balen, S Franks, R Homburg and S Kehoe. Proceedings of 59th RCOG Study Group, RCOG Press, London 2010.

6. Wild S, Pierpoint T, McKeigue P, Jacobs H. Cardiovascular disease in women with polycystic ovary syndrome at long-term follow-up: a retrospective cohort study. *Clin Endocrinol* 2000;**52**:595–600.

7. Fauser BCJM, Tarlatzis BC, Rerbar RW, Legro RS, Balen AH, Lobo R, Carmina E, Chang J, Yildiz B, Laven JSE, Boivin J, Petraglia F, Wijeyaratne C, Norman RJ, Dunaif A, Franks S, Wild RA, Dumesic D, Barnhart K. Consensus on women's health aspects of polycystic ovary syndrome (PCOS): the Amsterdam ESHRE/ASRM-Sponsored 3rd PCOS Consensus Workshop Group. Simultaneous Publication *Human Reproduction* 2012; **27**: 14–24. and *Fertility & Sterility* 2012; 97: 28–38.

Chapter 15

Ovulation Induction for Anovulatory Infertility

Adam H. Balen

1 Pretreatment Considerations

Folic acid should be taken at a daily dose of 400 mcg or, in those who are obese, 5 mg. There is debate about the restriction of fertility treatment to women who are overweight, although there is no doubt that obesity has a significant adverse impact on reproductive outcome. It influences not only the chance of conception but also the response to fertility treatment and increases the risk of miscarriage, congenital anomalies and pregnancy complications [1]. The British Fertility Society guidance suggests that treatment should be deferred until the BMI is less than 35 kg/m², although in those with more time (e.g. less than 37 years, normal ovarian reserve) a weight reduction to a BMI of less than 30 kg/m² is preferable [2]. Even a moderate weight loss of 5–10% of body weight can be sufficient to restore fertility and improve metabolic parameters.

A semen analysis should be performed before ovulation induction therapy is commenced. We recommend that tubal patency should be assessed by either hysterosalpingography (HSG) or laparoscopy before embarking upon ovulation induction therapy. There are some who believe that, if there are no firm indications (e.g. past history of pelvic infection, pelvic pain) a test of tubal patency can be delayed until there have been up to three or six ovulatory cycles. In order to minimize the risks of therapy, however, and also to ensure a cost-effective approach to treatment, we feel that an assessment of tubal patency is appropriate in every woman before commencing therapy.

2 Pituitary and Hypothalamic (WHO Group I Disorders)

Pituitary and hypothalamic causes of anovulation constitute about 5–10% of all cases of anovulation (see Chapter 4 on female fertility). In women with low body weight (e.g. anorexia nervosa), restoration of body weight may help to resume natural ovulation. A vast majority of cases presenting to a fertility clinic however, do not have frank anorexia but are usually underweight and/or exercising a little too much. There may be a delay of several months or even years before cycles are re-established after a gain in weight and many also have underlying ovulatory problems secondary to PCOS. Drugs should not be used to stimulate ovulation until a regain of weight in order to reduce the risks to the fetus of miscarriage, stillbirth and intrauterine growth restriction.

For patients with idiopathic hypogonadotrophic hypogonadism or Kallmann's syndrome and an intact pituitary gland, ovulation may be induced with either pulsatile gonadotrophin releasing hormone (GnRH) or gonadotrophin therapy. Pulsatile GnRH may be administered subcutaneously by a miniature infusion pump, with a pulse of 15 mcg being released every 90 minutes. This is the most physiological way to achieve unifollicular ovulation, but unfortunately the therapeutic preparations of GnRH are no longer available and so we are currently unable to use these pumps.

As an alternative, parenteral gonadotrophin therapy with both FSH and LH activity can be administered as a daily injection. Urinary human menopausal gonadotrophins (hMG) contain a combination of FSH and LH while the recombinant preparations usually contain only FSH or LH activity, although newer preparations with combined recombinant FSH and LH in a single injection are now available. In women with hypothalamic hypogonadism, recombinant FSH (rFSH) alone stimulates follicular growth, but results in inadequate oestrogen production confirming the need for LH to fulfil the 'two cell, two gonadotrophin' requirement for ovarian steroidogenesis [3]. Therefore, in practice, hMG preparations are usually administered.

The aim of ovulation induction is to select a single antral follicle that will be able to reach the preovulatory stage with appropriate endometrial development.

Serial ultrasound scanning to monitor the ovarian response is an integral part of treatment. When the follicle reaches a preovulatory size (17–18 mm diameter), a human chorionic gonadotrophin (hCG) injection is administered for oocyte maturation and to trigger ovulation. In order to minimize the chances of multifollicular development and thereby to reduce risks of multiple pregnancy and ovarian hyperstimulation syndrome (OHSS), low-dose step-up regimens are usually employed [4]. Luteal support after ovulation induction is not required. It has been suggested that adjuvant therapy with human growth hormone is of benefit to some women in this group who had a previous poor response to gonadotrophin ovulation induction but its use is not recommended as it does not improve live birth rates [5].

3 Hyperprolactinaemia

The management of hyperprolactinaemia centres around the use of a dopamine agonist, of which bromocriptine and cabergoline are the most widely used. Of course, if the hyperprolactinaemia is drug induced, stopping the relevant preparation should be commended. This may not, however, be appropriate if the cause is a psychotropic medication, for example a phenothiazine being used to treat schizophrenia. In these cases, careful discussion is required on appropriate fertility management with the patient's psychiatrist.

Most patients show a fall in prolactin levels within a few days of commencing bromocriptine therapy and a reduction of tumour volume within six weeks. Side effects can be troublesome (nausea, vomiting, headache, postural hypotension) and are minimized by commencing the therapy at night for the first three days of treatment and taking the tablets in the middle of a mouthful of food. The longer-acting preparation cabergoline appears to have fewer side effects and is more commonly used these days. Indeed not only does cabergoline appear to be better tolerated and more efficacious than bromocriptine but it is also now the drug of choice for hyperprolactinemia. It is not licensed for women who wish to conceive and so the recommendation has been to switch to bromocriptine if fertility is desired, although there is some debate as to whether this is still appropriate advice [6].

Longer-term side effects include Raynaud's phenomenon, constipation and psychiatric changes – especially aggression, which can occur at the start of treatment. Bromocriptine and cabergoline have been associated with pulmonary, retroperitoneal and pericardial fibrotic reactions and so echocardiography is recommended before starting treatment in order to exclude valvulopathy and this should be repeated after 3–6 months and then annually – although young patients are less at risk than older patients who may be prescribed higher doses for the management of Parkinson's disease. The maintenance dose should be the lowest that reduces prolactin to normal levels and is often lower than that needed initially to initiate a response.

Surgery, in the form of a transsphenoidal adenectomy, is reserved for cases of drug resistance and failure to shrink a macroadenoma or if there are intolerable side effects of the drugs (the most common indication). Nonfunctioning tumours should be removed surgically and are usually detected by a combination of imaging and a serum prolactin concentration of < 3000 mIU/L. When the prolactin level is between 3000 and 8000 mIU/L, a trial of bromocriptine is warranted, and if the prolactin level falls it can be assumed that the tumour is a prolactin-secreting macroadenoma (Figure 15.1a). Operative treatment is also required if there is suprasellar extension of the tumour that has not regressed during treatment with bromocriptine and a pregnancy is desired. With the present-day skills of neurosurgeons in transsphenoidal surgery, it is seldom necessary to resort to pituitary irradiation, which offers no advantages and requires long-term surveillance to detect consequent hypopituitarism (which is immediately apparent if it occurs after surgery).

Women with a microprolactinoma who wish to conceive can be reassured that they may stop bromocriptine when pregnancy is diagnosed and require no further monitoring, as the likelihood of significant tumour expansion is very small (less than 2%). On the other hand, if a patient with a macroprolactinoma is not treated with bromocriptine, the tumour has a 25% risk of expanding during pregnancy. This risk is probably also present if the tumour has been treated but has not shrunk, as assessed by CT or MRI scan (Figure 15.1b, c & d). The first-line approach to treatment of macroprolactinomas is therefore with bromocriptine combined with barrier methods of contraception. In cases with suprasellar expansion, a follow-up CT (or MRI) scan should be performed after three months of treatment to ensure tumour regression before it is safe to embark upon pregnancy. Bromocriptine can be discontinued during pregnancy,

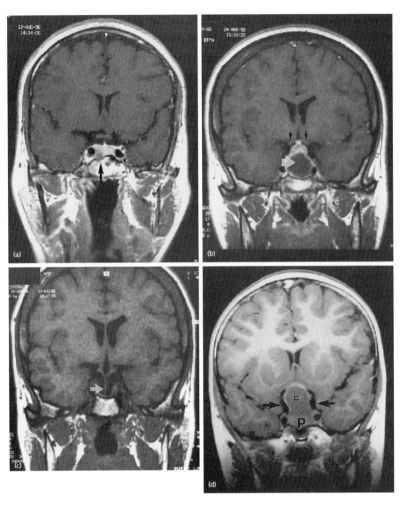

Fig. 15.1 (a) Pituitary microadenoma: Cranial magnetic resonance imaging (MRI). A coronal section T1-weighted spin echo sequence after i.v. gadolinium. The normal pituitary gland is hyperintense (bright) while the tumour is seen as a 4 mm area of non-enhancement (grey) in the right lobe of the pituitary, encroaching up to the right cavernous sinus. It is eroding the right side of the sella floor (arrow). Pituitary macroadenoma: MRI scans of a pituitary macroadenoma before and after bromocriptine therapy. (b) T1-weighted image post gadolinium enhancement demonstrating a macroadenoma with a large central cystic component (large arrow). There is suprasellar extension with compression of the optic chiasm (small arrows). (c) After therapy the tumour has almost completely resolved and there is tethering of the optic chiasm (arrow) to the floor of the sella.
(d) Craniopharyngioma: Cranial MRI. Coronal T1-weighted section after gadolinium enhancement. The tumour signal intensity on the T1 image and only part of the periphery of the tumour enhances. The carotid arteries have a low signal intensity (black arrows) due to the rapid flow within them and are deviated laterally and superiorly by the mass (C), which arises out of the pituitary fossa (P). Reproduced from Balen AH. *Infertility in Practice*, 4th edn. London: Informa Healthcare, 2014, with permission.

although an MRI scan should be performed if symptoms suggestive of tumour re-expansion occur, and it is necessary to recommence bromocriptine therapy if there is continuing suprasellar expansion. These patients also require expert assessment of their visual fields during pregnancy.

4 Polycystic Ovary Syndrome (WHO Group II)

PCOS accounts for approximately 80–90% of women with anovulatory infertility, which in turn comprises about a third of those attending the infertility clinic. A number of guidelines have been written for the management of anovulatory PCOS [7,8], the most recent by the World Health Organisation.

Various factors influence ovarian function and fertility, the most important being obesity. A patient's weight correlates with both an increased rate of cycle disturbance and infertility secondary to disturbances in insulin metabolism. Monitoring treatment is also harder in obese women because their ovaries are more difficult to see on ultrasound scans, thus raising the risk of missing multiple ovulation and multiple pregnancy. Hypersecretion of LH is found in 40% of women with PCOS and is associated with a reduced chance of conception and an increased risk of miscarriage, possibly through an adverse effect of LH on oocyte maturation. Elevated LH concentrations are more often found in slim women with PCOS, whilst those who are overweight are more likely to be hyperinsulinemic.

4.1 Obesity and Lifestyle

Obesity worsens both symptomatology and the endocrine profile and so obese women (BMI > 30 kg/m2) should be encouraged to lose weight, by a combination of calorie restriction and exercise. Weight loss improves the endocrine profile and the likelihood of ovulation and of a healthy pregnancy. There is no evidence that women with PCOS benefit from a specific diet compared with obese women without PCOS [9]. The right diet for an individual is one that is practical, sustainable and compatible with her lifestyle. It is sensible to reduce glycemic load by lowering sugar content in favour of more complex carbohydrates and to avoid fatty foods. Meal replacement therapy or low calorie diets may be appropriate: it is often helpful to refer to a dietitian, if available. An increase in physical activity is essential, preferably as part of the daily routine. Thirty minutes per day of brisk exercise is encouraged to maintain health, but to lose weight, or sustain weight loss, 60 to 90 minutes per day is advised. Concurrent behavioural therapy improves the chances of success of any method of weight loss. There are no medications that have been shown to assist with long-term weight reduction. Bariatric surgery is used increasingly because of the global epidemic of obesity and certainly has a role in the management of obese women with PCOS [10]. It is recommended by some that anyone with a BMI of greater than 40 kg/m2 should be referred for consideration of bariatric surgery. If there are comorbidities, such as Type 2 diabetes (DM2), then the BMI cut-off for surgery is lower at 30–35 kg/m2.

4.2 Ovulation Induction Therapies

Strategies to induce ovulation include weight loss, oral anti-oestrogens (principally clomifene citrate), parenteral gonadotrophin therapy and laparoscopic ovarian surgery. There have been no adequately powered randomized studies to determine which of these therapies provides the best overall chance of an ongoing pregnancy when used as first-line therapy. Women with PCOS are at risk of OHSS and so ovulation induction has to be carefully monitored with serial ultrasound scans. The realization of an association between hyperinsulinemia and PCOS has resulted in the use of insulin-sensitizing agents such as metformin, although results have been disappointing.

Carefully conducted and monitored ovulation induction can achieve good cumulative conception rates, and, furthermore, multiple pregnancy rates can be minimized with strict adherence to criteria that limit the number of follicles that are permitted to ovulate.

4.3 Clomifene Citrate Therapy

The anti-oestrogen clomifene citrate (CC) has traditionally been used as first-line therapy for anovulatory PCOS [7–8,11]. Clomifene citrate therapy is usually commenced on day 2 of the cycle and given for five days. If the patient has oligo/amenorrhea, it is necessary to exclude pregnancy and then induce a withdrawal bleed with a short course of a progestogen, such as medroxyprogesterone acetate 20 mg/day for 5 to 10 days. The starting dose of CC is 50 mg/day, for 5 days beginning on days 3–5 of the menstrual cycle (the first day of bleeding is considered day 1 of the cycle). If the patient has not menstruated by day 35 and she is not pregnant, a progestogen-induced withdrawal bleed should be initiated. The dose of CC may be increased to 100 mg if there is no response. Doses of 150 mg/day or more appear not to be of benefit. If there is an exuberant response to 50 mg/day, as in some women with PCOS, the dose can be decreased to 25 mg/day. Discontinuation of CC therapy should be considered if the patient is anovulatory after the dose has been increased up to 100 mg/day. If the patient is ovulating, conception is expected to occur at a rate determined by factors such as the patient's age. Clomifene citrate induces ovulation in approximately 70–85% of patients and approximately 60–70% should be pregnant by six cycles of therapy.

Clomifene citrate may cause an exaggeration in the hypersecretion of LH and have anti-oestrogenic effects on the endometrium and cervical mucus. We suggest measuring LH on day 8 of the cycle and if persistently elevated then move on to alternative therapy as the chance of conception is reduced and the risk of miscarriage increased [12,13]. All women who are prescribed CC should be carefully monitored with a combination of endocrine and ultrasonographic assessment of follicular growth and ovulation because of the risk of multiple pregnancies, which is approximately 10%. Clomifene therapy should therefore be prescribed and managed by specialists in reproductive medicine.

If pregnancy has not occurred after 6–9 normal ovulatory cycles, it is then reasonable to offer the couple assisted conception (that is in vitro fertilization (IVF)).

Patients with anovulatory infertility who are resistant to anti-oestrogens may be prescribed parenteral gonadotrophin therapy or treated with laparoscopic ovarian surgery. The term 'clomifene-resistance', strictly speaking, refers to a failure to ovulate rather than failure to conceive despite ovulation, which should be termed 'clomifene-failure'.

4.4 Aromatase Inhibitors

For completeness we need to consider the use of aromatase inhibitors such as letrozole that are used for advanced breast cancer and have been introduced as a treatment option for ovulation induction. Inhibition of the aromatase enzyme decreases the aromatization of androgens to oestrogens that in turn releases the hypothalamic–pituitary axis from negative feedback of oestrogen. Adverse effects on the endometrium and cervical mucus are considerably less than with CC and there are reports of good pregnancy rates with a lower incidence of multiple pregnancies [14].

Despite the potential advantages over CC, the use of letrozole was discouraged following a report at a meeting (that has not been published in a peer-reviewed journal) that suggested a significant increase in congenital malformations in newborns in letrozole-treated pregnancies. However, more recent studies have not supported the teratogenic effect of letrozole and a recent randomized controlled trial demonstrated a significantly higher live birth rate when compared with CC [15]. In this study, 750 women were randomized to receive letrozole or CC for up to five treatment cycles. The mean BMI of participants was 35 kg/m2. Each drug was taken for five days starting on day 3 of either a natural cycle or a progestogen-induced bleed. The starting doses were 50 mg of CC or 2.5 mg of letrozole; each was increased if there was no response to 100 mg and 5 mg respectively, to a maximum of 150 mg and 7.5 mg. There was a higher cumulative ovulation rate with letrozole, 61.7% versus 48.3% ($p < 0.001$). Live births were achieved in 103 of 374 patients (27.5%) taking letrozole and 72 of 376 (19.1%) in the CC group (rate ratio 1.44, 95% CI 1.10–1.87) [15].

A 2014 Cochrane review of 26 randomized controlled trials (RCTs) (5,560 women) compared letrozole with placebo, CC or laparoscopic ovarian drilling [16]. In 9 studies comparing letrozole with CC (4,783 women), the odds ratio for live birth favoured letrozole (OR 1.64, 95% CI 1.32–2.04) and there was a reduction in the rate of multiple pregnancy (OR 0.38, 95% CI 0.17–0.84) [16].

Therefore, the WHO guidance has supported the use of letrozole as first- line therapy for those countries where its use is permitted for this indication (which currently does not include the United Kingdom) [7]. It is still prudent to perform more research to assess the safety and efficacy of aromatase inhibitors for ovulation induction.

4.5 Gonadotrophin Therapy

Gonadotrophin therapy is indicated for women with anovulatory PCOS who have been treated with anti-oestrogens if they have failed to ovulate or if they have a response to clomifene that is likely to reduce their chance of conception (e.g. persistent hypersecretion of LH, anti-oestrogenic effect on endometrium).

In order to prevent the risks of overstimulation and multiple pregnancy, a low-dose step-up regimen should be used with a daily starting dose of 25–50 IU of FSH or hMG. This is only increased after 14 days if there is no response and then by only half an ampoule every 7 days. Treatment cycles using this approach can be quite long – up to 28–35 days – but the risk of multiple follicular growth is low and the multiple pregnancy rate is less than 5%. It can be extremely difficult to predict the response to stimulation of a woman with polycystic ovaries – indeed this is the greatest therapeutic challenge in all ovulation induction therapies. The polycystic ovary is characteristically quiescent, at least when viewed by ultrasound, before often exhibiting an exuberant and explosive response to stimulation. It can be very challenging to stimulate the development of a single dominant follicle.

Ovulation is triggered with a single subcutaneous injection of hCG 5000 units, when there has been the development of at least one follicle of at least 17 mm in its largest diameter. In order to reduce the risks of multiple pregnancy and OHSS, the exclusion criteria for hCG administration are the development of a total of two or more follicles larger than 14 mm in diameter. In overstimulated cycles hCG is withheld, and the patient counselled about the risks and advised to refrain from sexual intercourse. The cumulative conception and live birth rates after six months should be 65–70% and 55–60%, respectively. If conception has failed to occur after six ovulatory cycles in a woman younger than 25 years or after 12 ovulatory cycles in women older than 25, then it can be assumed that anovulation is unlikely to be the cause of the couple's infertility and assisted conception (usually IVF) is now indicated [7–8].

4.6 Insulin-Sensitizing Agents

It is logical to assume that therapy that achieves a fall in serum insulin concentrations should improve the symptoms of PCOS. The biguanide metformin both inhibits the production of hepatic glucose, thereby decreasing insulin secretion and also enhances insulin sensitivity at the cellular level. Many studies have now been carried out to evaluate the reproductive effects of metformin in patients with PCOS. Initial studies appeared to be promising, suggesting that metformin could improve fertility in women with PCOS, however, more recent large RCTs have observed limited benefit from metformin as either first-line therapy or in combination with other drugs in enhancing the chance of a live birth [7–8, 17].

Metformin, whilst associated with initial gastrointestinal side effects, is usually well tolerated and not complicated by hypoglycaemia. It also has a good safety profile, with no evidence of teratogenicity. The latest update of the Cochrane review of insulin-sensitizing agents and PCOS included 46 trials with a total of 4,227 participants [17]. Forty of these studies investigated metformin, involving 3,848 patients, with a median daily dose of metformin of 1500 mg and durations ranging from 4 to 60 weeks [17]. This systematic review concluded that metformin may improve menstrual frequency and ovulation rate, which may result in a marginal improvement in live birth rate when compared with placebo. Clinical pregnancy rates were improved for metformin versus placebo (OR 1.93, 95% CI 1.42 to 2.64, 9 RCTs, 1,027 women). This was also reflected in higher live birth rates with metformin versus placebo across 2 studies (OR 1.64; (1.02, 2.63), 385 women, p = 0.04). This review update includes a recent large Scandinavian study of 329 women, who received metformin (1500–2000 mg/day) or placebo for three months prior to fertility treatment and then for a further nine months during treatment and up to 12 weeks of gestation. They showed an increase in pregnancy rate from 40.4% to 53.6% (OR 1.61, 95% CI 1.13–2.29), with the greatest benefit seen in obese women [18]. Whilst there was no reduction in miscarriage rate, the live birth rate was increased in those who received metformin (41.9% vs 28.8%, p = 0.014) [18].

When metformin is added to CC in women with CC-resistance, clinical pregnancy rate is increased in both obese and non-obese patients (OR 1.59, 95% CI 1.25–2.02, 14 trials, I2 42%) [17]. However, the addition of metformin to CC did not improve live birth rates (OR 1.21, 95% CI 0.91–1.61, 8 trials, I2 30%). However, in the studies that compared metformin versus CC, there was evidence of an improved live birth rate (OR 0.3, 95% CI 0.17–0.52, 2 trials, 500 women) and clinical pregnancy rate (OR 0.34, 95% 0.21–0.55, 2 trials, 500 women) in the women (BMI > 30 kg/m2) taking CC [17].

Given the varied risk benefit ratio of other insulin sensitizing agents, metformin remains the main therapy in the management of infertility in PCOS women and there is insufficient evidence to recommend the use of other insulin sensitizers such as thiazolidinediones, d-chiro-inositol and myo-inositol in the treatment of anovulatory PCOS. Newer insulin sensitizing agents such as glucagon-like peptide-1 analogues have been studied more recently in women with PCOS. These agents include exenatide and liraglutide and are currently licensed for the treatment of DM2 and the latter also for obesity.

In summary, metformin has limited value in the management of anovulatory PCOS but could be used alone to improve ovulation rate and pregnancy rate, if facilities are not available for monitoring of CC or letrozole (which are more effective). Metformin combined with CC for CC-resistant patients may improve pregnancy rates but has not been shown to increase live births. A recent systematic review has also indicated that metformin therapy combined with lifestyle modification in women with PCOS may improve body weight [19]. For those women with PCOS and impaired glucose tolerance or DM2, metformin has a better defined role combined, of course, with lifestyle modification.

4.7 Surgical Ovulation Induction

An alternative to gonadotrophin therapy for CC-resistant PCOS is laparoscopic ovarian diathermy (LOD) (often referred to as 'ovarian drilling' or laparoscopic electrocautery 'LEO'), which has replaced the more invasive and damaging technique of ovarian wedge resection [7–8]. Laparoscopic ovarian surgery is free of multiple pregnancy risk and OHSS and does not require intensive USS monitoring. In addition, laparoscopic ovarian surgery is a useful therapy for anovulatory women with PCOS who fail to respond to CC and who persistently hypersecrete LH, need a laparoscopic assessment of their pelvis or who live too far away from the clinic to be able to attend for the intensive monitoring required of gonadotrophin therapy. Only fully trained laparoscopic surgeons should perform laparoscopic ovarian surgery.

After LOD, with restoration of ovarian activity, serum concentrations of LH and testosterone fall. Response depends on pretreatment characteristics, with those who are slim and with high basal LH concentrations having a better clinical and endocrine response. Commonly employed methods for laparoscopic surgery include monopolar or bipolar electrocautery (diathermy) and laser. The larger the amount of damage to the surface of the ovary, the greater is the risk of peri-ovarian adhesion formation. This has led to a strategy of minimizing the number of diathermy points to 4 per ovary for 4 seconds at 40 watts [7–8]. The risk of adhesion formation is far less after laparoscopic ovarian diathermy (10–20% of cases) than with wedge resection (100% in some series) and the adhesions that do form are usually fine and of limited clinical significance. The instillation of 500–1000 mLs of an isotonic solution into the pouch of Douglas, cools the ovaries in order to prevent heat injury to adjacent tissues and reduce the risk of the adhesion formation.

The largest RCT to date is the multicentre study performed in the Netherlands in which 168 CC-resistant patients, were randomized to either LOD (n = 83) or ovulation induction with recombinant FSH (rFSH, n = 65) [20]. The initial cumulative pregnancy rate after six months was 34% in the LOD arm versus 67% with rFSH. Those who did not ovulate in response to LOD were then given first CC and then rFSH so by 12 months the cumulative pregnancy rate was similar in each group at 67% [20]. Thus, those treated with LOD took longer to conceive and 54% required additional medical ovulation induction therapy. Furthermore the duration of effect may be limited to a few months, although some report more prolonged efficacy.

4.8 IVF in Women with Polycystic Ovaries

In vitro fertilization is not the first-line treatment for PCOS, but many patients with the syndrome may be referred for IVF, either because there is another reason for their infertility or because they fail to conceive despite ovulating (whether spontaneously or with assistance) – i.e. their infertility remains unexplained. Furthermore, approximately 25–30% of women have polycystic ovaries as detected by ultrasound scan. Many will have little in the way of symptoms and may present for assisted conception treatment because of other reasons (for example tubal factor or male factor). When stimulated, these women with asymptomatic polycystic ovaries have a tendency to respond sensitively and are at increased risk of developing OHSS. Care must therefore be taken and there is evidence of reduced risk if protocols using a GnRH antagonist are employed (see Chapter 21 'The Risks of Assisted Reproduction').

4.9 Complications of Ovulation Induction

Multiple pregnancy and OHSS are the most serious complications that should be avoided in ovulation induction treatment. Multiple pregnancy, even twins, is undesirable due to increased risk of perinatal mortality and morbidity. Women with PCOS are at an increased risk of developing OHSS. This occurs if many follicles are stimulated, leading to ascites, pleural and, sometimes, pericardial effusions with the symptoms of abdominal distension, discomfort, nausea, vomiting and difficult breathing. Hospitalization is sometimes necessary in order for intravenous fluids (colloids preferable to crystalloids) and heparin to be given to prevent dehydration and thromboembolism. Although this condition is rare it is a potentially fatal complication and should be avoidable with appropriate monitoring of treatment.

4.10 Pregnancy Outcomes

Women with PCOS may conceive naturally or, if they have anovulatory infertility, by ovulation induction. In addition to anovulation there may be other factors that contribute to subfertility in women with PCOS including the effects of obesity, metabolic, inflammatory and endocrine abnormalities on oocyte quality and fetal development. Women who are obese are also more likely to experience miscarriage and pregnancy complications. A number of studies have compared pregnancy outcomes in women with PCOS compared with controls and have found that women with PCOS demonstrated a significantly higher risk of developing gestational diabetes, pregnancy-induced hypertension, pre-eclampsia, adverse neonatal outcomes and preterm birth [21]. Their babies had a significantly higher risk of admission to a neonatal intensive care unit and a higher perinatal mortality, unrelated to multiple births. The potential mechanisms for these problems include obesity, altered glucose metabolism and disturbances in uterine blood flow and so careful monitoring of pregnancy is required.

5 Hypergonadotrophic Hypogonadism (WHO Group III)

Women in this group constitute 5% of all the causes of anovulation. They are amenorrhoeic and have low serum oestradiol and anti-Mullerian hormone (AMH) concentrations and elevated serum FSH concentrations indicating ovarian failure. The only realistic treatment option for these patients is egg donation. In addition, these women will require long-term hormone replacement (HRT) to prevent deleterious effects of hypo-oestrogenism on their bones. Occasional ovulations may occur unpredictably in some women who have just entered a state of premature ovarian insufficiency and so if pregnancy would be a disaster they should be advised to take the combined oral contraceptive pill (COCP); if, however, pregnancy is desired, the use of a standard HRT preparation should not inhibit ovulation.

6 Conclusion

The underlying principle of ovulation induction should be to use the lowest effective dose of drugs for achieving mono-follicular ovulation and to avoid the risk of multiple pregnancy and OHSS. The key to successful ovulation induction is determined by appropriate patient selection whereby health is optimized by modification of lifestyle before medical treatment is offered.

References

1. Balen AH, Dresner M, Scott EM, Drife JO. Should obese women with polycystic ovary syndrome (PCOS) receive treatment for infertility? *BMJ* 2006: 332: 434–435

2. Balen AH, Anderson R. Impact of obesity on female reproductive health: British Fertility Society, Police and Practice Guidelines. *Hum Fertil* 2007; 10: 195–206.

3. Shoham Z, Balen AH, Patel A, Jacobs HS. Results of ovulation induction using human menopausal gonadotropins or purified follicle-stimulating hormone in hypogonadotropic hypogonadism patients. *Fertil Steril* 1991; 56: 1048–53.

4. White DM, Polson DW, Kiddy D et al. Induction of ovulation with low-dose gonadotropins in polycystic ovary syndrome: an analysis of 109 pregnancies in 225 women. *J Clin Endocrinol Metab* 1996; 81: 3821–4.

5. European and Australian Multicentre Study. Co-treatment with growth hormone and gonadotrophin for ovulation induction in hypogonadotrophic patients: a prospective randomized, placebo controlled, dose response study. *Fertil Steril* 1995; 64: 917–23.

6. Colao A, Abs R, Bárcena DG, Chanso P, Paulus W, Kleinberg DL. Pregnancy outcomes following cabergoline treatment: extended results from a 12-year observational study. *Clin Endocrinol* 2008; 68: 66–71.

7. Balen AH, Morley LC, Misso M, Franks S, Legro RS, Wijeyaratne CN, Stener-Victorin E, Norman RJ, Fauser BJCM, Teede H. WHO recommendations for the management of anovulatory infertility in women with polycystic ovary syndrome (PCOS). *Hum Reprod Update* 2016; doi: 10.1093/humupd/dmw025.

8. *Current Management of Polycystic Ovary Syndrome.* Edited by Adam Balen, Steve Franks, Roy Homburg and Sean Kehoe. Proceedings of 59th RCOG Study Group, RCOG Press, London 2010.

9. Moran LJ, Hutchison SK, Norman RJ, Teede HJ. Lifestyle changes in women with polycystic ovary syndrome. *Cochrane Database Syst Rev* 2011; Issue 2. Art. No.: CD007506.

10. Scholtz S, Le Roux C, Balen AH. The role of bariatric surgery in the management of female fertility. RCOG Scientific Impact Paper number 17, October 2015. www.rcog.org.uk/globalassets/documents/guidelines/scientific-impact-papers/sip_17.pdf

11. Beck JI, Boothroyd C, Proctor M, Farquhar C, Hughes E. Oral anti-oestrogens and medical adjuncts for subfertility associated with anovulation. *Cochrane Database Syst Rev* 2005; Issue 1. Art. No.: CD002249; doi: 10.1002/14651858.CD002249.pub3.

12. Kousta E, White DM, Franks S. Modern use of clomifene citrate in induction of ovulation. *Hum Reprod Update* 1997; 3: 359–65.

13. Shoham Z, Borenstein R, Lunenfeld B, Pariente C. Hormonal profiles following clomifene citrate therapy in conception and non-conception

cycles. *Clin Endocrinol* 1990; 33: 271–8.

14. Casper RF, Mitwally MF. 2006 Review: aromatase inhibitors for ovulation induction. *J Clin Endocrinol Metab* 2006 Mar; 91(3): 760–71

15. Legro RS, Brzyski RG, Diamond MP, Coutifaris C, Schlaff WD, Casson P, Christman GM, Huang H, Yan Q, Alvero R, Haisenleder DJ, Barnhart KT, Bates GW, Usadi R, Lucidi S, Baker V, Trussell JC, Krawetz SA, Snyder P, Ohl D, Santoro N, Eisenberg E, Zhang H, Network NRM. Letrozole versus clomiphene for infertility in the polycystic ovary syndrome. *N Engl J Med* 2014; 371: 119–29.

16. Franik S, Kremer JA, Nelen WL, Farquhar C. Aromatase inhibitors for subfertile women with polycystic ovary syndrome. *Cochrane Database Syst*

Rev. 2014; Issue 2. Art. No.: CD010287. doi: 10.1002/14651858.CD010287.pub2.

17. Morley LC, Tang T, Yasmin E, Lord JM, Norman RJ, Balen AH. Insulin-sensitising drugs (metformin, rosiglitazone, pioglitazone, D-chiro-inositol) for women with polycystic ovary syndrome, oligo amenorrhoea and subfertility. *Cochrane Database Syst Rev.* 2015; Issue 9. Art. No.: CD003053. doi: 10.1002/14651858.CD003053.pub6.

18. Morin-papunen L, Rantala AS, Unkila-Kallio L, Tiitinen A, Hippeläinen M, Perheentupa, A, Tinkanen H, Bloigu R, Puukka K, Ruokonen A, Tapanainen, JS. Metformin improves pregnancy and live-birth rates in women with polycystic ovary syndrome (PCOS): a multicenter, double-blind, placebo-controlled

randomized trial. *J Clin Endocrinol Metab* 2012; 97: 1492–500.

19. Naderpoor N, Shorakae S, de Courten B, Misso ML, Moran LJ, Teede HJ. Metformin and lifestyle modification in PCOS: systematic review and meta-analysis. *Human Reprod Update* 2015; 21: 560–574.

20. Bayram N, van Wely M, Kaaijk EM, Bossuyt PMM, van der Veen F. Using an electrocautery strategy or recombinant FSH to induce ovulation in polycystic ovary syndrome: a randomised controlled trial. *BMJ* 2004; 328: 192–5.

21. Boomsma, CM, Eijkemans, MJ, Hughes, EG, Visser, GH, Fauser, BC, Macklon, NS. A meta-analysis of pregnancy outcomes in women with polycystic ovary syndrome. *Hum Reprod Update* 2006; 12, 673–83.

The Role of Regulation in Reproductive Medicine

Nick Jones

Debra Bloor

1 Background

The Human Fertilisation and Embryology Authority (HFEA) started work on 1 August 1991. However, its formation was the result of a long process of discussion and development of in vitro fertilization (IVF) regulation in the United Kingdom in summary:

- 1982 – Warnock Committee Inquiry starts. The Warnock Committee was established in July 1982 'to consider recent and potential developments in medicine and science related to human fertilisation and embryology; to consider what policies and safeguards should be applied, including consideration of the social, ethical, and legal implications of these developments; and to make recommendations'.
- 1984 – Warnock Report published 18 July. It highlighted the 'special status' of the embryo and proposed the establishment of a regulator.
- 1987 – Human Fertilisation and Embryology: A framework for legislation (Cm 259). White paper picking up the recommendations of the Warnock Report.
- 1990 – Human Fertilisation and Embryology Act
- 1991 – Human Fertilisation and Embryology Act 1990 comes into force
- The HFEA officially starts work on the 1st of August 1991.
- 2007 – Human Fertilisation and Embryology Bill: Major review of fertility legislation, updating and amending the 1990 Act.
- 2009 – Human Fertilisation and Embryology Act 2008[1] comes into force. New provisions come into force in April and October 2009, additional changes in April 2010.

The HFEA licenses all clinics and establishments in the United Kingdom undertaking assisted reproduction and human embryo research. It issues types of licences, depending on which activities are carried out. For example, a clinic carrying out IVF or associated treatments will need to obtain a 'Treatment and Storage' licence. If it wishes to extend or change the range of activities carried out, it would need to apply to vary its licence.

The main types of licences are as follows:

- Storage
- Treatment – for clinics offering intrauterine insemination (IUI) and other basic fertility treatments which do not involve the creation of embryos
- Treatment and storage – for clinics offering IVF, intracytoplasmic sperm injection (ICSI) and gamete and embryo storage
- Treatment (including embryo testing) and storage – for clinics offering IVF, ICSI, gamete and embryo storage and embryo testing
- Research – for laboratories carrying out research on human embryos

The HFEA monitors clinics' performance, expects clinics to report adverse incidents and checks compliance with standards at inspection. Most clinics are granted a four-year licence, and are usually inspected every two years. If there are concerns about a clinic, inspections may be more frequent – particularly if it is considered the safety of patients, embryos and gametes are at risk. The purpose of an inspection is to assess a clinic's compliance with the Human Fertilisation and Embryology Act 1990 (as amended), licence conditions, General Directions and the provisions of the Code of Practice [2]. Inspection is intended to

- provide an independent and professional perspective on the running of the clinic
- promote good practice so that clinics can improve the quality of service they provide to patients and donors
- provide clinics with a positive learning experience

- provide clinics with the opportunity to feed back on their experience of the inspection process, to assist the HFEA improve its procedures
- give patients reliable information about a clinic's compliance with statutory and other obligations, and about the quality and safety of licensed activities undertaken at that centre
- be evidence-based, consistent, proportionate and focused on risk – to add value for clinics and people using services.

The clinic is provided an opportunity by the inspector to prepare for the inspection to minimise potential disruption to activities being carried out on the day. Some inspections are unannounced or, where relevant, with short notice (where clinics have low activity levels) providing an opportunity to see things as they are. The onus is on clinics to demonstrate compliance, not on inspectors to find fault. There is a focus on quality and safety of patient care and the protection of the embryo. Most of the time is spent on direct observation of practice, with some sampling of documentation and records.

The inspection team usually consists of two to four inspectors, depending on the size of the clinic and the services it offers. The inspectors are HFEA staff members, supplemented by external advisors (doctor, nurse, embryologist, counsellor working in licensed centres) who occasionally form part of the inspection team.

During the inspection of new clinics or clinics applying to renew their licence, the inspection team evaluates compliance with all relevant standard licence conditions. A focused *interim* inspection takes place midway through the four-year inspection cycle and is usually unannounced. During the interim inspection the inspection team gathers information without spending too much time talking to clinic staff or reviewing documentation. Instead, practice is observed and patients are asked about their experiences of care. The inspection team also evaluates

- the actions taken by the clinic to address any areas of non-compliance identified either at the previous inspection, or through continuous monitoring;
- compliance with the following inspection areas:
  - quality of service (including outcomes and multiple pregnancy rates);
  - patient experience;
  - effectiveness of witnessing;

  - staffing levels;
  - management of stored gametes and embryos;
  - the suitability of the premises and facilities for surgical procedures;
  - medicines' management practices;
  - infection prevention and control practices;
  - compliance with requirements to use CE marked medical devices (particularly culture medium and reagents);
  - effectiveness of the quality management system and review of the centre's website;
- The inspection report will also comment on information from on-going monitoring of clinics' performance and on information in self assessment questionnaires.

Feedback is provided to the Person Responsible (PR) on the day of inspection. After the inspection, the HFEA inspector writes a report, which includes areas of good practice and those areas of practice which require improvement. The inspection report comments on the actions taken by the clinic to address areas of non-compliance identified. Areas of practice that require improvement are divided into the following categories:

- A critical area of non-compliance – a critical area of non-compliance is an area of practice which poses a significant risk of causing harm to a patient, donor, embryo or to a child who may be born as a result of treatment services.
- A major area of non-compliance – a major area of non-compliance is an area of practice which

  - poses an indirect risk of causing harm to a patient, donor, embryo or to a child who may be born as a result of treatment services;
  - indicates a major shortcoming from the statutory requirements;
  - indicates a failure of the Person Responsible to carry out his/her legal duties;
  - is a combination of several 'other' areas of non-compliance, none of which on their own may be major but which together may represent a major area of non-compliance.

- An 'other' area of non-compliance – a departure from non-major statutory requirements or good practice.

The Person Responsible is given two weeks to share the report with the team and to comment on the report.

A final report is presented to a HFEA licensing committee, which decides whether the licence should be renewed or continued (depending on the type of inspection) and if there are any conditions that must be fulfilled. The final report and minutes from the licensing committee meeting are published on the HFEA website *Choose a Fertility Clinic* section. The inspection team continues to monitor the actions taken by the clinic, to ensure that all actions are addressed.

2 Analysis

The HFEA adopts a high-trust model – a model in which trust is earned through disclosure of problems (incidents and material events), implementation of recommendations for improvements from inspections and a belief that clinics strive for and are motivated by quality and improvement.

The regulatory landscape in which the HFEA operates changes continually and in response it must expect to adapt and change.

For example, a raft of new requirements was transposed into the Act in 2007. Notably at this time, it became a mandatory requirement for clinics to have documented and validated processes and procedures and to establish a quality management system (QMS) to support continuous improvement. In response, the HFEA's inspection regime had a greater focus on clinics' documentation. Moreover, further changes to the Act in 2009 significantly updated the consent regime and introduced complex new consent requirements which in turn resulted in a continued focus on clinics' consent procedures and documentation of consent. And in 2012 the HFEA extended its remit to inspect a number of additional clinical activities (safeguarding, infection control, medicines management and the pre-, peri- and post-operative pathway) so that clinics in England that only carry out HFEA licensable activity could be exempted from the requirement to be registered with the Care Quality Commission (the health and social care regulator in England).

It was (and remains) straightforward to inspect documentation. It is harder to assess the quality of processes themselves and to evaluate the quality of services provided and experienced by patients.

The HFEA seeks to learn from its clinical governance and inspection activities and its assessment is that while clinics 'tick the box' in carrying out audits and in conducting root cause analysis to identify the causes of incidents, complaints and/or poor

> **Box 16.1**
>
> **Grade A:** involves severe harm to one person (such as a death, being implanted with the wrong embryo or birth of an affected child following genetic testing) or major harm to many (such as the failure of a frozen storage unit containing the embryos of many patients).
>
> **Grade B:** involves serious harm to one person (such as the loss or damage of embryos for one patient) or moderate harm to many (such as sensitive personal data about more than one patient being sent to the wrong recipient).
>
> **Grade C:** involves minor harm, such as one of many eggs being rendered unusable in the laboratory.

performance, in common with the healthcare sector in general, these activities may not always be effective in identifying *opportunities* for improvement.

In consideration of this, since 2014 the HFEA has phrased recommendations for improvement to encourage clinics to consider why a non-compliance has evaded their QMS; why an incident has occurred; or why a patient has experienced poor service. Having identified the *root cause*, clinics are encouraged to identify corrective actions specific to their own circumstances and then to assess the effectiveness of the corrective actions. Additionally, the HFEA is working closely with clinics that see recurrence of C grade incidents (Box 16.1) or whose root cause analysis is deficient. This approach aims to support the continued development of a 'learning culture' that is intended to be more effective in driving improvement. Since early 2015, the HFEA has also focused on whether clinics have learned from incidents (both their own and those documented in the HFEA annual review), complaints and guidance in the course of interim inspections.

The culture in clinics may not be susceptible to such incentives or such approaches may not bring about fast results. However, the HFEA believes that a change in approach is warranted to continue to raise the bar to encourage continuous improvement in the quality of service provided by clinics.

The rest of this chapter summarises the results of a recent analysis of the HFEA's activities relating to its core activities leading to this assessment. It addresses three principal activities:

1. Ongoing monitoring of clinic performance using the 'risk-based assessment tool';

2. a review of adverse incidents reported by clinics to the HFEA;
3. findings from inspection.

2.1 Risk-Based Assessment Tool

The HFEA's ability to undertake 'on-going' monitoring of a clinic's performance between inspection visits was enhanced by the introduction, in April 2011, of a risk-based assessment tool (RBAT) [3] that provides information about licensed clinics' performance in near to real time. Clinics have been able to access their own RBAT outputs through the HFEA's clinic portal since April 2012 and information from RBAT analysis has routinely been included in inspection reports since then. The risk tool measures performance in relation to

- outcomes in terms of both clinical pregnancy rates and clinical multiple pregnancy rates;
- submission of critical register information relating to treatments using donor gametes;
- timeliness of payment of monthly HFEA invoices.

Where the trend analysis performed by RBAT suggests that there may be a dip in performance, an automated alert is sent to the Person Responsible and clinics are expected to act on these alerts to investigate any possible causal factors and take corrective action if appropriate.

Analysis of risk tool outputs (Figure 16.1) suggests that clinics had fewer alerts related to success rates in 2014/15. While it is difficult to establish a cause and effect of regulatory activities in respect of this improvement, the ongoing reduction suggests that centres are taking action to continually improve success rates. It is likely that the HFEA's proactive real time monitoring – most significantly interventions should performance trends continue on a negative trajectory – plays a role in encouraging this.

Only four clinics received four or more alerts relating to multiple pregnancies. Although a small number of clinics continue to struggle to meet the 10% multiple birth target, the HFEA discusses and motivates these clinics to encourage change; ultimately however, if these interventions fail to have an impact, then it is recognised that the significant risk posed by multiple births are such that regulatory action may be initiated in line with the HFEA Compliance and Enforcement Policy [4].

Alerts related to errors in the submission of information to the HFEA register about treatments involving donor gametes increased in 2014/15: the HFEA's Information for Quality programme is expected to have a significant impact on improving the quality of data submission although it is likely to be some time before this work has a measurable impact.

By providing the information required for clinics to monitor their own performance in comparison to national norms, the HFEA targets and helps clinics that may be struggling to improve the quality of care given to patients. Overall, clinics respond positively to requests to act on these alerts.

2.2 A Review of Adverse Incidents Reported by Clinics to the HFEA

An estimated 1% of the 60,000 cycles of IVF treatment that are carried out in the United Kingdom each

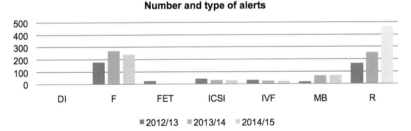

Number and type of alerts

■ 2012/13 ■ 2013/14 ▪ 2014/15

Fig. 16.1 The number and type of risk tool alerts in each of the last three years

F: Finance; the sum of all alerts related to delay or non-payment of invoices
R: Register; the sum of all alerts related to errors in reporting of treatments involving donor gametes
MB: Multiple births; the sum of all alerts related to trends in clinical multiple pregnancy rates as measured against the relevant target
ICSI: the sum of all alerts related to trends in clinical pregnancy rates following ICSI treatments
IVF: the sum of all alerts related to trends in clinical pregnancy rates following IVF treatments
DI: the sum of all alerts related to trends in clinical pregnancy rates following DI treatments
FET: the sum of all alerts related to trends in clinical pregnancy rates following frozen treatment cycles (IVF and ICSI).

year are affected by some sort of adverse incident. The Person Responsible for an HFEA licensed clinic has a statutory duty to report and analyse the causes of incidents. Similarly, the Authority has a duty to investigate and take appropriate control measures in relation to reported incidents.

The primary reason for reporting and investigating incidents is to improve safety for patients, embryos and clinic staff. Reporting an incident is not enough on its own; to be most effective, learning should be extracted from each and every incident to minimise the risk of it happening again.

In December 2014, the HFEA published its first annual report, looking at incidents reported by clinics between 1 January 2013 and 31 December 2013. The second annual report for incidents reported in 2014 was published in September 2015 [5] and a third in 2018 [6].

To promote transparency and information sharing the HFEA provides a dedicated governance section on its website since 2014. This includes links to all published A grade incident (Box 16.1) investigation reports and the accompanying Licence Committee minutes, the risk grading matrix, relevant definitions and descriptions of the types of incidents that fall into the different incident categories.

HFEA inspectors have also adjusted the focus of inspection to look for evidence that clinics have learnt from incidents rather than focussing on clinics' processes for incident reporting. Moreover, the HFEA's clinical governance lead provides bespoke incident training sessions where clinics seem to be struggling to recognise when an incident should be reported to the HFEA to individual clinics, or where a high number of incidents are reported. This encourages clinics to carry out an in-depth analysis of the causes of incidents (root cause analysis using the 'five-why' technique) [6]. This work is in the early stages; however, one clinic has managed to reduce its administration incidents from nine in 2014 to two this year following a focussed site visit.

The HFEA's monthly email for licensed clinics (clinic focus) is being used as a platform to share ad hoc lessons from incidents and also to disseminate good practice advice on handling complaints and learning disseminated by other professional bodies.

The HFEA has a national role in gathering information on incidents, identifying patterns and disseminating learning across the sector so that clinics can learn from the mistakes of others. Analysis of incidents suggests that clinics may need more time to embed learning and more support to extract learning from incidents. On this basis the HFEA has refreshed its approach to inspection and clinical governance activities in an attempt to support and encourage clinics in the continued development of a learning culture.

2.3 Findings from Inspection

In 2014/15 there were 59 inspections of treatment and/or storage clinics:

- 28 renewal inspections
- 14 interim inspections and
- 17 inspections of other types (initial/new premises/additional/clinical governance).

All inspections in 2014/15 identified areas of non-compliance (Figure 16.2), although three inspections identified only 'other' areas of non-compliance. When critical and major areas of non-compliance are considered, 32 inspections identified fewer than 10 areas of non-compliance while six inspections identified more than 10 areas of non-compliance. Management review meetings, within the terms of the HFEA Compliance and Enforcement policy, were held with respect to four of the clinics where more than 10 areas of non-compliance were observed and licences of less than the usual four years were issued in all four cases. With respect to the two clinics having more than 10 areas of non-compliance but where licences for four years were issued, the risks associated with the areas of non-compliance were not considered serious enough to warrant a management review.

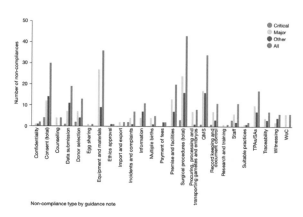

Fig. 16.2 The areas of non-compliance, by severity, identified at inspections in 2014/15

The most frequently observed types of areas of non-compliance observed in the two years from 2013 to 2015 were as follows:

- The quality management system (QMS)
- Consent
- Equipment and materials
- Procuring, processing and transporting of gametes and embryos
- Witnessing
- Traceability

QMS: A clinic is required to have a QMS and is the mechanism by which it is expected to achieve continuous improvement. Clinics struggled initially to implement all of the requirements, introduced in 2007, and subsequently inspections tended to focus on clinics' quality management systems and processes. Because of the pivotal role of the QMS in ensuring quality of care, the HFEA continues to focus on this aspect of practice. However, since April 2015 it has refreshed its approach, reviewing the impact and effectiveness of a clinic's *audits* of practice.

Consent: This is at the heart of the regulatory regime and consent failure is a significant risk of fertility treatment. Consent requirements are complex, changing significantly in 2009. Resultantly, the HFEA continues to scrutinise a clinic's procedures for taking consent and common recommendations include those relating to the storage of gametes and embryos after the gamete provider's consent to storage has expired, problems with reporting of consent to disclosure intentions and in relation to legal parenthood. The observation of these anomalies (accounting for 6 of 22 critical areas of non-compliance observed has had a wider impact beyond regulatory action – and the HFEA held a set of workshops for clinic staff relating to consent across the country in 2014.

Equipment and materials: Common areas of non-compliance here include failure to validate new and/or repaired equipment and using non-CE marked medical devices. The requirements relating to CE marking are often poorly understood although collaborative working between the HFEA and the UK Medicines & Healthcare products Regulatory Agency has served to clarify requirements. Clinics are working through the

implementations of these requirements – hence the frequency of recommendations for improvement.

Procuring, processing and transporting gametes and embryos: Common areas of non-compliance here include inadequacy of process validation and poor practice around the screening of gamete providers. Validation requirements were often poorly understood following introduction in 2007 and the HFEA continues to clarify these encouraging clinics to not only 'tick the boxes' with respect to validation documentation but also to demonstrate the effectiveness of their validation in ensuring the quality of services. With respect to viral screening the frequency of this area of non-compliance has arisen as a result of changes in guidance.

Witnessing: Risk of misidentification is (with consent) the most significant risk of fertility treatment and effective witnessing is key to minimising it. As a result the HFEA scrutinises this area of practice closely. Clinics largely have good procedures in place to minimise these risks and common areas of non-compliance (for example, the absence of witnessing at the disposal of sperm after treatment and errors in the documentation of witnessing) tend to carry an extremely low level of risk.

Although this is a common area of non-compliance, there were no critical witnessing areas of non-compliance.

Traceability: The most common areas of non-compliance observed in traceability were failures to label tubes used during egg collection – as clinics generally only carry out one egg collection at a time there are no significant opportunities for misidentification. However, due to the potential impact, the HFEA continues to prompt clinics to be robust in the documentation of the measures taken to minimise all possible risks.

The HFEA asks the clinic Person Responsible to provide feedback to the HFEA regarding the inspection process (through the completion of a questionnaire on the HFEA website). Feedback has been provided with respect to 42 renewal inspections and 36 interim inspections carried out between 2013 and 2015. Seventy two of the 78 respondents (92%) considered that their inspection visit had promoted improvement to the way the clinic carries out its work and >95% of the

78 respondents were satisfied with their inspection report and with the recommendations and timescales for implementation within it. There was some negative feedback. Two of 42 respondents experiencing renewal inspections and three of 29 experiencing interim inspections did not agree that patients were not inconvenienced and/or their care was not jeopardised by the inspection. Furthermore, five of 29 respondents experiencing an unannounced interim inspection did not agree that staff were able to take the inspection in their stride and carry on with their work while the inspection took place. Although these respondents are in a minority, the HFEA remains mindful of this feedback and continues to endeavour to minimise any negative impact of the inspection visit on patient treatment. Of 78 respondents, three said that they did not have enough time to discuss the inspection findings on inspection and two felt they did not understand an issue of non-compliance. It is noted that inspection team leaders telephone clinics, where required, after an inspection and all but one respondent was satisfied with this interaction.

3 Conclusion

Analysis of inspection findings supports a conclusion that HFEA licensed clinics and research centres are generally compliant and areas of serious non-compliance and the need for the application of regulatory sanctions are rare. But mistakes do happen and sometimes performance is poor. The regulatory regime aims to be sensitive to trends and responsive to risks so that improvement can be encouraged quickly to minimise the impact on quality of service. The regime also aims to continually raise the bar. In the next phase the HFEA will want to see clinics challenging themselves to deliver even better quality of service. It expects clinics to ensure their expectations in terms of quality are clearly documented and that metrics for quality (quality indicators) should not be restricted to the laboratory or pregnancy outcomes. Clinics should aim to document the quality they expect to achieve with respect to all of their activities – administrative, clinical laboratory and counselling. Clinics should audit their work to check they achieve the quality they expect. Where they do not, there should be an in-depth root cause analysis to identify the reason and how improvement can be achieved. The assisted reproduction sector is continually evolving – the regulatory regime will continue to evolve too.

References

1. The Human Fertilisation and Embryology Act 1990 (as amended) www.legislation.gov.uk/ukpga/2008/22/contents

2. *HFEA Code of Practice* 8th Edition www.hfea.gov.uk/code.html

3. The HFEA Risk Tool www.hfea.gov.uk/6674.html

4. The HFEA Compliance and Enforcement Policy www.hfea.gov.uk/6681.html

5. Adverse Incidents in Fertility Clinics: Lessons to Learn January-December 2014 www.hfea.gov.uk/9870.html

6. The 'Five Why' Methodology https://improvement.nhs.uk/documents/2156/root-cause-analysis-five-whys.pdf

Common Stimulation Regimens in Assisted Reproductive Technology

Sesh K. Sunkara

1 Introduction

Since the early days of in vitro fertilisation (IVF), the results of IVF treatment have much improved with a 32.8% live birth rate being reported for women aged under 35 years in the United Kingdom in the year 2012 [1]. The paradigm shift from natural unifollicular IVF treatment cycles to multifollicular stimulated IVF treatment cycles has been an important contributing factor to this improvement, largely enabled by the availability of ovulation induction drugs. It has led to the evolution of the concept of superovulation whereby the ovaries are stimulated to produce high numbers of good quality oocytes that will compensate in part for the deficiencies in IVF and cleavage, and facilitate a yield of good numbers of high quality embryos available for transfer, thereby increasing the probability of pregnancy. Ovarian stimulation is now an essential part of IVF with 98.3% of IVF in the United Kingdom being stimulated cycles in 2013 [1].

The use of superovulation regimens led to the introduction of controlled ovarian stimulation (COS) in order to achieve better cycle control by the avoidance of a premature luteinising hormone (LH) surge. A premature LH surge leads to high cycle cancellation and poor pregnancy rates as a result of either premature ovulation or inappropriate luteinisation before oocyte retrieval. In conjunction with the drugs that cause multifollicular stimulation of the ovaries, pituitary suppression with gonadotrophin releasing hormone (GnRH) analogues which eliminate endogenous gonadotrophin interference caused by exogenous superovulation regimens and timed ovulation trigger control all events in the process of COS.

An understanding of the physiology of ovulation is important to comprehend the use of stimulation regimens in IVF treatment. During a normal menstrual cycle following the involution of the corpus luteum and the consequent fall in oestrogen production, follicle stimulating hormone (FSH) levels rise during the luteo-follicular transition [2]. This rise in FSH stimulates the recruitment of a cohort of follicles. Further development of these follicles during the follicular phase is dependent on continued stimulation by gonadotrophins. According to the concept of an FSH 'threshold' postulated by Brown in 1978, FSH concentrations need to exceed a certain level for follicular development to proceed [3]. When the FSH 'threshold' is surpassed in a normal cycle, it stimulates the growth of a cohort of small antral follicles and ensures further preovulatory follicular development [4]. The duration of this period in which the threshold is exceeded (FSH 'window') is limited in the normal cycle as there follows a decrease in FSH during the early-mid follicular phase [2]. Extension of the 'window' period leads to multiple follicular development. In a normal menstrual cycle, a single follicle continues to develop despite falling levels of FSH due to an increased sensitivity to the hormone [5], but the remaining follicles undergo atresia in response to the declining levels of FSH. Ovulation is triggered by a sharp and transient surge in LH as a result of the positive feedback from oestrogen produced by the dominant growing preovulatory follicle.

Thus the duration of elevated FSH plays an important role in determining the number of follicles that will undergo further development. In superovulation regimens, a supra-physiological dose of FSH is used to recruit multiple ovarian follicles with higher 'threshold' FSH requirements. Exogenous administration of FSH stimulates the granulosa cells of the ovarian follicles and induces multiple follicular growth.

Ovarian stimulation is important as it enhances the oocyte yield and the number of oocytes retrieved is an important prognostic variable for IVF success [6]. The aim of COS is to optimise the number of oocytes with individualised stimulation regimens by fine tuning the different stages of COS to achieve maximum efficacy and safety [7].

The components of COS are pituitary suppression, ovarian stimulation and ovulation triggering preparing for oocyte retrieval. The various events of COS in relation to the hypothalamic pituitary ovarian axis and the commonly used drugs at each stage are represented schematically in Figure 17.1.

2 Pituitary Suppression Regimens

The commonly employed COS regimens in IVF are the long GnRH agonist regimen, the short GnRH agonist regimen, the GnRH antagonist regimen and modifications of these.

2.1 Long GnRH Agonist Regimen

With the GnRH agonist long regimen, pituitary down-regulation with GnRH agonist is commenced in the follicular phase or more commonly in the mid luteal phase of the menstrual cycle. Menstruation usually follows within two weeks of starting GnRH agonist. Pituitary down-regulation is confirmed by transvaginal ultrasound scan demonstrating quiescent ovaries with follicles of size $\leq$ 10 mm diameter and endometrium $\leq$ 5 mm in thickness. On confirmation of down-regulation, ovarian stimulation is commenced with gonadotrophin injections. Ultrasound monitoring is performed during ovarian stimulation to assess follicular recruitment and growth. Gonadotrophin and GnRH agonist administration are continued until ovulation trigger. Human chorionic

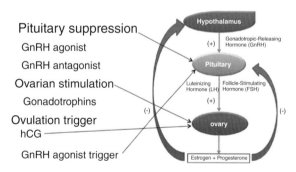

Fig. 17.1 Stages of COS

gonadotrophin (hCG) is administered subcutaneously when the criteria for triggering final oocyte maturation is met. Figure 17.2a is a schematic representation of events in the long GnRH agonist regimen.

A modification of the long agonist regimen is the long stop regimen where the GnRH agonist is stopped on commencement of ovarian stimulation. The use of this regimen is based on the rationale that prolonged pituitary down-regulation with continuous GnRH agonist administration during ovarian stimulation with gonadotrophins suppresses ovarian response. However, current evidence does not favour the use of the long stop regimen over the standard long GnRH agonist regimen [8].

2.2 Short GnRH Agonist Regimen

With the short GnRH agonist regimen, treatment is started in the early follicular phase (days 1 to 3 of the menstrual cycle) after a transvaginal ultrasound scan confirming quiescent ovaries and a thin endometrium $\leq$ 5 mm in thickness. Gonadotrophin injections are commenced one day following the start of the GnRH agonist. Ultrasound monitoring is performed during ovarian stimulation to assess follicular recruitment and growth. Gonadotrophin and GnRH agonist administration are continued until ovulation trigger. hCG is administered subcutaneously when the criteria for triggering ovulation is met. Figure 17.2b is a schematic representation of events in the short GnRH agonist regimen.

A modification of the short agonist regimen is the ultra-short regimen where the GnRH agonist is stopped following commencement of ovarian stimulation with gonadotrophins.

2.3 GnRH Antagonist Regimen

With the GnRH antagonist regimen, ovarian stimulation with gonadotrophin injections is commenced in the early follicular phase of the menstrual cycle after a transvaginal ultrasound scan confirming quiescent ovaries and a thin endometrium ($\leq$ 5 mm). The GnRH antagonist is commenced on day 6 of stimulation (fixed administration) or when the leading follicle is $\geq$14 mm (flexible administration). Both the gonadotrophin and the GnRH antagonist are continued until the day of ovulation triggering. Figure 17.2c is a schematic representation of events in the GnRH antagonist regimen. In an antagonist cycle the trigger is either hCG as above or GnRH agonist.

3 Gonadotrophin Dose and Type

It is imperative to use the right gonadotrophin dose to optimise the number of oocytes retrieved, maximise

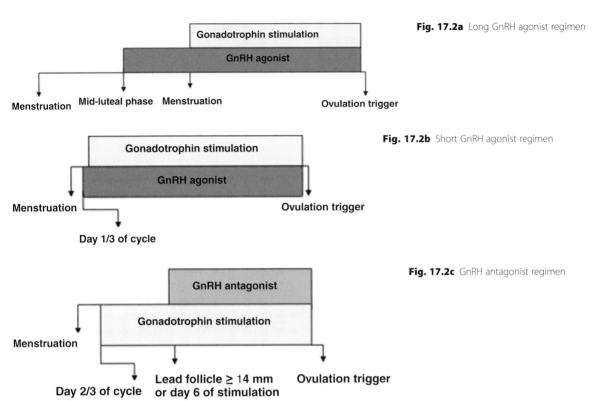

Fig. 17.2a Long GnRH agonist regimen

Fig. 17.2b Short GnRH agonist regimen

Fig. 17.2c GnRH antagonist regimen

live birth rates following IVF and at the same time minimise risks such as ovarian hyperstimulation syndrome (OHSS) and cycle cancellation. When exogenous gonadotrophin is administered, the number of mature follicles recruited largely depends upon the number of follicles attaining FSH sensitivity. Hence administration of a high gonadotrophin dose may induce excessive ovarian response consequently leading to a high risk of OHSS. On the other hand, administration of an inappropriately low gonadotrophin dose may lead to the growth of a low number of follicles resulting in an 'iatrogenic' poor response.

The successful therapeutic use of urinary gonadotrophins started with the first generation product human menopausal gonadotrophin (hMG) or menotropin, which contained 75 IU of FSH and 75 IU of LH in each standard ampoule. This was followed in the early 1980s by the development of urofollitropin, the second generation product from which the LH activity had been reduced to 0.1 IU/ 75 IU FSH. Subsequently, the third generation product, highly purified urofollitropin (Metrodin HP®) with practically no residual LH activity was developed in the early 1990s. Due to its enhanced purity with very small amount of protein, Metrodin HP® could be administered subcutaneously

which was an advantage over the previous generations which had to be administered intramuscularly. The more recent fourth generation gonadotrophin is produced in vitro through recombinant deoxy ribo nucleic acid (DNA) technology, by genetically engineered Chinese hamster ovary cells. This is recombinant human FSH (r-FSH or follitropin) which is free of LH and contains less than 1% of contaminant proteins. There are two preparations of r-FSH that are commercially available for clinical use, follitropin-α and follitropin-β, both of which have the advantage of subcutaneous administration. Over the years there have been numerous randomised controlled trials (RCTs) comparing urinary gonadotrophins versus recombinant FSH for COS. Current evidence suggests that the two gonadotrophin preparations are comparable in IVF outcomes [9].

4 Ovulation Trigger

Following recruitment and growth of follicles to the mature stage resulting from ovarian stimulation, the next step is maturation of oocytes facilitated by the ovulation trigger in COS regimens. The LH surge that induces germinal vesicle breakdown and ovulation in a natural menstrual cycle is not suppressed in stimulated multifollicular cycles necessitating artificial triggering of ovulation. hCG which is naturally produced by the human placenta and excreted in large quantities in the urine of pregnant women bears a close molecular resemblance to LH and has a similar effect on the LH receptor. hCG is used because of this molecular resemblance and also due to its longer serum half-life (36 hours) compared to the short serum half-life of LH (108–148 minutes) [10], which avoids the inconvenience of repeated administrations. Administration of hCG results in luteinisation of the granulosa cells, progesterone biosynthesis, resumption of meiosis, oocyte maturation and subsequent follicular rupture 36–40 hours later. It is administered after the stimulated development of mature preovulatory follicles in order to induce maturation, but oocyte retrieval is undertaken before ovulation. The usual criteria for the administration of hCG is the presence of ≥ 3 follicles of ≥ 18 mm in diameter. The preparations of hCG that are available for clinical use are the urinary and recombinant forms and are comparable for IVF outcomes [11]. The usual dose of hCG for final ovulation triggering is between 5000 IU and 10,000 IU as a single dose.

The GnRH agonist trigger has been proposed as an alternative to the hCG trigger by virtue of inducing a rise in endogenous LH and FSH due to its initial flare effect. The specific mode of action of the antagonist by competitive blockade of the pituitary receptors and a shorter half-life means that the pituitary remains responsive to the GnRH agonist thus enabling its use for triggering ovulation. The mechanism of action of the GnRH agonist in causing down-regulation and desensitisation of the pituitary receptors precludes the use of agonist trigger in those cycles. Use of the GnRH agonist trigger significantly lowers the incidence of OHSS compared to the hCG trigger [12].

5 Individualised COS

The main objective of individualisation of treatment in IVF is to offer every single woman the best treatment tailored to her own unique characteristics, thus maximising the chances of pregnancy and eliminating the iatrogenic and avoidable risks resulting from ovarian stimulation. It is therefore important to categorise women based on their predicted response in order to individualise COS regimens. Women can be identified as having a poor response, normal response

or a hyper-response based on individual characteristics and ovarian reserve tests (ORTs). Among the various ORTs including basal FSH, basal oestradiol, inhibin B, antral follicle count (AFC) and anti-mullerian hormone (AMH), AFC and AMH have the highest accuracy for the prediction of either a poor or an excessive response following ovarian stimulation [13]. Results from individual patient data (IPD) meta-analyses of patient characteristics and ORTs demonstrated age as being the most important among patient characteristics for the prediction of poor or excessive response and AFC or AMH as having the highest predictive accuracy among ORTs [14,15]. The cut-off levels of AFC and AMH for prediction of poor response is an AFC of < 5 to <7 and AMH of <0.5 ng/ml to <1.1 ng/ml [16]. The cut-off levels for AFC and AMH for the prediction of hyper-response is an AFC of >14 to >16 [17,18] and AMH of 3.5 ng/ml to 3.9 ng/ml [19,20]. Individualisation involves tailoring the different stages of COS to suit each woman.

With regards to the optimal gonadotrophin dosage an RCT, comparing a gonadotrophin dose of 225 IU daily versus 150 IU daily in women aged 23–41 years undergoing IVF demonstrated the number of oocytes to be significantly higher with 225 IU daily compared to 150 IU daily [21]. This study excluded women with basal FSH > 10 IU/L, polycystic ovary syndrome (PCOS), previous poor response and previous OHSS. Another RCT comparing a daily gonadotrophin dose of 225 IU versus 300 IU daily among women predicted as normal responders based on a total AFC of 8–21 showed no significant difference in the number of oocytes retrieved between the two doses [22]. This evidence would therefore suggest that the ideal gonadotrophin dose for women predicted as normal responders is 225 IU daily. An RCT comparing gonadotrophin doses of 300 IU versus 375 IU versus 450 IU daily among women predicted as poor responders based on a total AFC of <12 showed no significant difference in the number of oocytes retrieved nor live birth rates between the three arms suggesting an unlikely benefit with gonadotrophin doses > 300 IU daily [23]. Women with PCOS and those predicted to have a hyper-response should be stimulated with a lower gonadotrophin dose of ≤ 150 IU daily to avoid excessive stimulation. Excessive response (>20 oocytes) is associated with a decrease in live birth rate in a fresh embryo transfer IVF cycle [6] in addition to a higher incidence of OHSS.

Updated evidence has demonstrated comparable pregnancy rates with the GnRH antagonist and GnRH agonist regimens in unselected women in addition to a lower risk of OHSS with the antagonist regimen [24]. Between the long and the short GnRH agonist regimens, the long agonist regimen has better outcomes in terms of the number of oocytes retrieved and pregnancy rates compared to the short agonist regimen [8]. The GnRH antagonist and long GnRH agonist regimens are therefore suitable options for pituitary suppression. An RCT comparing the long GnRH agonist regimen versus short GnRH agonist regimen versus GnRH antagonist regimen in women with a previous poor ovarian response demonstrated the long agonist and antagonist regimens to be suitable for these women with regards to the number of oocytes retrieved [25]. A recent meta-analysis of studies comparing GnRH antagonist versus GnRH agonist regimes in women with PCOS showed comparable pregnancy rates between the two groups and a significantly lower incidence in severe OHSS in the GnRH antagonist group [26]. An added advantage of the use of GnRH antagonist based protocols is the use of GnRH agonist as a substitute for hCG in triggering of final oocyte maturation, potentially eliminating the risk of OHSS [12]. The Cochrane review comparing the GnRH agonist versus the hCG trigger however, demonstrated significantly reduced live birth rates in fresh autologous cycles with the use of the GnRH agonist trigger although there was no reduction in live birth rates in oocyte donor/recipient cycles [12]. Following initial use of the GnRH agonist trigger the need to modify the standard luteal support to obtain reliable reproductive outcomes was soon recognised. Study groups have since endeavoured to fine tune the luteal phase support in IVF cycles using the GnRH agonist trigger to optimise clinical outcomes. Recent suggestions and developments in overcoming luteal insufficiency which occurs in such cycles are use of (i) a 'dual trigger' [27], (ii) low dose hCG supplementation [28], (iii) intensive luteal oestradiol and progesterone supplementation [29], (iv).rec-LH supplementation [30] and (v) luteal GnRH agonist administration [31]. Alternatively, all the available embryos are frozen for transfer in a subsequent cycle.

6 Minimal Stimulation Regimens

Minimal stimulation regimens are advocated as a cost-effective alternative to conventional stimulation. Currently there is no standardised regimen for minimal stimulation with the use of antioestrogens such as clomiphene citrate with or without lower doses of gonadotrophins or use of gonadotrophins alone. It is however important to evaluate cost-effectiveness in relation to the efficiency in achieving the desired outcome of a live birth, and hence it is crucial to assess robust evidence in resorting to such regimens.

7 Conclusion

After decades of IVF practice, it is now recognised that individualisation in IVF is the way forward following categorisation of women as normal responders, poor responders and hyper-responders. The long GnRH agonist and antagonist regimens are effective in normal responders and the ideal gonadotrophin dose is 225 IU daily. The GnRH antagonist regimen is ideal for women with PCOS and women categorised as hyper-responders. Whilst the pregnancy rates are comparable to those of the GnRH agonist regimen, the antagonist regimen significantly lowers the risk of OHSS in addition to enabling the use of the GnRH agonist trigger which potentially eliminates OHSS. A lower gonadotrophin dose $\leq$150 IU daily is recommended in these women. The long GnRH agonist and antagonist regimens are ideal for poor responders. Higher gonadotrophin doses >300 IU daily are unlikely to be beneficial in poor responders, simply increasing costs, and hence the maximal gonadotrophin dose should not exceed 300 IU daily. It is important to establish the right COS regimen and gonadotrophin starting doses which is better than later dose adjustments for achieving best outcomes. Figure 17.3 is a schematic representation of individualisation of COS regimens.

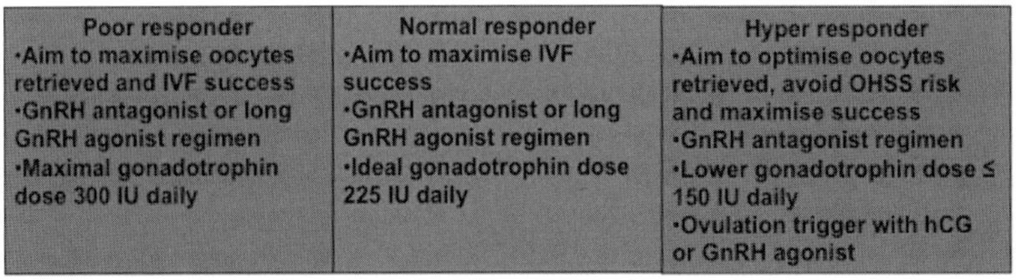

Poor responder	Normal responder	Hyper responder
•Aim to maximise oocytes retrieved and IVF success •GnRH antagonist or long GnRH agonist regimen •Maximal gonadotrophin dose 300 IU daily	•Aim to maximise IVF success •GnRH antagonist or long GnRH agonist regimen •Ideal gonadotrophin dose 225 IU daily	•Aim to optimise oocytes retrieved, avoid OHSS risk and maximise success •GnRH antagonist regimen •Lower gonadotrophin dose ≤ 150 IU daily •Ovulation trigger with hCG or GnRH agonist

Fig. 17.3 Individualised controlled ovarian stimulation

References

1. Human Fertilisation and Embryology Authority. www.hfea.gov.uk/9461.html. Last accessed on 26 September 2015.

2. le Nstour E, Marraoui J, Lahlou N, Roger M, De ZD, Bouchard P. Role of estradiol in the rise in follicle-stimulating hormone levels during the luteal-follicular transition. *J Clin Endocr Metab* 1993:77;439–42.

3. Brown JB. Pituitary control of ovarian function: concepts derived from gonadotrophin therapy. *Aust N Z J Obstet Gynaecol* 1978:18;47–54.

4. Fauser BCJM and Van Heusden AM. Manipulation of human ovarian function: Physiological concepts and clinical consequences. *Endocr Rev* 1997:18;71–106.

5. Hsueh AJW. Paracrine mechanisms involved in granulosa cell differentiation. *J Clin Endocrinol Metab* 1986:15;117–34.

6. Sunkara SK, Rittenberg V, Raine-Fenning N, Bhattacharya S, Zamora J, Coomarasamy A. Association between the number of eggs and live birth in IVF treatment: an analysis of 400 135 treatment cycles. *Hum Reprod* 2011;26:1768–74.

7. La Marca A and Sunkara SK. Individualization of controlled ovarian stimulation in IVF using ovarian reserve markers: from theory to practice. *Hum Reprod Update* 2014;20:124–40.

8. Siristatidis CS, Gibreel A, Basios G, Maheshwari A, Bhattacharya S. Gonadotrophin-releasing hormone agonist protocols for pituitary suppression in assisted reproduction. *Cochrane Database Syst Rev* 2015; Issue 11. Art. No.: CD006919. DOI: 10.1002/ 14651858.CD006919.pub4.

9. van Wely M, Kwan I, Burt AL, Thomas J, Vail A, Van der Veen F, Al-Inany HG. Recombinant versus urinary gonadotrophin for ovarian stimulation in assisted reproductive technology cycles. *Cochrane Database Syst Rev* 2011: Issue 2. Art. No.: CD005354. DOI: 10.1002/14651858.CD005354. pub2.

10. Wide L, Eriksson K, Sluss PM, Hall JE. The common genetic variant of luteinizing hormone has a longer serum half-life than the wild type in heterozygous women. *J Clin Endocrinol Metab* 2010;95:383–9.

11. Youssef MA, Al-Inany HG, Aboulghar M, Mansour R, Abou-Setta AM. Recombinant versus urinary human chorionic gonadotrophin for final oocyte maturation triggering in IVF and ICSI cycles. *Cochrane Database Syst Rev* 2011a: Issue 4. Art. No.: CD003719.

12. Youssef MA, Van der Veen F, Al-Inany HG, Griesinger G, Mochtar MH, Aboulfoutouh I, Khattab SM, van Wely M. Gonadotropin-releasing hormone agonist versus HCG for oocyte triggering in antagonist assisted reproductive technology cycles. *Cochrane Database Syst Rev* 2011b: Issue 10. Art. No.: CD008046.

13. Broekmans FJ, Kwee J, Hendriks DJ, Mol BW, Lambalk CB. A systematic review of tests predicting ovarian reserve and IVF outcome. *Hum Reprod Update*. 2006;12:685–718.

14. Broer SL, van Disseldorp J, Broeze KA, Dolleman M, Opmeer BC, Bossuyt P, Eijkemans MJ, Mol BW, Broekmans FJ; IMPORT study group. Added value of ovarian reserve testing on patient characteristics in the prediction of ovarian response and ongoing pregnancy: an individual patient data approach. *Hum Reprod Update* 2013;19:26–36.

15. Broer S, Madeleine D, Disseldorp J, Broeze KA, Opmeer BC, Patrick MM. Bossuyt P Eijkemans MJ.C, Mol BW, Broekmans FJM; on behalf of the IPD-EXPORT Study Group. Prediction of an excessive response in in vitro fertilization from patient characteristics and ovarian reserve tests and comparison in subgroups: an individual patient data meta-analysis. *Fertil Steril* 2013;100:420–9.

16. Ferraretti AP, La Marca A, Fauser BC, Tarlatzis B, Nargund G, Gianaroli L; ESHRE working group on Poor Ovarian Response Definition. ESHRE consensus on the definition of 'poor response' to ovarian stimulation for in vitro fertilization: the Bologna criteria. *Hum Reprod* 2011;26:1616–24.

17. Ng EH, Tang OS, Ho PC. The significance of the number of antral follicles prior to stimulation in predicting ovarian responses in an IVF programme. *Hum Reprod* 2000;15:1937–42.

18. Aflatoonian A, Oskouian H, Ahmadi S, Oskouian L. Prediction of high ovarian response to controlled ovarian hyperstimulation: anti-Mullerian hormone versus small Antral follicle count (2–6 mm). *J Assist Reprod Genet* 2009;26:319–25.

19. Arce JC, La Marca A, Mirner Klein B, Nyboe Andersen A, Fleming R. Antimullerian hormone in gonadotropin releasing-hormone antagonist cycles: prediction of ovarian response and cumulative treatment outcome in good-prognosis patients. *Fertil Steril* 2013;99:1644–53.

20. Polyzos NP, Tournaye H, Guzman L, Camus M, Nelson SM. Predictors of ovarian response in women treated with corifollitropin alfa for in vitro fertilization/ intracytoplasmic sperm injection. *Fertil Steril* 2013;100:438–44.

21. Yong PY, Brett S, Baird DT, Thong KJ. A prospective

randomized clinical trial comparing 150 IU and 225 IU of recombinant follicle-stimulating hormone (Gonal-F*) in a fixed-dose regimen for controlled ovarian stimulation in in vitro fertilization treatment. *Fertil Steril* 2003;79:308–15.

22. Jayaprakasan K, Hopkisson J, Campbell B, Johnson I, Thornton J, Raine-Fenning N. A randomised controlled trial of 300 versus 225 IU recombinant FSH for ovarian stimulation in predicted normal responders by antral follicle count. *BJOG*. 2010;117:853–62.

23. Berkkanoglu M and Ozgur K. What is the optimum maximal gonadotropin dosage used in microdose flare-up cycles in poor responders? *Fertil Steril* 2010;94:662–5.

24. Al-Inany HG, Youssef MA, Aboulghar M, Broekmans F, Sterrenburg M, Smit J, Abou-Setta AM. Gonadotrophin-releasing hormone antagonists for assisted reproductive technology. *Cochrane Database Syst Rev*. 2011; Issue 5. Art. No.: CD001750.

25. Sunkara SK, Coomarasamy A, Faris R, Braude P, Khalaf Y. Long

gonadotropin-releasing hormone agonist versus short agonist versus antagonist regimens in poor responders undergoing in vitro fertilization: a randomized controlled trial. *Fertil Steril* 2014;101:147–53.

26. Lin H, Li Y, Li L, Wang W, Yang D, Zhang Q. Is a GnRH antagonist protocol better in PCOS patients? A meta-analysis of RCTs. *PLoS One*. 2014;9:e91796.

27. Shapiro BS, Daneshmand ST, Garner FC, Aguirre M, Thomas S. Gonadotropin-releasing hormone agonist combined with a reduced dose of human chorionic gonadotropin for final oocyte maturation in fresh autologous cycles of in vitro fertilization. *Fertil Steril*. 2008;90:231–3.

28. Humaidan P, Ejdrup Bredkjaer H, Westergaard LG, Yding AC. 1,500 IU human chorionic gonadotropin administered at oocyte retrieval rescues the luteal phase when gonadotropin-releasing hormone agonist is used for ovulation induction: a prospective, randomized,

controlled study. *Fertil Steril* 2010;93:847–54.

29. Engmann L, DiLuigi A, Schmidt D, Nulsen J, Maier D, Benadiva C. The use of gonadotropin-releasing hormone (GnRH) agonist to induce oocyte maturation after cotreatment with GnRH antagonist in high-risk patients undergoing in vitro fertilization prevents the risk of ovarian hyperstimulation syndrome: a prospective randomized controlled study. *Fertil Steril* 2008;89:84–91.

30. Papanikolaou EG, Verpoest W, Fatemi H, Tarlatzis B, Devroey P, Tournaye H. A novel method of luteal supplementation with recombinant luteinizing hormone when a gonadotropin-releasing hormone agonist is used instead of human chorionic gonadotropin for ovulation triggering: a randomized prospective proof of concept study. *Fertil Steril* 2011; 95:1174–7.

31. Pirard C, Donnez J, Loumaye E. GnRH agonist as luteal phase support in assisted reproduction technique cycles: results of a pilot study. *Hum Reprod* 2006;21:1894–900.

Chapter 18

Oocyte Retrieval and Embryo Transfer

Julia Kopeika
Tarek El-Toukhy

1 Oocyte Retrieval

The oocyte retrieval procedure has undergone a substantial evolution over almost forty years moving from the abdominal to vaginal approach. Ultrasound-guided oocyte retrieval is performed now as a routine procedure worldwide.

1.1 Pre-retrieval Biological Processes

1.1.1 Background Characteristics of Patient

The purpose of controlled ovarian stimulation (COS) is to achieve multi-follicular development culminating in a collection of a number of fertilisable oocytes. However, this may not always be possible, especially in patients with poor ovarian reserve. Patient background characteristics such as age, antral follicle count, anti-Mullerian hormone (AMH), body mass index (BMI) and previous response to COS are important not only for choosing an appropriate individually tailored stimulation protocol but also for counselling regarding the expected outcome of oocyte retrieval.

It is important to assess accessibility to the ovaries in advance of stimulation. If a patient had previous abdominal or pelvic surgeries which could compromise transvaginal access to the ovaries, an alternative route for oocyte retrieval (e.g. transabdominal retrieval) and the associated risks should be considered and discussed with the patient.

1.1.2 Oocyte Triggering Medication

Stimulation protocols are considered in detail in Chapter 17. Key considerations for triggering pre-oocyte collection are when to trigger in relationship to follicular development, the type and dose of trigger as well as the interval between trigger and oocyte retrieval.

1.2 Retrieval

1.2.1 Technical Aspects

1.2.1.1 Route of Egg Retrieval

The first in vitro fertilisation (IVF) baby was derived from laparoscopically aided oocyte retrieval scheduled in the natural menstrual cycle. Laparoscopic oocyte retrieval, however, yielded oocytes from only one third of follicles [1]. The next breakthrough in oocyte retrieval was almost a decade later, when the transabdominal ultrasound-guided technique was developed. Even though the yield was similar to the laparoscopic method, the transabdominal route offered easier access and a lower risk of complications. Whilst the transabdominal ultrasound transducer was used, access to the ovaries was attempted transvesically, per-urethrally and finally transvaginally [1]. The transvaginal ultrasound-guided approach is currently the main route used for oocyte retrieval.

1.2.1.2 The Physics of Oocyte Retrieval

Length and Size of Needle, and Aspiration Pressure
During the dawn of IVF, a needle and syringe were used to provide suction manually to retrieve follicular fluid and oocytes from the ovary. Subsequently, aspiration devices were developed to provide continuous suction. The vacuum used did not usually exceed 120 mmHg. A foot operated 'on-off' valve at 200 mmHg was utilised. Currently the aspiration pressure used by the majority of IVF unit ranges between 120 and 200 mmHg.

The evaluation of the physics of oocyte retrieval in relation to aspiration pressure, length and gauge of needle and velocity of follicular fluid aspiration has been studied mostly in animal models. It has been suggested that oocytes may be damaged during the process of collection by turbulence and velocity of the follicular fluid [2]. The authors argued that a large vacuum gradient could potentially damage the

138

oocytes and that a high velocity of laminar flow or turbulent flow would increase the chance of stripping the cumulus cells off the oocyte. Changes in vacuum pressure or needle gauge or length would influence the flow rate in the system. Raised pressure increases the volume of flow and velocity of the fluid much more rapidly in a larger gauge needle. The size of the bevel can also exacerbate fluid turbulence. Turbulent flow occurs over a longer distance in long bevel compared to short bevel needles. The turbulence on entry into the needle exerts randomly directed forces on the cumulus oocyte complex, which may overcome the adherence of the cumulus cells to the oocyte. Early studies suggest that oocyte pick up is better when larger gauge needles are used. Needles of 14= and 16-gauge were considered the best choices for oocyte recovery; however, a smaller needle is likely to result in less tissue trauma and thus less bleeding and balance needs to be achieved.

An optimal combination of the above variables has been shown to improve the oocyte retrieval rate in animals. How relevant these findings are to human practice is difficult to ascertain since no similar studies have been carried out.

Temperature, pH and Osmolarity Control It is well-established that fluctuations in environmental factors such as temperature, pH and osmolarity can influence oocyte quality. Hence, effort should be put into minimising unwanted fluctuation during the transportation period of oocytes from follicles to lab incubator dish via the oocyte collecting system. For example, the oocyte is known to be very sensitive to reduced temperature [3], pH or osmotic stress [4]. The maintenance of 37 °C is important during IVF manipulations therefore all equipment (test tube heater, table incubators, plates and media that come into direct contact with oocyte during retrieval) should be pre-warmed. Heating devices must be regularly calibrated and monitored. Prevention of harmful pH fluctuation can be achieved by using appropriate buffers. The team involved in the egg retrieval procedure should ensure that all equipment and media are ready to use before commencing the retrieval procedure.

1.2.2 Pain-Relief

Effective analgesia is an essential part of any surgical procedure. The purpose is not only to improve the patient's experience and eliminate the perception of pain but also to help the surgeon to perform the procedure safely and efficiently. Ideally, the chosen method of analgesia should be short-acting with a good safety profile and minimal impact on gametes. As the technique of oocyte retrieval was evolving into being minimally invasive, so was the choice of anaesthetic, starting from general anaesthesia for a laparoscopic approach to paracervical block and/or conscious sedation for a transvaginal approach.

A recent meta-analysis [5] showed that no one particular modality of conscious sedation or analgesia was superior in providing effective pain relief for transvaginal oocyte retrieval. The use of more than one method simultaneously, such as when combined with acupuncture or paracervical block, resulted in better pain relief than a single modality alone [5].

1.2.3 Variables of the Procedure

1.2.3.1 Vaginal Disinfection prior to Egg Retrieval

Early studies raised concern that if traditionally used vaginal antiseptics (e.g. povidine iodine or betadine) are trapped in tissue after cleaning, these could contaminate the follicular aspirate and damage oocytes [6]. This result was not confirmed in larger studies [7,8] where the pregnancy rates were comparable in both groups of patients with or without saline washing after betadine cleaning of vagina. These authors argue that it is unlikely that betadine found in the vagina could come into contact with oocytes while retrieving them in the closed system of the needle and tubing. No studies on vaginal preparation with chlorhexidine have been published.

1.2.3.2 Antibiotic Administration

Pelvic infection is a rare complication following transvaginal egg retrieval with an incidence ranging from 0.5% to 4% [7]. The theoretical mechanism of infection is either due to inoculation of vaginal microbiological flora into the peritoneal cavity or reactivation of pre-existing chronic infection in the pelvis. Routine use of prophylactic antibiotics during transvaginal oocyte retrieval has questionable benefit. For example, the incidence of infection in a cohort of 2,670 patients was 0.6% with no routine antibiotics [9], while in another cohort of 674 patients with routine antibiotics the incidence was 1.3% [10].

Due to the relative rarity of infection after transvaginal oocyte retrieval, a sample size of around 4,000 patients would be required to provide a meaningful answer regarding the benefit of routine administration of prophylactic antibiotics. Until such a large study is undertaken, it would be sensible to provide antibiotics cover only to patients at higher risk of infections, such as those with previous history of pelvic inflammatory disease, complex pelvic surgery and/or endometriosis.

1.2.3.3 Other Variables of Successful Oocyte Retrieval

Once the vulva and vagina are cleaned, the ultrasound probe is introduced and the ovaries are visualised and inspected. Gentle pressure on the probe usually achieves a good application of the vaginal wall to the ovary, in order to minimise the chance of visceral organs, such as bowel loops, being trapped between. The probe should be aligned in such a way that the aspiration needle enters the nearest follicle at the right angle. A gentle stabbing movement should achieve penetration of the follicle, after which aspiration of the follicular fluid can be achieved by applying suction pressure. Maintenance of suction during the entry to the follicle may prevent fluid and oocyte loss caused by the sudden increase of intra-follicular pressure during needle penetration [2]. Once the follicle has been completely drained, if pressure has been released, it is possible for negative pressure to pull an oocyte back into a follicle from the needle, particularly if the oocyte is in the last portion of fluid in the needle [2].

Some authors suggested that rotating the needle in a follicle during aspiration increases the number of oocytes obtained [11]. This potential benefit should be balanced however, against the theoretical concern of causing damage to cumulus oocyte complex if it is still attached to the follicle wall that is scraped by the needle. Furthermore, depending on the speed of the surgeon, prolonged residence of the aspirate in the dead space of the needle and tubing may lead to clotting in the needle and loss of oocytes or to exposure of oocytes to non-optimal environmental conditions.

In summary, careful needle entry into the follicle, avoidance of blockage of the needle lumen and timed application of aspiration pressure should theoretically optimise the oocyte retrieval technique [11].

1.2.4 Follicular Flushing

Follicular flushing was introduced with the purpose of increasing oocyte retrieval rates. Even though some studies suggested possible benefits of flushing with an apparent increase in retrieval rate from 40% at first aspiration to 97% after four flushes, systematic review

of the literature revealed no benefits in terms of number of retrieved eggs or pregnancy rate in normal responders [1]. Many clinics do not practice routine follicle flushing except for poor responders. Even in this group of patients however, the benefit of follicular flushing is uncertain. A recent study suggested that flushing might have a detrimental effect on the pregnancy rate [12]. A theoretical problem created by flushing is inadvertently pushing the oocyte out of the follicle. The needle tip may have tracked through the posterior follicle wall or may have created a large opening in the anterior follicle wall. Fluid can easily be injected into the ovary outside of the follicle, theoretically losing an oocyte from the follicle and also leading to impaired visualisation. Creation of high-speed turbulent flow could also be harmful for the oocyte–cumulus complex.

1.3 Post-retrieval Monitoring of the Patient

A short period (1–2 hrs) of observation is generally advised to monitor the woman for possible complications. As a result of significant advances in the technique of oocyte retrieval, the risk of complications is rare. Serious complications such as intra-peritoneal bleeding, uretero-vaginal fistula and ovarian abscess have been reported very rarely and mostly in the form of case reports. Minor complications such as mild vaginal bleeding have been reported in up to 6% of women [13]. Such bleeding usually settles with vaginal pressure and requires no further intervention.

2 Embryo Transfer

The first successful embryo transfer was performed in 1891 by Heape, when a spear-headed needle was used to transport fertilised eggs into a foster uterus in rabbits. It was a further 87 years before the first successful embryo transfer had occurred in a human [14]. The main method of transfer in early animal studies was a surgical trans-fundal approach under anaesthetic. Originally, the trans-cervical approach seemed to give a much inferior pregnancy rate of 2–4% in comparison with surgical trans-myometrial (50%) in different animal species. However, refinement of the trans-cervical method soon produced similar good results and became the mainstream technique in humans. Embryo transfer is the final success-determining step in an IVF cycle and also depends on a number of variables.

2.1 Patient Preparation

2.1.1 Full Bladder

It is thought that a full bladder could straighten the utero-cervical angle during embryo transfer and facilitate entry into the uterine cavity with a soft catheter. In 2007, a systematic review [15] suggested that a full bladder could be associated with a higher pregnancy rate (OR 1.44, 95% CI 1.04–2.04). This review derived its conclusion based on two studies. The larger of the two studies was not a true randomised controlled trial since allocation to the different treatment groups was based on alternate days. A subsequent Cochrane review [16] showed no difference in pregnancy rate between full or empty bladder (OR 0.98, 95% CI 0.57–1.68) when only two small randomised controlled trials with no power calculation were included. Further research into the effect of a full bladder at the time of embryo transfer on the live birth rate after IVF is warranted.

2.1.2 Role of Uterine Relaxants

Uterine contractility during embryo transfer has been thought to be associated with lower implantation rate. There is evidence that uterine contractions in stimulated IVF cycles are increased at least six-fold in comparison with natural cycles. It was speculated that administration of pharmacological agents that reduce uterine contractility could have a positive influence on embryo implantation rates. Administration of prostaglandin synthesis inhibitors just before embryo transfer showed variable effects on pregnancy rates in two studies of moderate quality [17,18].

Data from a prospective cohort study suggested that administration of atosiban (oxytocin/vasopressin receptor antagonist) at the time of embryo transfer was associated with a higher implantation rate [19]; however, when the same group conducted a multi-center randomised controlled trial, no difference was found in live birth rate between atosiban and placebo group in a general IVF population [20]. The role of similar drugs in patients with recurrent implantation failure or with adenomyosis remains unknown.

2.1.3 Mock Embryo Transfer

The aim of embryo transfer is to deliver an embryo into optimal location in the uterine cavity causing minimal disturbance to the surrounding environment. Mock Embryo Transfer (MET) can be undertaken prior to the actual procedure in order to establish if there are any potential difficulties that could be addressed in timely manner in order to reduce uterine trauma and avoid the risk of depositing the embryo in a suboptimal location. Since uterine and cervical anatomy has a great degree of variability, MET may help to assess variables such as uterine cavity position, measurement, ease of access and the choice of catheter. However the possible disadvantage of MET is the possibility of causing irritation, trauma or increased contractility of the uterus. There are, as yet, no randomised controlled trials assessing the potential advantages of MET.

A relatively small study of 135 patients randomly allocated to MET before starting IVF showed that MET was associated with higher implantation and pregnancy rate [21]. The timing of MET, whether before starting controlled ovarian stimulation, at the time of egg collection or just before the actual embryo transfer, did not seem to influence IVF outcome [21].

2.2 Variables during Embryo Transfer

2.2.1 Technical Aspects

Each step of the embryo transfer procedure should be aimed at minimisation of patient discomfort or pain, since it is plausible that pain caused by pelvic examination may cause undue uterine contractions that could increase the chance of embryo expulsion. In 6 to 16% of embryo transfers, the embryo could be found in the fluid at the external os after completion of the procedure [22]. The choice of the right speculum size and gentle speculum introduction into the vagina could help to minimise discomfort and patient distress. Excessive opening of vaginal speculum valves could alter the cervical-uterine angle and cause pain.

One randomised controlled trial suggested that mechanical closure of the cervix with vaginal speculum valves after introducing the embryo transfer catheter can be associated with increase in the clinical pregnancy rate [23]. These results were not substantiated by a subsequent quasi-randomised study, which did not demonstrate any significant benefit in mechanical closure of cervix during embryo transfer [24].

2.2.2 Vaginal/Cervical Disinfection during Embryo Transfer and Cleaning of the Cervix

The cervical canal contains mucus that plays an important physiological role in protecting the reproductive system from ascending bacterial contamination via mechanical and bacteriostatic means. Even though this mucus becomes thinner under the influence of increased oestrogen, it may at least in theory, interfere with embryo transfer since it can block the tip of catheter, increase the risk of embryo retention or interfere with deposit of an embryo into the correct place in the endometrial cavity. If an embryo gets embedded in cervical mucus, it might be dislodged more easily from the original site during withdrawal of the catheter. A number of studies have, however, failed to demonstrate any benefit in rigorous removing or flushing of cervical mucus during embryo transfer [25,16].

Another risk is contamination of the catheter and uterus by cervical flora. It has been demonstrated in earlier studies that the transfer catheter tip had positive microbial growth in 49.1% of cases [26]. It has been suggested at the time that microbial contamination at embryo transfer may be associated with reduced pregnancy [26] and live birth rates. It would be reasonable to speculate that if microbial contamination is associated with reduction in pregnancy rates, then prevention of such contamination with antibacterial treatment would be reasonable to undertake.

A Cochrane review [27] based on one randomised study demonstrated no improvement in pregnancy rate in patients treated with co-amoxiclav in spite of confirmed reduced genital tract microbial colonisation.

2.2.3 Type of Transfer Catheters

There is a wide variety of embryo transfer catheters available for clinical use. They vary in diameter, length, malleability and stiffness. The ideal catheter should cause minimum trauma to the endometrium but be firm enough to pass the cervical canal and mucus. Several studies have looked at the difference in pregnancy rate between different types of catheter. A systematic review [28] showed that the use of soft catheters was associated with a higher pregnancy rate (OR 1.49, 95% CI 1.26–1.77). There appears to be little difference between the different types of soft catheters in chance of clinical pregnancy.

2.2.4 Role of Ultrasound Guidance

Ultrasound is an essential part of many steps during an IVF cycle. The use of ultrasound-guided embryo transfer has the potential benefit of visualisation of the tip of the catheter to allow confirmation that placement of the embryo has occurred beyond the internal os into the optimal place in uterine cavity.

The disadvantages of ultrasound-guided transfer are the need for a second operator, inconvenience of having a full bladder and the occasional need to move the catheter tip for the purpose of visualisation [29]. A Cochrane review [30] concluded that ultrasound guidance appears to improve the likelihood of clinical pregnancies and live birth when compared with clinical touch method. However, there was substantial heterogeneity amongst the studies included. A more recent systematic review [29] attempted to adjust for the type of catheter used. They concluded that ultrasound guidance during embryo transfer improves the chance of achieving a live birth and the likelihood of a clinical pregnancy compared with clinical touch, when using the same catheters and techniques. Clinical touch however involves contact of the catheter with the fundus and drawing back into the cavity – a technique little used since it is more likely to induce unwanted uterine activity.

2.2.5 The Site of Embryo Deposition

The site of embryo placement in the uterine cavity has been suggested to directly influence the implantation rate with better outcome if the tip of the catheter is placed close to the middle area of cavity [31] or 15 to 20 mm from the fundus [32] compared to 10 mm from the fundus.

2.2.6 Role of Operator

Even though, the pregnancy rate after embryo transfer is strongly dependent on patient clinical characteristics and quality of the transferred embryo, the impact of embryo transfer technique should not be underestimated. Both retrospective and prospective studies have demonstrated significant differences in pregnancy rate between different operators [1, 33].

2.2.7 Troubleshooting

The impact of a difficult embryo transfer on pregnancy rate has been examined in various studies. A difficult embryo transfer can be defined as a procedure that may require additional manoeuvres, instruments, force and/or where it results in the presence of blood at the catheter tip on its removal. A recent systematic review demonstrated that a difficult embryo transfer was associated with a reduced clinical pregnancy rate (OR 0.75, 95% CI 0.66–0.86) [34]. The presence of blood at catheter tip after transfer however, was not associated with a reduction in clinical pregnancy rate. Once an operator is faced with difficulties in passing the catheter through the cervical canal, the following measures could be undertaken to overcome such difficulties: use of a malleable stylet catheter or tenaculum and, in some cases, performance of transmyometrial transfer under sedation. One or more members of the clinical team in any IVF unit should be skilled in performing transmyometrial embryo transfer.

2.3 Post-embryo Transfer

2.3.1 Catheter Examination (Retained Embryo)

Once the clinician has finished the procedure, the catheter should be returned to the embryologist to check for embryo retention. Retention of an embryo is reported in 3 to 4% of embryo transfers but does not appear to influence IVF outcome. It is more likely to occur when the catheter has mucus or blood on the tip. If the embryo was found to be retained in the catheter, the patient needs to be reassured and the procedure repeated.

2.3.2 Rest after Embryo Transfer

Historically, bed rest was encouraged following embryo transfer for a variable amount of time that often used to last for more than 24 hours. However, a recent meta-analysis demonstrated no benefit of bed rest on the rate of ongoing pregnancy (OR 0.88, 95% CI 0.60–1.31, $I^2 = 0\%$), [35].

2.4 QC

It is important to have arrangements in place for regular audit of transfer practitioner performance. This should be an integral part of the quality assurance system implemented in any successful IVF unit. There are multiple variables that can interfere with success but only by robust monitoring of the different aspects of the process of IVF will there be meaningful analysis to help improve and maintain favourable pregnancy results.

2.5 Summary

In summary, based on current evidence the following steps of embryo transfer are shown to improve the clinical pregnancy rate:

- Thorough cleaning of the cervix
- Gentle manipulation
- Use of soft embryo transfer catheters
- Use of ultrasound guidance
- Placement of embryos 2cm below the fundus into the cavity
- Robust quality assurance system

References

1. Healy MW, Hill MJ, Levens ED. Optimal oocyte retrieval and embryo transfer techniques: where we are and how we got here. *Semin Reprod Med.* 2015;33:83–91

2. Horne R, Bishop CJ, Reeves G, Wood C, Kovacs GT. Aspiration of oocytes for in-vitro fertilization. *Hum Reprod Update.* 1996 Jan–Feb;2(1):77–85.

3. Pickering SJ, Braude PR, Johnson MH, Cant A, Currie J. Transient cooling to room temperature can cause irreversible disruption of the meiotic spindle in the human oocyte. *Fertil Steril.* 1990;54:102–8.

4. Mullen SF, Agca Y, Broermann DC, Jenkins CL, Johnson CA, Critser JK. The effect of osmotic stress on the metaphase II spindle of human oocytes, and the relevance to cryopreservation. *Hum Reprod.* 2004;19:1148–54.

5. Kwan I, Bhattacharya S, Knox F, McNeil A. Pain relief for women undergoing oocyte retrieval for assisted reproduction. *Cochrane Database Syst Rev.* 2013 Jan 31; Issue 1. Art. No.: CD004829. doi: 10.1002/14651858.CD004829. pub3

6. Van Os HC, Roozenburg BJ, Janssen-Caspers HA, Leerentveld RA, Scholtes MC, Zeilmaker GH, Alberda AT. Vaginal disinfection with povidon iodine and the outcome of in-vitro fertilization. *Hum Reprod.* 1992 Mar;7(3): 349–50.

7. Hannoun A, Awwad J, Zreik T, Ghaziri G, Abu-Musa A. Effect of betadine vaginal preparation during oocyte aspiration in in vitro fertilization cycles on pregnancy outcome. *Gynecol Obstet Invest.* 2008;66(4): 274–8.

8. Funabiki M, Taguchi S, Hayashi T, Tada Y, Kitaya K, Iwaki Y, Karita M, Nakamura Y. Vaginal preparation with povidone iodine disinfection and saline douching as a safe and effective method in prevention of oocyte pickup-associated pelvic inflammation without spoiling the reproductive outcome: evidence from a large cohort study. *Clin Exp Obstet Gynecol.* 2014;41(6):689–90.

9. Bennett SJ, Waterstone JJ, Cheng WC, Parsons J. Complications of transvaginal ultrasound-directed follicle aspiration: a review of 2670 consecutive procedures. *J Assist Reprod Genet.* 1993 Jan;10(1):72–7.

10. Tureck RW, Garcia CR, Blasco L, Mastroianni L Jr. Perioperative complications arising after transvaginal oocyte retrieval. *Obstet Gynecol* 1993;81:590–3.

11. Rose B. Approaches to oocyte retrieval for advanced reproductive technology cycles planning to utilize in vitro maturation: a review of the many choices to be made. *J Assist Reprod Genet*. 2014 Nov;31(11):1409–19.

12. Mok-Lin E, Brauer AA, Schattman G, Zaninovic N, Rosenwaks Z, Spandorfer S. Follicular flushing and in vitro fertilization outcomes in the poorest responders: a randomized controlled trial. *Hum Reprod*. 2013 Nov;28(11):2990–5.

13. Siristatidis C, Chrelias C, Alexiou A, Kassanos D. Clinical complications after transvaginal oocyte retrieval: a retrospective analysis. *J Obstet Gynaecol*. 2013 Jan;33(1):64–6.

14. Buster J. Historical Evolution of Oocyte and Embryo Donation as a Treatment for Intractable Infertility. In *Principals of Oocyte and Embryo Donation*. Ed. Sauer MV, Springer, New York, 1998.

15. Abou-Setta AM. Effect of passive uterine straightening during embryo transfer: a systematic review and meta-analysis. *Acta Obstet Gynecol Scand*. 2007; 86(5):516–22.

16. Derks RS, Farquhar C, Mol BW, Buckingham K, Heineman MJ. Techniques for preparation prior to embryo transfer. *Cochrane Database Syst Rev*. 2009 Oct 7; Issue 4. Art. No.: CD007682. doi: 10.1002/14651858.CD007682. pub2.

17. Moon HS, Park SH, Lee JO, Kim KS, Joo BS. Treatment with piroxicam before embryo transfer increases the pregnancy rate after in vitro fertilization and embryo transfer. *Fertil Steril*. 2004 Oct; 82(4):816–20.

18. Dal Prato L, Borini A. Effect of piroxicam administration before embryo transfer on IVF outcome: a randomized controlled trial. *Report Biomed Online*. 2009 Oct;19(4):604–9.

19. Lan VT, Khang VN, Nhu GH, Tuong HM. Atosiban improves implantation and pregnancy rates in patients with repeated implantation failure. *Reprod Biomed Online*. 2012 Sep; 25(3):254–60.

20. Ng EH, Li RH, Chen L, Lan VT, Tuong HM, Quan S. A randomized double blind comparison of atosiban in patients undergoing IVF treatment. *Hum Reprod*. 2014 Dec;29(12):2687–94. doi: 10.1093/humrep/deu263. Epub 2014 Oct 21.

21. Mansour R, Aboulghar M, Serour G. Dummy embryo transfer: a technique that minimizes the problems of embryo transfer and improves the pregnancy rate in human in vitro fertilization. *Fertil Steril*. 1990 Oct;54(4):678–81.

22. Ghazzawi IM1, Al-Hasani S, Karaki R, Souso S. Transfer technique and catheter choice influence the incidence of transcervical embryo expulsion and the outcome of IVF. *Hum Reprod*. 1999 Mar;14(3):677–82.

23. Mansour R. Minimizing embryo expulsion after embryo transfer: a randomized controlled study. *Hum Reprod*. 2005 Jan;20(1): 170–4.

24. Amui J, Check JH, Brasile D. Speculum retention during embryo transfer does not improve pregnancy rates following embryo transfer–a randomized study *Clin Exp Obstet Gynecol*. 2011;38(4): 333–4.

25. Ruhlman C, Bisioli C, Terrado G, Rolla ED, Nicholson RE, Gnocchi D, et al. The inefficacy of cervical mucus aspiration prior to embryo transfer. A prospective randomized trial. ASRM/CFAS Conjoint Annual Meeting. *Fertil Steril*. 1999;72 Suppl 1(3):154.

26. Egbase PE, al-Sharhan M, al-Othman S, al-Mutawa M, Udo EE, Grudzinskas JG. Incidence of microbial growth from the tip of the embryo transfer catheter after embryo transfer in relation to clinical pregnancy rate following in-vitro fertilization and embryo transfer. *Hum Reprod*. 1996 Aug;11(8):1687–9.

27. Kroon B, Hart RJ, Wong BM, Ford E, Yazdani A. Antibiotics prior to embryo transfer in ART. *Cochrane Database Syst Rev*. 2012; Mar 14:Issue 3. Art. No.: CD008995. doi: 10.1002/14651858.CD008995.pub2.

28. Abou-Setta AM, Al-Inany HG, Mansour RT, Serour GI, Aboulghar MA. Soft versus firm embryo transfer catheters for assisted reproduction: a systematic review and meta-analysis. *Hum Reprod*. 2005 Nov; 20(11):3114–21.

29. Teixeira DM, Dassunção LA, Vieira CV, Barbosa MA, Coelho Neto MA, Nastri CO, Martins WP. Ultrasound guidance during embryo transfer: a systematic review and meta-analysis of randomized controlled trials. *Ultrasound Obstet Gynecol*. 2015 Feb;45(2):139–48. doi: 10.1002/uog.14639. Epub 2015 Jan 5.

30. Brown J, Buckingham K, Abou-Setta AM, Buckett W. Ultrasound versus 'clinical touch' for catheter guidance during embryo transfer in women. *Cochrane Database Syst Rev*. 2010 Jan 20;Issue 1. Art. No.: CD006107.

31. Oliveira JB, Martins AM, Baruffi RL, Mauri AL, Petersen CG, Felipe V, Contart P, Pontes A, Franco Júnior JG. Increased implantation and pregnancy rates obtained by placing the tip of the transfer catheter in the central area of the endometrial cavity. *Reprod Biomed Online*. 2004 Oct; 9(4):435–41.

32. Coroleu B, Barri PN, Carreras O, Martínez F, Parriego M, Hereter L, Parera N, Veiga A, Balasch J. The influence of the depth of embryo replacement into the uterine cavity on implantation rates after IVF: a controlled, ultrasound-guided study. *Hum Reprod*. 2002 Feb;17(2):341–6.

33. Yao Z, Vansteelandt S, Van der Elst J, Coetsier T, Dhont M, De Sutter P. The efficacy of the embryo transfer catheter in IVF and ICSI is operator-dependent: a randomized clinical trial. *Hum Reprod*. 2009 Apr; 24(4):880–7.

34. Phillips JA, Martins WP, Nastri CO, Raine-Fenning NJ. Difficult embryo transfers or blood on catheter and assisted reproductive outcomes: a systematic review and meta-analysis. *Eur J Obstet Gynecol Reprod Biol*. 2013 Jun; 168(2):121–8.

35. Abou-Setta AM, Peters LR, D'Angelo A, Sallam HN, Hart RJ, Al-Inany HG. Post-embryo transfer interventions for assisted reproduction technology cycles. *Cochrane Database Syst Rev*. 2014 Aug 27;Issue 8. Art. No.: CD006567.

Gamete Preparation and Embryo Culture

Karen Schnauffer

1 How It All Started

The pioneers of in vitro fertilisation (IVF) were Robert Edwards, a scientist working at Cambridge University, and Patrick Steptoe, a gynaecologic surgeon from Oldham, who collaborated together to develop the techniques required to collect human eggs from the ovary and fertilise them in the laboratory. The birth of Louise Brown in 1978 is regarded as the single most important milestone in the world of assisted conception as it revealed that babies could be born as a result of eggs and sperm being mixed together in a laboratory to create embryos which were then transferred back into the patient's uterus to create a pregnancy; a process known as IVF [1].

Robert Edwards' interest in human fertilisation began in the 1960s; as a physiologist he had the theoretical background to develop culture media and appropriate culture condition, and in 1968 achieved fertilisation of human eggs.

2 Culture Media

Although the modified Tyrode's medium (T6) was one of the original culture media used, the first major breakthrough in the world of assisted conception was the development of human tubal fluid (HTF) medium in 1985 [2]. This medium was formulated based on the composition of the fluid in the fallopian tubes, and this resulted in higher pregnancy rates than embryos cultured in T6. Overnight, this became the medium of choice for virtually every clinic; they used a basic recipe to make the medium in-house and then tested its suitability for use with a mouse embryo assay. If there was >80% blastocyst rate, the medium was deemed suitable for use.

If we fast forward to the current day, the compositions of media are more complex (Table 19.1) and are now commercially available. Although each brand is similar in terms of its basic composition there are various supplements that are unique to some

companies, some of which are considered confidential and the exact recipe not shared with the customers. Culture media can be purchased as a series of different media that meet the requirements of the embryo at different stages in its development known as sequential media, or, the more recently introduced, single-step media which avoids the embryo having to be removed from the incubator during its culture to have the medium replaced.

3 Mimic in vivo Conditions

For obvious reasons it is essential that the environment that the gametes and/or embryos are exposed to mimics the in vivo conditions as best as it can in terms of sterility, temperature, pH and osmolality.

4 Sterility

In 2007 the EU Tissues and Cells Directive (EUTD) [3] was introduced, covering all procedures involving donation, procurement, testing, processing, preservation, storage and distribution of human tissues and cells, for human application. This Directive also extended the Human Fertilisation and Embryology Authority's remit to include the licensing of services involving fresh gametes and meant that all IVF labs had to raise the bar to ensure they met certain air quality requirements to minimise the chance of contamination between gametes and embryos and the ambient environment. Prior to this, embryology laboratories were effectively a room with the lights dimmed down and/or blinds on the windows. Many laboratories introduced mobile air purifiers to upgrade the air quality but this was not a requirement. The EUTD was interpreted differently in different EU member states. In the United Kingdom, the requirement is for laboratories to carry out procedures involving the manipulation of gametes and/or embryos in an environment where the air quality is at least Grade C in the critical work area supported by a

Table 19.1 Examples of composition of modern culture media

Supplement	Example of addition
Water	Ultrapure
Bicarbonate pH buffer	
Protein source	HAS, Synthetic Replacement, recombinant albumin
Salts	NaCl, KCl, KH2PO4, CaCl2, MgSO4
Energy	Pyruvate, lactate, glucose
Amino acids	Non-essential aa's (proline, serine, alanine, aspargine, glycine, glutamate) Essential aa's (cystine, histadine, leucine, lysine, methionine, glutamine etc)
Antibiotics	Penicillin, streptomycin, gentamycin
Chelators	EDTA
Hyaluronic acid	EmbryoGlue (Vitrolife)
... and many others	

background environment of at least Grade D. The Directive, however, does not require micromanipulation procedures such as intracytoplasmic sperm injection (ICSI) or embryo biopsy to be carried out within a hood. However, as with all handling of gametes or embryos, documented procedures should be in place at all times to keep the risk of contamination minimal.

5 Temperature

We all understand the importance of keeping gametes and embryos at the correct physiological temperature, but this does not only apply to the temperature within the incubators but also to everything the gametes and embryos come into contact with i.e. culture media, hot blocks, work surfaces and consumables (such as Petri dishes, test tubes, catheters).

It has been well documented that the meiotic spindle which segregates chromosomes during cell division is highly temperature dependant. In order for the chromosome segregation to be successful it is crucial that eggs and embryos remain as close to the physiological temperature as possible. We know that the microtubular organisation in oocytes held at lower temperature is disrupted, and with extended exposure the spindle is irreversibly disrupted [4]. In order to avoid this damage to the spindle it is critical that laboratories ensure that everything that comes into contact with the gametes and embryos is kept at 37^0C. This process however, is not as simple as setting all the equipment to 37^0C; all equipment needs to be

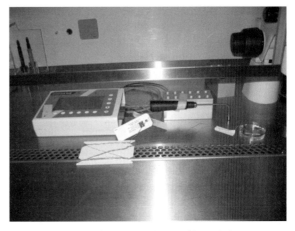

Fig. 19.1 Example of process validation of heated plate – thermocouple recording the temperature of the heated surface of a class II safety cabinet and the temperature within a droplet of culture medium that holds an egg/embryo (image courtesy of Hewitt Fertility Centre)

validated to ensure that the temperature where the gametes and embryos will be situated is set correctly to 37^0C (Figure 19.1).

Validation not only applies to the equipment but also to the processes; for example the temperature within the egg collection dish throughout an egg collection procedure. This temperature mapping allows the temperature changes within the dish during the egg collection procedure to be assessed and allows the process to be optimised to ensure that the temperature changes were minimised.

6 pH

All culture media are made up of a balanced salt solution backbone, and this salt solution has many purposes including helping to maintain the physiological pH of media. In mammals the optimal range is 7.2–7.4, and therefore an appropriate buffer should be used to achieve the required pH. Sodium bicarbonate is the most commonly used buffer for maintaining pH in culture media but in order to maintain the physiological pH it relies on a constant supply of carbon dioxide (CO_2). This buffering system is ideal for culturing gametes and embryos in a carbon dioxide incubator for long periods of time. In order to determine the pH of a medium based on the amount of bicarbonate and CO_2 present, the Henderson–Hasselbalch equation (Figure 19.2) is applied. The bicarbonate concentration in culture media varies but is approximately 25 mmol and, as such, you will usually see incubators set at 5–6% CO_2 to achieve the correct pH. If there is not enough CO_2 present, the pH increases and the medium turns a pinky/purple colour and cell growth is inhibited.

Certain procedures such as egg collection, ICSI and embryo biopsy require gametes and embryos to be in an atmospheric environment for fairly long periods of time thus potentially affecting the pH of the medium. Bicarbonate buffered media are not suitable for holding gametes and embryos during these procedures for the reasons described earlier and therefore alternatives to a bicarbonate buffer are used. HEPES (4-(2-hydroxyethyl)-1-piperazineethanesulfonic acid) and more recently MOPS (93-(N-morpholino) propanesulfonic acid) are two examples of zwitterions (organic chemical buffering agents) that do not require a CO_2-enriched atmosphere to maintain the required physiological pH despite changes in the CO_2 concentration, and therefore are suitable for culture of gametes and embryos for short periods of time.

7 Osmolality

Another area to consider for successful culture is the osmolality of the culture medium that gametes and

$$pH = pKa - \log_{10}\left(\frac{[Acid]}{[Base]}\right)$$

Fig. 19.2 The Henderson–Hasselbalch equation to determine the pH of culture media

embryos will be exposed to. The physiological osmolality of human plasma is 275–295 mOsm/kg and although mammals can tolerate small variations in their osmolality, maintaining the appropriate level is essential for successful culture. Areas to consider when maintaining osmolality are minimising medium evaporation by ensuring that the correct volume of medium or oil overlay is used, the use of humidified incubators and wherever possible using dish lids to minimise evaporation effects. These again would require validating as part of the laboratory set-up.

8 Gamete Preparation

8.1 Sperm Prep

Various studies have described that sperm quality is affected by the duration and type of arousal the male is exposed to whilst producing a sample [5,6,7]. Gone are the days when the male partner would be handed a magazine and sent off to use a hospital toilet cubicle to produce a sample. Nowadays there are designated rooms; fully equipped with reclining chair, sample hatch directly through to the laboratory and, more frequently, a video system including headphones to enhance privacy (Figure 19.3). Magazines pose significant infection control issues and feedback from patients describes how unpleasant it is to be given the same magazine that the man before was handed!

In some circumstances patients may prefer to produce their samples at home and must be provided with clear guidance to ensure that the quality of the semen sample is not affected by fluctuations in temperature and must ideally arrive at the laboratory within one hour of ejaculation.

All patients are instructed to have between 2–7 days sexual abstinence. Samples are produced by masturbation and ejaculated into a clean, non-toxic, wide-mouthed container. A sample may, in exceptional circumstances (i.e. an inability to produce a sample by masturbation) be collected into a special non-toxic

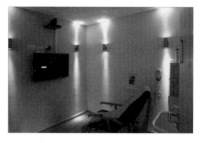

Fig. 19.3 Example of a male room equipped with DVD, reclining chair and hatch (image courtesy of the Hewitt Fertility Centre)

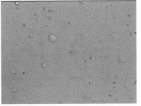

Fig. 19.4 Examples of good and poor sperm samples (images courtesy of the Hewitt Fertility Centre)

condom designed for semen collection. This type of condom should be provided by the laboratory with the manufacturer's instructions as to how it should be used (NB. contraceptive condoms are highly spermotoxic) [8].

Once the sample has been produced, it is passed immediately through to the laboratory where it is allowed to liquefy for approximately 30 minutes prior to analysis and/or preparation. After the liquefaction period, the sample is assessed for degree of liquefaction, pH and appearance before the volume is calculated. A wet preparation is prepared for microscopic appearance and motility assessment (Figure 19.4). For therapeutic preparations this initial assessment will help inform the most appropriate preparation method; density gradient, swim-up, or wash and resuspend [8].

Increased sperm progression and sperm concentration have been associated with higher pregnancy rates [9]. Sperm motility is assessed either manually or with the use of a computer-aided semen analysis (CASA) system within one hour of a semen sample being produced. Evaluation of at least 200 sperm is undertaken and the sperm are graded as progressive motility (PR), non-progressive motility (NP) or immotility (IM) and an average percentage reported for each category. Sperm concentration is calculated using a haemocytometer chamber (e.g. Improved Neubauer) and after allowing the sperm to settle, counting at least 200 spermatozoa.

The importance of sperm morphology with regards to pregnancy rates is fairly contentious as the assessment of morphology is difficult due to the variability of human sperm; however, studies looking at sperm recovered from the female reproductive tract and from around the zona pellucida of an egg have facilitated derivation of 'normal' morphology parameters [10].

For therapeutic treatment, the sperm sample is prepared by one of a number of procedures depending on the initial assessment of the sample. Discontinuous density gradient works on the principle that there are density differences between live and dead sperm, cells and debris. Density gradient solutions (such as PureSperm™ or Isolate™) are added to a centrifuge tube to form layers with the lowest density at the top (Figure 19.5). The sperm sample is then added as a top layer and the sample centrifuged. These commercially available density gradient solutions are specifically developed to minimise any pH and osmolarity changes that could have a detrimental effect on sperm function. This process effectively filters out dead sperm, cells and debris, leaving a pellet of 'good' sperm to be collected at the bottom of the tube.

An alternative sperm preparation procedure is a swim-up and is suitable for good quality samples. The principle of this technique is that some motile sperm in a sample will inevitably swim upwards. The sperm sample is added to the bottom of a round bottom test tube and culture medium is carefully layered over the top creating a clean interface between the two layers. After 30–60 minutes, the top part of the culture medium containing all the 'best' sperm is gently aspirated.

These methods can also be used to prepare sperm samples from viral discordant patients which effectively remove the virus leaving a negative sample which can then be used for treatment (i.e. IUI, IVF, ICSI). As

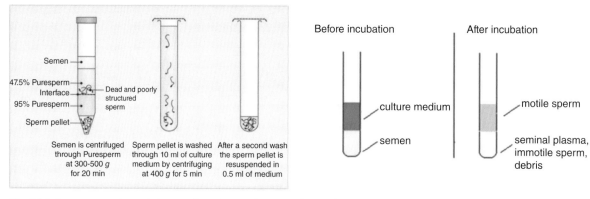

Fig. 19.5 Sperm preparation techniques – discontinuous density gradient and swim-up

the HIV virus is carried in the seminal fluid and not on the sperm, a process known as Sperm Washing can be used to separate the virus from the infected seminal fluid. This is achieved by first performing a density gradient and then a series of washes. The final prepared sample is then sent for PCR testing and if negative, can be used for treatment.

8.2 Egg Preparation

The preparation of eggs is much simpler. During an egg collection the requirement is for the removal of follicular fluid and blood which can be achieved by washing the eggs through a series of medium droplets before incubating them prior to insemination (either by IVF or ICSI). Although human eggs are microscopic the oocyte–cumulus complex (OCC) can be seen with the naked eye (Figure 19.6). The eggs are graded during an egg collection; however, this grading system only provides a description of the OCC and not the actual grade of the egg (i.e. immature, mature, post mature).

Other egg preparation techniques include denudation prior to ICSI and artificial oocyte activation. Preparation of eggs for ICSI involves placing the eggs in a diluted hyaluronidase solution and for a short period of time (approximately 30 seconds) to dissolve the cells in the cumulus and the corona radiata. This process allows the egg maturity to be assessed with regards to the suitability for the ICSI procedure. Only eggs with an extruded polar body (MII) are suitable for ICSI, those at the metaphase I (MI) and germinal vesicle (GV) stage have not fully undergone the maturation process and maintain a full complement of DNA and therefore are not suitable for ICSI (Figure 19.7).

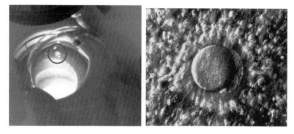

Fig. 19.6 Oocyte cumulus complex seen in a Petri dish during the egg collection procedure.

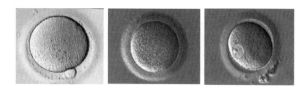

Fig. 19.7 Egg grading - MII oocyte (suitable for ICSI); MI oocyte (immature); Germinal vesicle (GV) (immature)

Oocyte activation is an essential early event during the fertilisation process. If the oocyte fails to activate then the fertilisation process will not proceed and the egg will not fertilise properly. Oocyte activation is caused by factors on the sperm which cause an increase in calcium levels in the oocyte. If the sperm are lacking these factors, or the oocytes do not respond to the factors properly, then the oocytes may fail to activate and not fertilise. Artificial oocyte activation (AOA) is a relatively new technique that uses calcium ionophore to help increase the calcium levels within the egg and promote activation. Immediately after the eggs have been injected using conventional ICSI, they are placed in a calcium ionophore solution. After 15 minutes exposure the eggs are removed from the calcium ionophore solution and rinsed through a series of culture medium droplets, to remove the calcium ionophore, before being placed in conventional culture. The eggs are then left overnight and checked for fertilisation the following morning.

9 New Technologies

There have been relatively few major breakthroughs in the world of assisted conception since its inception, with the introduction of ICSI in 1991 and to a lesser extent pre-implantation genetic diagnosis (PGD) in 1997 being notable. However, even with these so-called game changers the embryologists were still left with the same dilemma as to which was the best embryo to choose for embryo transfer, and replacing numerous embryos in an attempt to achieve a pregnancy is clearly not the answer as producing a multiple birth is not the desirable outcome [11].

Conventional incubation of embryos involves placing embryos in droplets of culture medium in a culture dish, under an oil overlay. This dish is then placed in an incubator for the duration of the treatment (2–6 days) and the embryos are removed from the incubator (usually only once per day) to observe their development. These observations provide a 'snap-shot' of how the embryo is developing at the time of the observation and does not account for the continuing changes and developments of an embryo as it grows. In order to minimise the disturbances and protect the embryo, it is essential that the dish is only removed from the incubator briefly during the culture period.

As such, a wealth of information about early embryo development has remained untapped. With the introduction of timelapse imaging systems, there is now the potential for constant surveillance of embryo development without having to remove the dish from the stable, controlled environment of the incubator. The timelapse systems provide images every 5 or 10 minutes and enable the observation of key events to help select the 'best' embryos. The embryologist can record the exact time at which the embryo divides and can monitor in detail the way this development occurs. The key timings of developmental embryo events, known as morphokinetics, has enabled the development of algorithms that assist with the selection of the 'best' embryo [12]. There is now evidence that the use of systems such as the EmbryoScope^{TM} may result in an increase in pregnancy rates [13] and a reduction in early pregnancy loss [14]. De-selection of embryos is now regarded as another benefit of timelapse systems as embryos that develop abnormally are identified and therefore can be excluded from the embryo selection cohort [15]. Furthermore, there is emerging evidence that particular morphokinetic patterns might be associated with the genetic 'normality' of the embryo perhaps providing, at last, a non-invasive marker of aneuploidy [16].

References

1. Steptoe PC, Edwards RG. Birth after the reimplantation of a human embryo. *Lancet*. 1978; 12 (8085):366.

2. Quinn P, Kerin JF, Warnes GM. Improved pregnancy rate in human in vitro fertilization with the use of a medium based on the composition of human tubal fluid. *Fertil Steril*. 1985 Oct;44(4): 493–498.

3. Commission Directive 2006/17/ EC of 8 February 2006 implementing Directive 2004/23/ EC of the European Parliament and of the Council as regards certain technical requirements for the donation, procurement and testing of human tissues and cells.

4. Pickering SJ, Braude PR, Johnson MH, Cant A, Currie J. Transient cooling to room temperature can cause irreversible disruption of the meiotic spindle in the human oocyte. *Fertil Steril*. 1990;54:102–108.

5. Roijen JH, Slob AK, Gianotten WL, Dohle GR, van der Zon ATM, Vreeburg JTM., Weber RFA. Sexual arousal and the quality of semen produced by masturbation. *Hum Reprod*. 1996;11(1):147–151.

6. Kilgallon SJ, Simmons LW. Image content influences men's semen quality. *Biol Lett*. 2005; 22(3):253–255.

7. Pound N, Javed MH, Ruberto C, Shaikh MA, Del Valle AP. Duration of sexual arousal predicts semen parameters for masturbatory ejaculates. *Physiol Behav*. 2002;76:685–689.

8. WHO. Laboratory manual for the examination and processing of human semen 5th edition, 2010.

9. Zinamen M, Brown C, Selevan G, Clegg E. Semen quality and human fertility: a prospective study with healthy couples. *J Androl*. 2000;21(1): 14–53.

10. Menkveld R, Stander FS, Kotze TJ, Kruger TF, van Zyl JA. The evaluation of morphological characteristics of human spermatozoa according to stricter

criteria. *Hum Reprod.* 1990 Jul; 5(5):586–592.

11. HFEA. One Child at a Time, 2006. https://ifqlive.blob.core.windows.net/umbraco-website/1311/one-child-at-a-time-report.pdf.

12. Meseguer M, Herrero J, Tejera A, Hilligsøe K, Ramsing NB, Remohı́ J. The use of morphokinetics as a predictor of embryo implantation. *Hum Reprod.* 2011;26(10): 2658–2671.

13. Rubio I, Galán A, Larreategui Z, Ayerdi F, Bellver J, Herrero J, Meseguer, M. Clinical validation of embryo culture and selection by morphokinetic analysis: a randomized, controlled trial of the EmbryoScope. *Fertil Steril.* 2014 Nov;102(5):1287–1294.

14. Barrie A, Schnauffer K, Kingsland C, Troup S. Treatment outcome and early pregnancy loss – a comparison of conventional and embryoscope® systems. *Fertil Steril.* 2013;100(3): Supplement, S248.

15. Athayde Wirka K, Chen AA, Conaghan J, Ivani K, Gvakharia M, Behr B, Suraj V, Tan L, Shen S. Atypical embryo phenotypes identified by time-lapse microscopy: high prevalence and association with embryo development. *Fertil Steril.* 2014 Jun; 101(6):1637–1648.

16. Chavez SL, Loewke KE, Han J, Moussavi F, Colls P, Munne S, Behr B, Reijo Pera RA. Dynamic blastomere behaviour reflects human embryo ploidy by the four-cell stage. *Nat Commun.* 2012;(3):1251.

Chapter 20

Single Embryo Transfer

Martine Nijs

1 Assisted Reproduction Worldwide: Availability and Outcomes

Worldwide 95% of the adults express their desire for a child. Between 8 and 12% of reproductive-aged couples worldwide have problems conceiving. The probable global average for infertility is estimated to affect 9% of women. In some regions of the world, the rates of infertility are much higher, reaching up to 30% in some populations [1]. Over the past decade, there has been a significant increase in the number of centres offering Assisted Reproduction Techniques (ART). The number of ART cycles performed worldwide has increased clearly over time: a 5–10% increase per annum. The International Committee for Monitoring Assisted Reproductive Technologies reported >1,251,881 procedures with ART in their World Report on Assisted Reproductive Technologies for 2007 [2]. This Committee yearly summarises the data collection set from 2,419 of 3,354 (72.1%) known ART clinics in 55 countries. In 2007, in the United Kingdom, availability of ART was estimated to have been at 766 cycles per million inhabitants. Availability of ART treatments varies by country from 12 (Guatemala) to 4,140 (Israel) treatments per million population. The latter is the result of substantial economic support for patients undergoing in vitro fertilisation (IVF). Australia, New Zealand, and European countries, especially northern Europe, also strongly support ART treatments. The overall worldwide delivery rate per fresh aspiration stood at 20.3% in 2007, ranging from 8% to 33%. For frozen-embryo transfer (FET), delivery rates were 18.4%, resulting in a cumulative delivery rate of 25.8%. In the United Kingdom in 2013, a delivery rate of 26% per cycle started was noted [3]. In Europe, the delivery rate after cycle of intrauterine insemination (IUI) with husband's semen was 8.9% and 13.8% after IUI with donor semen [4].

With wide regional variations, single embryo transfer (SET) represented 23.4% of the fresh transfers, with 5 countries in which SET rates were >50%: Sweden (69.9%), New Zealand (61.3%), Australia (59.6%), Finland (57.8%), and Belgium (50.2%). In South Korea and several countries in Latin America and the Middle East, the mean number of embryo transfers (ETs) remained at >3 embryos. In the United Kingdom, the proportion of elective single ETs (eSETs) has increased substantially: in 2008, fewer than 5% of embryo transfers were eSET, but by 2014 this had increased to 29% [3, 5].

Worldwide, the proportion of deliveries with twins and triplets from fresh transfers was 22.3% and 1.2%, respectively [2]. In the United Kingdom, the overall multiple pregnancy rate was 27% in 2008 and fell to 16% in the first half of 2014 [3]. In Europe, twin and triplet delivery rates associated with IUI cycles were 9.6%/0.5% and 8.5%/0.2%, following treatment with husband and donor semen, respectively [4].

In 2007, 229,442 babies born as a result of an ART treatment were reported worldwide. In the United Kingdom in 2013, live birth rate per cycles started (fresh and frozen treatment cycles) was 26% [3]. Overall in 2014, 4% of the babies born in Europe were from ART; in the United Kingdom, this was 2%.

2 Multiple Pregnancies

Multiple pregnancies are the most common in patients who are being treated with fertility medication to induce ovulation (up to 10% multiples and 1% have triplets or more). The use of drugs to induce superovulation with multiple oocytes produced, caused the vast majority of the increase in multiple pregnancies (up to 30% of pregnancies after gonadotrophin treatments are multiples). IVF and Intracytoplasmic sperm injection (ICSI) treatment also contributed in the increase of multiple pregnancies because of transfer of more than one embryo. The single biggest risk of a fertility treatment is a multiple pregnancy; hence the single most important factor responsible for the increase in specific risks for mother, babies and the family. Mothers have an increased risk of hypertension (20% vs. 1–2%); pre-eclampsia (30% vs. 2–10%); and diabetes (12% vs. 4%) during the twin pregnancy. Risks during or after birth include C-section, death of the mother ($\times 2$ increase), and a higher incidence of stress and depression after giving birth.

Vanishing twin pregnancies are associated with pregnancies with an adverse perinatal outcome like lower birth weight or small for gestational age, lower Apgar scores, and higher risk for perinatal mortality.

Babies from a twin or triplet pregnancy have an increased risk: very premature and premature birth (twins: 50% before 37 weeks; triplets: 90% increase); extremely low and low birth weight; admission to a neonatal intensive care unit (40–60% vs. 20%); perinatal mortality (3–6 times higher for twins; 9 times higher for triplets); cerebral palsy (1 in 80 twins versus 1 in 434 for singletons). All complications result in an increased cost for pregnancy care and more care after birth because of increase of learning difficulties, slower language development, impaired sight, and congenital heart disease (7.4% of twin pregnancies). A family with twins or triplets will endure higher costs for pregnancy care, for the delivery, and for care after birth. A higher stress level has been observed in these families as well as intense bereavement support to cope with loss or handicaps [6–11]. With approximately 13,000 IVF babies being born each year in the United Kingdom, this contributes significantly and disproportionately to the national multiple birth rates and presents a significant public health concern.

3 Strategies to Prevent Multiple Pregnancies

The main strategy to reduce the multiple birth rate is to transfer one single healthy embryo at a time, even when more are available. Only with a collaborative and multidisciplinary approach that involves clinicians, laboratory staff, nurses, counsellors, professional bodies, governments, and patients, this can be achieved.

3.1 Clinic

It is imperative that prevention of multiple pregnancies starts with the correct diagnosis of infertility and the correct choice of treatment mode for infertility: non-ART, cycle monitoring with planned intercourse,

IUI, IVF, or ICSI. Health and lifestyle advice should to be part of the clinical advice.

Clinicians should identify those patients who are at risk of multiple pregnancies. The National Institute for Health and Care Excellence (NICE) guidelines [12] clearly advocate eSET and propose several identifiers: For women under the age of 37 years undertaking their first treatment cycle, these include maternal age, obstetric and gynaecological, history, previous treatment history, ovarian response or reserve, the number of embryos created and quality of embryos or blastocysts available for transfer, and cryopreservation. Maximising oocyte and embryo quality is an essential part of an effective eSET strategy.

A focus should remain on optimising superovulation regimens: the optimal number of good quality oocytes and embryos to achieve a live birth is between 6 and 15 mature oocytes [13]. A Cochrane review of GnRH antagonists in assisted reproduction suggests that overall the antagonist protocol gave a 1.5% lower LBR and 2% lower CPR compared with the agonist protocol. Care should be taken since GnRH antagonist use is associated with a lower risk of ovarian hyper stimulation syndrome (OHSS) compared with GnRH agonist. However, excellent cumulative success rates following mild IVF stimulation protocols and SET can be obtained [14].

Patients entering an oocyte donation programme should only have a single embryo transferred; studies demonstrate that delivery rates for these patients are similar to double embryo transfer (DET), but with fewer risks. NICE therefore recommends using an embryo transfer strategy based on the age of the oocyte donor. However, care should be taken since even with SET for these patients, an increased risk for pre-eclampsia during the pregnancy is observed [12, 13].

3.2 Laboratory

Single embryo transfer is only possible when IVF is performed under the best conditions and when optimal embryo culture and embryo selection systems are in place. It is essential that pre-selection of gametes (spermatozoa and oocytes) is in place, since a clear association exists between some sperm and oocyte aberrant morphologies and genetic normality and fertilising potential [15]. As for the culture system for embryos, a systematic review of randomised controlled trials describing the effect of embryo culture media on IVF/ICSI success rates did not reveal a superior culture medium [16]. Different embryo culture systems are in place such as small and large volume box incubators, bench top incubators, and micro fluid systems. To date, no study has clearly demonstrated a distinct advantage of any specific incubator type regarding human embryo development or clinical outcomes [17]. Manual morphological embryo selection is still the most prevalent first-line method for embryo grading in IVF laboratories. The live birth rate is positively associated with increasing cell number up to eight cells on day 3. A negative correlation is demonstrated with miscarriage and increasing fragmentation, asymmetry scores and/or multi-nucleation. Although cryopreservation is a strong marker for good quality embryos, not having cryopreservation does not reliably indicate poor quality. Advances in embryo culture media and incubation systems have enabled the reliable extended culture of embryos to the blastocyst stage of development with transfer on day 5 or 6 of culture. A positive correlation with live birth was found with good quality blastocyst morphology: a large ICM, a pavoid structured trophectoderm, and presence of early hatching. There is a body of evidence that the number of supernumerary vitrified blastocysts correlates positively with the odds of implantation and live birth in good quality single-blastocyst transfers. Fresh transfer outcomes can predict the success of a subsequent cryopreserved transfer utilising blastocysts of the same cohort. Time-lapse monitoring (TLM) has recently emerged as a novel technology to perform a semi-quantitative evaluation of embryo morphology and developmental kinetics in culture. This technique permits the continuous evaluation of early embryo development by automated imaging every 5–20 min. Embryo scoring occurs without removal from the incubator, so embryos are not exposed to changes in light, humidity, temperature, pH, and gas phase that is necessary for serial manual morphological grading. A systematic review of TLM studies could not support the clinical use of this technology for selection of human preimplantation embryos [18].

However, it has been demonstrated that around 50% of morphological normal looking blastocysts on day 5 are genetically abnormal and are aneuploid. Perhaps preimplantation genetic screening (PGS) using the new generation technique genetic tests with comprehensive aneuploidy screening (PGD-A) of all 24 chromosomes could assist in selection of the healthy embryo for transfer. A systematic review of

the literature in 2015 showed potential benefits of using PGD-A techniques over morphology-based selection of embryos, in particular, a PGD-A screened embryo had a higher implantation rate than a morphologically screened embryo [19]. It is essential that more prospective randomised controlled studies are performed, to identify clearly which patients can benefit from PGD-A.

Embryo culture and embryo scoring clearly remains a significant challenge in IVF, since to date, none has been shown conclusively to yield improved implantation and live birth rates [15, 20]. The UK Best Practice Guidelines for Elective Single Embryo Transfer rightfully points out that further research is required to define the best embryo culture and embryo selection systems [15].

3.3 Government, Regulating Bodies, Professional Societies

Very few countries have legal restrictions on the number of embryos used per transfer. In Belgium, in the Province of Quebec, Canada, and in Sweden the number of embryos transferred in fresh or frozen embryo transfer cycles are cycle, age, and embryo-quality dependent. These countries are also funding IVF treatments for patients (e.g. Belgium: up to 6 full IVF/ICSI cycles). Since the implementation of the law, multiple pregnancy rates (MPRs) have dropped significantly: <10% in Belgium; <5% in the Province of Quebec, and in Sweden. Moreover a recent Swedish study following in excess of 25,000 women receiving eSET showed that the risk of neonatal death and morbidity was significantly reduced. In 2010, Turkey introduced a new legislation mandating SET in women less than 35 years of age in the first or second cycle of treatment and limiting clinics to the transfer of two embryos in the third or subsequent treatment cycles and in women over the age of 35 years. Since the implementation of this policy, a significant reduction in MPR is noted, with only a modest downward trend in clinical pregnancy rates (from 39.9% to 34.5%).

In Finland, Norway, Denmark, and Australia, SET is done on a voluntary non-funded basis. This has resulted in MPRs between 5 and 10%. In other countries, the professional bodies have developed specific guidelines to assist practitioners in selecting patients for SET. In Japan, mild stimulation and natural cycle protocols along with blastocyst transfer are highly recommended, resulting in an MPR of less than 6%.

In the United States, <1% of the fresh embryo transfers prior to 2002 were eSET. In 2010 only 9.6% of the transfers were eSET, resulting in a 32.4% twin rate. In 2012, the American Society for Reproductive Medicine [21] recommended the following as indications for SET in their Practice Committee Report on SET: female age <35, more than one 'top-quality embryo' available for transfer, first or second treatment cycle, previous successful IVF cycle and recipient of embryos created from donor oocytes. Most recent data from the United States (2013) show 22.5 % eSET in the good prognosis, <35 age group with a modest reduction in the twin rate to 28.3%.

In the United Kingdom, in October and November 2007, 21 parties, made up of professional bodies, patient groups, and the Human Fertilisation and Embryology Authority (HFEA) made a decision to adopt an outcome-based policy, to reduce the risk of multiple births from fertility treatment. This policy encouraged fertility centres to adopt eSET into routine use and required a phased reduction in the multiple birth rate (MBR) from 24% in 2009, 20% in 2010, 15% in 2011, to 10% in 2012, and thereafter. To monitor the trend in SET, clinics have to submit data about each treatment they carry out and its outcomes to the HFEA Register.

The 2015 HFEA report on the evolution of multiple pregnancies in the United Kingdom [3], shows how a collaborative approach from clinics, patient groups, and the HFEA can have dramatic effects on the multiple pregnancy rates. The conclusions of the 2015 report are the following:

- There has been a marked shift from patients having a double embryo transfer (DET) to having an eSET since 2008. This is most noticeable in younger patients on their first treatment cycle.
- As a result, the multiple pregnancy and multiple birth rates have dropped dramatically: overall, the multiple birth rate has dropped from one in four IVF live births in 2008 to only one in six in 2013.
- Despite this dramatic change, pregnancy and birth rates have been maintained and have recently started to rise.
- Blastocyst transfers appear to be associated with an increased risk of monozygotic (identical) twins compared to cleavage stage transfers.
- Women aged under 38 on their first fresh treatment cycle have a higher pregnancy rate after eSET than after DET.

This resulted in an encouraging and sustained trend in reduction of multiple pregnancy rates from 26.6% in 2008 to 16.3% in 2013. During this period, the gradual improvement in live birth rate from IVF and ICSI treatment, which has been observed since 1994, remained unaffected.

Several guidelines have been published to assist clinics in defining strategies for reducing multiple pregnancy rates.

In the NICE guidelines [12], several factors were recommended which should be considered when determining an individual patient's suitability for eSET. A summary can be found in Box 20.1.

The British Fertility Society (BFS) and the Association of Clinical Embryologists recently updated the 'UK Best Practice Guidelines for Elective Single Embryo Transfer' [15]. Practitioners should be guided by the following when allocating patients for SET: female partner's age, previous pregnancies, cause

Box 20.1 Embryo transfer strategy summary table (including fresh & frozen embryos) [12].			
Attempt at age	<37	37–39	40–42
First cycle	SET	>1 Top Quality embryo Available: SET	Consider DET
		no Top Quality embryo Available: consider DET	
Second cycle	>1 Top Quality embryo Available: SET	>1 Top Quality embryo Available: SET	*
	no Top Quality embryo Available: consider DET	no Top Quality embryo Available: consider DET	*
Third cycle	No more than 2 embryos	No more than 2 embryos	*

The NICE guidelines do not advise a 2nd or 3rd cycle for patients over 40 years old.

of infertility, number of previous IVF failures, response to follicular stimulation, number of oocytes, number of good-quality embryo, and number cultured to blastocyst. Where blastocyst transfer is performed, clinics should review their eSET data and criteria for extended embryo culture regularly.

3.4 Patients' Involvement

It is imperative that patients are involved in the decision taking for SET, eSET, or DET. Patients are less risk adverse and are not aware of the risks involved of multiple pregnancies. Some patients have the specific desire for twins and this is mostly driven by cost of treatment and reduced time to pregnancy. Other patients perceive patient selection (be it mandatory or voluntary) included in an eSET program as unfair. For counselling couples undergoing IVF treatment it is of paramount importance to be able to predict success. Several prediction models for the chance of success after IVF treatment have been developed and can be used for making decisions on SET or DET [26, 27, 28]. It is imperative the ART team follows the same strategy when counselling patients.

In those countries where ART is not funded, affordability of access to assisted reproductive technologies and embryo transfer practices can influence the decision making for SET or DET. Chamber et al. calculated that a 10-percentage-point decrease in affordability would predict a 5.1-percentage-point decrease in the percentage of fresh SET cycles (P < 0.01) and a 7.5-percentage-point increase in the percentage of fresh cycles transferring ≥3 embryos (P < 0.01) [22, 23]. In Australia, the dramatic reduction in multiple births has primarily occurred as a result of a voluntary shift to use of SET, after intensive counselling of the patient, since Australia has no legislation enforcing SET. Pregnancy rates did not change after the voluntary implementation of SET programme.

4 Cost Benefit

Sequential single ETs, when clinically appropriate, can reduce total ART treatment and pregnancy/infant-associated medical costs by reducing multiple births without lowering live birth rates. The Belgian funding system for IVF is based on this principle. It was calculated that the short- and long-term pregnancy/infant-associated medical costs saved by avoiding multiple pregnancies was sufficient to fund 6 IVF/ICSI cycles for the Belgian infertile population. Hence the Belgian government linked the funding to an enforced SET programme [24].

5 Challenges

A multiple pregnancy is one of the most significant risks of fertility treatment but can be avoided. Clinics must continue to show a sustained commitment to reduce their multiple pregnancy rates year-on-year to its lowest achievable value.

Challenges to the more universal acceptance of eSET are the imitations of our methods to select the best and safest stimulation scheme for our patients, to select the optimal culture system for the embryos, to improve the best selecting method for the embryo with the highest implantation potential for transfer, and to develop and implement safe cryopreservation supernumerary embryos with high survival rates after warming/thawing. Efforts to decrease the multiple pregnancy rates may also not be valued enough by patients, because of a lack of awareness of multiple pregnancy risks in the general public.

Ultimately, evidence-based education for clinicians, embryologists, and patients, and a thorough counselling discussion between the couple and their IVF specialist are crucial, so that the desired result of a pregnancy is achieved in as many patients as possible, while maximising the chances of a healthy outcome for the mother and her child.

References

1. Inhorn MC, Patrizio P. Infertility around the globe: new thinking on gender, reproductive technologies and global movements in the 21st century., *Hum Rep Update* 2015; 21: 411–26.

2. Ishihara O, Adamson GD, Dyer S, et al. International Committee for Monitoring Assisted Reproductive Technologies: World Report on Assisted Reproductive Technologies. *Fertil Steril* 2007; 103: 402–13.

3. HFEA Report, Improving outcomes for fertility patients: multiple births 2015. Available online www.hfea.gov.uk/docs/ Multiple_Births_Report_ 2015.pdf2015 (Accessed December 2015).

4. Kupka MS, Ferraretti AP, de Mouzon J, et al. Assisted reproductive technology in Europe, 2010: results generated from European registers by ESHRE. *Hum Reprod.* 2014; 10: 2099–113.

5. HFEA Fertility treatment in 2013: trends and figures. Available

online www.hfea.gov.uk/ 9463.html (Accessed December 2015).

6. Barrington KJ, Janvier A. The paediatric consequences of Assisted Reproductive Technologies, with special emphasis on multiple pregnancies Acta Paediatrica. *Int J Pediatr.* 2013; 102: 340–8.

7. Henningsen AA, Wennerholm UB, Gissler M. Risk of stillbirth and infant deaths after assisted reproductive technology: a Nordic study from the CoNARTaS group. *Hum Reprod.* 2014; 29: 1090–6.

8. Sejbaek CS, Pinborg A, Hageman I. Are repeated assisted reproductive technology treatments and an unsuccessful outcome risk factors for unipolar depression in infertile women? *Acta Obstet Gynecol Scand.* 2015; 94: 1048–55.

9. Society of Obstetricians and Gynaecologists of Canada, Pregnancy outcomes after assisted human reproduction. *Obstet Gynaecol Can.* 2014; 36: 64–83.

10. Jauniaux E, Ben-Ami I, Maymon R. Do assisted-reproduction twin pregnancies require additional antenatal care? *Reprod Biomed Online* 2013; 26: 107–19.

11. Evron E, Sheiner E, Friger M. Vanishing twin syndrome: is it associated with adverse perinatal outcome? *Fertil Steril.* 2015; 103: 1209–14.

12. National Institute for Health and Care Excellence. Fertility: assessment and treatment for people with Fertility problems. Clinical Guidelines CG156, 2013, Available online www.nice.org.uk/ guidance/cg156 (Accessed December 2015).

13. Masoudian P, Nasr A, De Nanassy J et al. Oocyte donation pregnancies and the risk of preeclampsia or gestational hypertension: a systematic review

and meta-analysis. *Am J Obstet Gynecol.* 2016; 214(3): 328–39.

14. Bodri D, Kawachiya S, De Brucker M, et al. Cumulative success rates following mild IVF in unselected infertile patients: a 3-year, single-centre cohort study. *RBM Online* 2014; 28: 572–81.

15. Harbottle S, Hughes S, Cutting R, et al. Elective single embryo transfer: an update to UK Best Practice Guidelines. *Hum Fertil.* 2015; 18: 165–183.

16. Mantikou E, Youssef M, Wely van M, et al. Embryo culture media and IVF/ICSI success rates: a systematic review. *Hum Rep Update.* 2014; 19: 210–20.

17. Swain JE Decisions for the IVF laboratory: comparative analysis of embryo culture incubators. *RBM Online.* 2014; 28: 535–47.

18. Kaser DJ and Racowsky C. Clinical outcomes following selection of human preimplantation embryos with time-lapse monitoring: a systematic review. *Hum Rep Update.* 2014; 20: 617–31.

19. Lee E, Illingworth P, Wilton L, et al. The clinical effectiveness of preimplantation genetic diagnosis for aneuploidy in all 24 chromosomes (PGD-A): systematic review. *Hum Reprod* 2015; 30: 473–83.

20. Bolton V, Leary C, Harbottle S, et al. How should we choose the 'best' embryo? A commentary on behalf of the British Fertility Society and the Association of Clinical Embryologists. *Hum Fertil.* 2015; 18: 156–164.

21. American Society for Reproductive Medicine Practice Committee of American Society for Reproductive Medicine; Practice Committee of Society for Assisted Reproductive Technology. Criteria for number of embryos to transfer: a

committee opinion. *Fertil & Steril.* 2012; 99: 44–6.

22. Chambers GM, Lee E, Hoang VP, et al. Hospital utilization, costs and mortality rates during the first 5 years of life: a population study of ART and non-ART singletons. *Hum Reprod.* 2014; 29: 601–10.

23. Chambers GM, Hoang VP, Sullivan EA, et al. The impact of consumer affordability on access to assisted reproductive technologies and embryo transfer practices: an international analysis. *Fertil Steril.* 2014; 101: 191–198.

24. Youssef MM, Mantikou E, van Wely M. Culture media for human pre-implantation embryos in assisted reproductive technology cycles. *Cochrane Database Syst Rev.* 2015; Issue 11. Art. No.: CD007876. DOI: 10.1002/14651858.CD007876. pub2.

25. De Neubourg D, Bogaerts K, Wyns C, et al. The history of Belgian assisted reproduction technology cycle registration and control: a case study in reducing the incidence of multiple pregnancy. *Hum Reprod.* 2013; 28: 2709–19.

26. Dhillon RK, McLernon DJ, Smith PP, et al. Predicting the chance of live birth for women undergoing IVF: a novel pretreatment counselling tool. *Hum Reprod.* 2016; 31: 84–92.

27. te Velde ER, Nieboer D, Lintsen AM, et al. Comparison of two models predicting IVF success; the effect of time trends on model performance. *Hum Reprod.* 2014; 29: 57–64.

28. Nelson SM, Lawlor DA, et al. Predicting live birth, preterm delivery, and low birth weight in infants born from in vitro fertilisation: a prospective study of 144,018 treatment cycles. *PLoS Med.* 2011; 8(1).

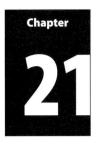

The Risks of Assisted Reproduction

Neil McClure

1 Introduction

Assisted reproductive techniques (ART) are now responsible for more than 2% of all human births in the United Kingdom and closer to 5% in mainland Europe. According to the Human Fertilisation and Embryology Authority (HFEA), 63,600 cycles of treatment were performed in 2013 alone in the United Kingdom [1]. Despite being so common, the ART 'industry' remains one of the most tightly regulated branches of medicine – and probably not without due reason as the consequences of error are potentially huge. This chapter deals, though, with the medical complications of the treatment process and not the 'social' complications of embryo mishandling.

There is surprisingly little published evidence on the complication rates of ART, probably because the treatment is actually so safe and the incidence of complication so low that it makes the collection of meaningful data, from any one unit, almost statistically pointless. Further, most medical complications of treatment are probably not managed by the individual ART unit, which would often not be equipped for this, but by general practitioners and the patients' local hospitals. However, Aragona et al published data on the incidence of severe complications in 2011, quoting a figure of 0.08% [2]. This, however, excluded ovarian hyperstimulation syndrome (OHSS) which, in its severe form, had a reported incidence of 0.08% in the HFEA figures for 2014 [3]. This is likely to represent considerable under-reporting and the true incidence is probably closer to 1%.

So what are the 'medical' complications of ART? Perhaps the easiest way is to categorise them 'chronologically' – as the cycle progresses from ovarian stimulation through to the birth of the child (Table 21.1).

2 Complications of Stimulation

An under-response to stimulation is hugely disappointing for couples undergoing treatment but it is neither physically dangerous nor life-threatening – unlike excessive ovarian stimulation. Technically, all patients undergoing ovarian stimulation for ART have ovarian 'hyperstimulation'; it is when this develops into ovarian hyperstimulation syndrome that problems arise. The risk factors for OHSS are listed in Box 21.1.

2.1 Definition and Pathophysiology

OHSS is a third-spacing phenomenon of intravascular fluids and proteins into the ovaries, peritoneal, pleural and, rarely, pericardial cavities. In normal, unstimulated ovarian cycles there is a natural increase in the volume of peritoneal fluid around the time of ovulation. Vascular Endothelial Growth Factor (VEGF) would appear to be central to this process. This cytokine is produced in response to the luteinising hormone (LH) surge and, in iatrogenic ovarian stimulation, to the human chorionic gonadotrophin (hCG) used to induce the final maturation of the follicle prior to oocyte retrieval [4]. Part of these peri-ovulatory changes is the neo-vascularisation of the granulosa cells in the follicle and part of that process is an increase in capillary permeability. When this process is exaggerated by the presence of a large number of follicles, the effects of the VEGF extend to the peritoneal capillaries resulting in an outpouring of a protein-rich exudate from the vascular compartment. OHSS will not occur in a stimulated cycle if there is no spontaneous LH surge or the hCG trigger is withheld. OHSS also appears to have two peaks of incidence: the first around 7 days after the ovulatory hCG injection and the second around 14 days later and thought to be in response to the hCG of pregnancy. The first group

Table 21.1 Complications of ART

POINT of COMPLICATION	COMPLICATION
Ovarian Stimulation	• Failure to respond • Over response and ovarian hyperstimulation syndrome (OHSS) • Hypercoagulation, deep vein thrombosis and pulmonary embolism • Cerebrovascular accident
Egg Collection	• Visceral damage • Internal haemorrhage • Infection
Embryo Transfer	• Infection
Pregnancy	• Multiple pregnancy • Ectopic pregnancy • Miscarriage – first and second trimester
Child	• Abnormality • Prematurity • Low birth weight

Box 21.1 Risk factors for ovarian hyperstimulation syndrome

- Age
- Previous history of OHSS
- Polycystic Ovarian Syndrome
- Elevated anti-mullerian hormone levels
- High antral follicle count
- High number of eggs collected
- Free fluid in Pouch of Douglas and ovarian oedema at egg collection
- Number of secondary follicles at egg collection

---

self-limits unless there is a pregnancy but in the second group the condition can persist for weeks.

The loss of protein-rich fluid from the vascular space results in significant haemoconcentration with a resultant rise in haematocrit and blood viscosity. This puts the patient at immediate risk of deep vein thrombosis, pulmonary embolism and, much more rarely, arterial thrombosis. In addition, the reduction in circulating volume results in a decrease in renal perfusion potentially leading to pre-renal failure. This induces an increase in anti-diuretic hormone, which lowers the serum sodium, and an activation of the renin–angiotensin–aldosterone system which results in hyperkalaemia.

The accumulation of the exudate in the peritoneal cavity can lead to considerable ascites and the abdomen gradually becomes increasingly tense, ultimately splinting the diaphragm and resulting in significant breathing difficulties. This is further compounded by a 'Meig's Syndrome'-like phenomenon with pleural effusion(s) and further compromise of respiratory efforts. As a result the patient can become markedly short of breath, even hypoxic at rest, ultimately developing Adult Respiratory Distress Syndrome which carries a high mortality rate.

2.2 Prediction and Prevention

In the past prediction relied on clinical history – age, PCOS, past history of OHSS etc. (Box 21.1). More recently it has become clear that patients with an elevated anti-mullerian hormone (AMH) level and/or a high antral follicle count are at markedly increased risk of developing the condition. As a result the stimulation protocol can be adjusted to decrease the risk. Metformin and dopamine agonists such as Cabergoline have also been reported to be helpful in reducing the incidence and severity of OHSS [5, 6]. However, the use of pure gonadotrophin releasing hormone (GnRH) antagonists rather than agonists has made the greatest inroad into reducing the incidence of the condition which is further decreased by using a GnRH agonist trigger instead of hCG. In a Cochrane review of 17 randomised controlled trials, Youssef et al reported that whilst trigger substitution resulted in a decrease in OHSS it also resulted in a decrease in live birth rate and an increase in miscarriage [7]. These poorer pregnancy outcomes were not seen in ovum recipients from such cycles.

Alternative strategies for decreasing the incidence of the condition include coasting – reducing or withdrawing the follicle-stimulating hormone (FSH) stimulation for a few days but with the attendant risk of collapsing estradiol levels and loss of the cycle; reducing the dose of hCG given or withholding it completely and abandoning the cycle; using progestogen/progesterone exclusively for endometrial support in the luteal phase instead of hCG – which 'rescues' the copora lutea by stimulation; and freezing all embryos to avoid pregnancy.

2.3 Diagnosis and Management

All patients should be warned to look out for the signs and symptoms of OHSS after oocyte retrieval. Ideally patients should weigh themselves daily: if their weight increases by more than 5kg, they are at high risk of OHSS. Equally, they may present with increasing abdominal bloating and discomfort or with increasing shortness of breath on even minimal exertion. Rarely they present with deep vein (or arterial) thrombosis and/or pulmonary embolism.

On presentation they should be weighed and their abdominal girth measured. Increases in both mark clinical deterioration. Apart from documenting a relevant history, the abdomen, chest and calf muscles must be examined and any shortness of breath noted. An ultrasound of the abdomen will confirm and quantify ascites and ovarian enlargement. A chest X-ray, an ECG and a ventilation perfusion scan may be ordered as appropriate. Blood should be drawn for measurement of serum sodium, potassium and albumin levels and also for evidence of renal or liver dysfunction. Similarly a full blood picture will show evidence of haemoconcentration, particularly with the haematocrit. The white cell count will also be raised and may be mistaken for evidence of an infection. Leucocytosis is part of OHSS; pyrexia is not. A baseline coagulation profile is also recommended at admission. If the case is thought to be in any way serious, a urinary catheter should be sited and fitted with a urinometer. The hourly renal output is key to the management of the condition.

The initial phase of management is rehydration to ensure that there is sufficient fluid in the vascular compartment to perfuse the kidneys and result in urine production. Only normal saline should be used for transfusion. There is no role for potassium containing fluids as the patients are likely to be (or to become) moderately hyperkalaemic. This will be corrected by normal saline infusion. The minimum renal output to ensure renal survival is 30mlhr^{-1}. To achieve this it may be necessary to infuse in excess of 200mlhr^{-1}.

Once rehydration has been achieved and the kidneys are working again, we enter the phase of fluid restriction. Clearly, with the capillaries leaking fluid so avidly, any excess fluid in the vascular compartment will leak into the third space. Therefore, fluids (usually intravenous) should be restricted to a rate sufficient to maintain renal function – i.e. to maintain the renal output between 30–50mlhr^{-1}. This maintenance phase is critical as the patient must not be over-transfused. It can also have quite a prolonged duration, particularly if the patient is pregnant. During this time it may be necessary to carry out paracentesis or a pleural tap as the clinical situation dictates. Eventually, there will be a spontaneous diuresis that heralds the resolution of the condition but not the resolution of the risk of deep venous thrombosis. Once the diuresis is underway, the intravenous fluids and fluid restriction can be stopped.

A key part of OHSS management is the prevention of thrombosis. Clearly, rehydration will help but it is mandatory to ensure that prophylactic doses of low molecular weight heparin are given and that compression stockings are worn. Where the patient is bedbound, intermittent pneumatic compression boots must be worn.

As the peritoneal fluid is an exudate it is rich in protein and patients may become albumin depleted. Albumin infusions may be given to correct this. In our own unit, if levels drop below 30gdl^{-1} we give 100ml of 20% albumen intravenously and repeat as necessary.

One of the great temptations in the management of OHSS is to administer diuretics; this is particularly true of intensive care specialists when they become involved. Diuretics are contraindicated as the diuresis they induce is from fluid taken from the vascular space. Therefore, in fact they make the condition significantly worse. They are only indicated in the rare circumstance where clearly the haematocrit has dropped and exudation is being spontaneously physiologically reversed but this is not being reflected in the renal output. Here a one-off bolus may be given to nudge the kidneys into activity.

One of the other more unusual and unpleasant complications of OHSS is vulval oedema. In truth there is little that can be done about this. It will resolve spontaneously, with the condition, and in the interim management involves the liberal application of an emollient and possibly some sort of local pressure.

3 Egg Collection and Embryo Transfer

3.1 Complications

Fortunately the risk of complications directly attributable to egg collection or embryo transfer is small.

Clearly, at vaginal oocyte retrieval the operator is passing a sharp needle into the peritoneal cavity under two-dimensional ultrasound guidance. What the needle is doing in the third dimension is anyone's guess. It is essential to identify a clear unobstructed path to the follicles and mandatory to avoid passing the needle through the bowel. It is, however, probably fantasy to think that this never happens. Yet in their review of 7,098 oocyte retrievals, Aragona et al only identified 4 cases of intraperitoneal bleeding and 2 cases of ovarian abscess (0.06% and 0.003% respectively) [2].

Risk factors for haemorrhage clearly include aberrant anatomy and the use of anticoagulants. Patients must be made aware of the risk of haemorrhage and must not take anticoagulants or even non-steroidal anti-inflammatory preparations – the latter being popular amongst those who perceive themselves to be at risk of miscarriage. One of the major problems in identifying internal haemorrhage is homeostatic compensation. In otherwise fit young women, internal bleeding can be concealed and a rising pulse and dropping blood pressure tend to happen only when matters have reached a very grave point and can be catastrophically sudden in onset. Where a patient complains of excessive abdominal pain after oocyte retrieval and if there are signs of worsening peritonism, the haematocrit should be checked. It is more than possible that ovarian haemorrhage will not present for 8–12 hours after retrieval. The decision about conservative versus surgical management is on a patient-by-patient basis.

By contrast, vaginal bleeding after oocyte retrieval is more common but it is almost always easily resolved by grasping the bleeding point with a pair of sponge-holding forceps and leaving them in place for 15 minutes.

The risk of pelvic infection is greatly increased where the patient has a history of pelvic infection. All patients should be screened for chlamydia and treated, if necessary, pre-collection. The role of prophylactic antibiotics remains controversial. Certainly, if a patient has a history of pelvic inflammatory disease (PID), has bilateral hydrosalpinges or if she has severe endometriosis (particularly if an endometrioma is inadvertently entered at egg collection) she should have antibiotic prophylaxis at the time of egg retrieval. Otherwise it is less clear and the majority of units do not administer antibiotic prophylaxis to all [8, 9]. Similarly, there is no evidence that cleansing

the vagina prior to oocyte retrieval significantly decreases the already very small incidence of post-retrieval pelvic infection. As it adds greatly to patient discomfort, it is probably unnecessary.

The same applies to embryo transfer. Whilst removing gross collections of clot/discharge or other vaginal deposits from the cervix is a good idea, the removal of cervical mucus is somewhat pointless. It is always contaminated with bacterial colonies yet the passage of the transfer catheter through the cervical canal does not seem to increase the incidence of pelvic infection. If, however, an embryo transfer has been difficult or traumatic, perhaps there is a prophylactic role for antibiotics.

4 Pregnancy

4.1 Miscarriage

Not infrequently couples are referred for ART on the basis of recurrent miscarriage. In vitro fertilisation (IVF) and intracytoplasmic sperm injection (ICSI) are not treatments for recurrent miscarriage as miscarriage rates after successful ART are not dissimilar to those in the general population. Sunkara et al interrogated the HFEA database from 1991 to June 2008 reviewing 402,185 stimulated fresh IVF cycles and 124,351 pregnancy outcomes [10]. They found that miscarriage rates fell with increasing oocyte numbers – presumably reflecting links between egg numbers and maternal age and between maternal age and miscarriage rates. However, they did not identify any increased rate of miscarriage where there were excessive numbers of oocytes collected.

4.2 Obstetric Complications

It has long been postulated that there is an increase in preterm birth (PTB) and low birth weight (LBW) in ART pregnancies, particularly if high numbers of oocytes were collected. Sunkara et al published a further interrogation of the HFEA data in 2015 [11]. They found that if more than 20 oocytes were collected the risk of both PTB and LBW were increased (adjusted odds ratios [OR] 1.15 and 1.17 respectively) but that the risk was not increased where low numbers of oocytes were collected. The HFEA database does not allow identification of subgroups, such as obese women or women with PCOS who are thought to have an increased tendency for these complications, whether conception is natural or by ART.

Women with PCOS may be over-represented in the >20 oocytes group as PCOS is clearly associated with excessive ovarian response.

4.3 Ectopic Pregnancy

The incidence of ectopic pregnancy is strongly linked with the presence of damaged fallopian tubes in both spontaneous and ART pregnancies. Using the Society for Assisted Reproductive Technologies (SART) database (2008–2011), Londra et al showed that in 103,070 clinical ART pregnancies, 1.38% were ectopic [12]. However, the odds of ectopic pregnancy were 65% lower in frozen compared with fresh transfer cycles. Donor oocyte transfers also had lower odds for ectopic pregnancy compared with autologous cycles and, further, the difference between fresh and frozen transfers disappeared. They suggested that there may be an abnormality in the tubal-uterine environment secondary to the hyperstimulation of the ovaries which contributes to abnormal implantation after ART.

5 Maternal Death

Maternal death is fortunately extremely rare as a result of assisted reproduction. Bratt et al reviewed all deaths related to IVF in the Netherlands from 1984–2008 [13]. They found an incidence of 6/100,000 for deaths directly related to IVF and 42.5/100,000 for deaths in IVF pregnancies. Thus, the overall mortality in patients undergoing IVF procedures was lower than that in the general population but the overall mortality related to IVF pregnancies was higher than the maternal mortality in the general population. They attributed the decreased mortality to the 'healthy female effect' in women undergoing IVF and the higher maternal mortality in IVF pregnancies to the high number of multiple pregnancies and to the fact that donor egg IVF results in pregnancies in women who are older. In the United Kingdom, the 2007 Confidential Enquiry into Maternal Deaths reported four deaths from OHSS between 2003 and 2005 [14]. However, the same publication in 2014, covering 2009–2012, fortunately reported no such deaths [15]. Nor does the most recent maternal mortality statistics publication [16].

6 Conclusions

Assisted reproduction is a remarkably common, remarkably tightly controlled and a remarkably safe procedure – in trained hands. Dangers abound throughout the process but advances in training – particularly the sub-specialty training programme of the RCOG; refinements in the prediction of OHSS – particularly the use of AMH; advances in monitoring and refinements of stimulation protocols – particularly the use of GnRH antagonists with a GnRH agonist trigger, have all contributed to increasing safety as witnessed by the complete absence of assisted reproduction–related deaths in the most recent Confidential Enquiry into Maternal Deaths.

Complacency, though, is inappropriate and it is essential that we all strive to make ART ever safer both for the potential mother and any resulting child.

References

1   HFEA. Fertility Treatment in 2013: Trends and Figures. 2015.

2   Aragona C, Mohamed MA, Espinola MS, Linari A, Pecorini F, Micara G, Sbracia M. Clinical complications after transvaginal oocyte retrieval in 7,098 IVF cycles. *Fertil Steril* 2011; **95**(1): 293–4

3   HFEA. Adverse Incidents in Fertility Clinics 2014: Lessons to Learn. 2015.

4   McClure N, Healy DL, Rogers PA, Sullivan J, Beaton L, Haning RV Jr, Connolly DT, Robertson DM. Vascular endothelial growth factor as capillary permeability agent in ovarian hyperstimulation syndrome. *Lancet* 1994; **344** (8917): 235–6.

5   Tso LO, Costello MF, Albuquerque LT, Andriolo RB, Macedo CR. Metformin in women with polycystic ovary syndrome for improving fertility. *Cochrane Database Syst Rev* 2014; Issue 11. Art. No.: CD006105. DOI: 10.1002/14651858.CD006105. pub3.

6   Tang H, Hunter T, Hu Y, Zhai S-D, Sheng X, Hart RJ. Cabergoline for preventing ovarian hyperstimulation syndrome. *Cochrane Database Syst Rev* 2012; Issue 2. Art. No.: CD008605. DOI: 10.1002/14651858.CD008605. pub2.

7   Youssef MA, Van der Veen F, Al-Inany HG, Mochtar MH, Griesinger G, Nagi Mohesen M, Aboulfoutouh I, van Wely M. Gonadotropin-releasing hormone agonist versus HCG for oocyte triggering in antagonist-assisted reproductive technology. *Cochrane Database Syst Rev*. 2014 Oct; Issue 10. Art. No.: CD008046. DOI: 10.1002/14651858.CD008046.pub4.

8   Brook N, Khalaf Y, Coomarasamy A, Edgeworth J, Braude P. A randomized controlled trial of

prophylactic antibiotics (co-amoxiclav) prior to embryo transfer. *Hum Reprod* 2006; **21**(11):2911–15.

9   Kroon B, Hart RJ, Wong BMS, Ford E, Yazdani A. Antibiotics prior to embryo transfer in ART. *Cochrane Database Syst Rev.* 2012; Issue 3. Art. No.: CD008995. DOI: 10.1002/14651858.CD008995. pub2.

10 Sunkara SK, Khalaf Y, Maheshwari A, Seed P, Coomarasamy A. Association between response to ovarian stimulation and miscarriage following IVF: an analysis of 124 351 IVF pregnancies. *Hum Reprod* 2014; **29**(6): 1218–24.

11 Sunkara SK, La Marca A, Seed PT, Khalaf Y. Increased risk of preterm birth and low birthweight with very high number of oocytes following IVF: an analysis of 65 868 singleton live birth outcomes. *Hum Reprod* 2015; **30**(6): 1473–80

12 Londra L, Moreau C, Strobino D, Garcia J, Zacur H, Zhao Y. Ectopic pregnancy after in vitro fertilization: differences between fresh and frozen-thawed cycles. *Fertil Steril* 2015; **104**(1): 110–18.

13 Braat DD, Schutte JM, Bernardus RE, Mooij TM, van Leeuwen FE. Maternal death related to IVF in the Netherlands 1984–2008. *Hum Reprod* 2010; **25**(7): 1782–6.

14 Lewis G (ed.). The Confidential Enquiry into Maternal and Child Health (CEMACH). Saving Mothers Lives; Reviewing Maternal Deaths to Make Motherhood Safer 2003–2005. The Seventh Report of the United Kingdom Confidential Enquiries into Maternal Deaths in the United Kingdom. London: CEMACH, 2007.

15 Knight M, Kenyon S, Brocklehurst P, Neilson J, Shakespeare J, Kurinczuk JJ (eds.) on behalf of MBRRACE-UK. Saving Lives, Improving Mothers' Care - Lessons learned to inform future maternity care from the UK and Ireland Confidential Enquiries into Maternal Deaths and Morbidity 2009–2012. Oxford: National Perinatal Epidemiology Unit, University of Oxford 2014.

16 Knight M, Bunch K, Tuffnell D, Jayakody H, Shakespeare J, Kotnis R, Kenyon S, Kurinczuk JJ (eds.) on behalf of MBRRACE-UK. Saving Lives, Improving Mothers' Care - Lessons learned to inform maternity care from the UK and Ireland Confidential Enquiries into Maternal Deaths and Morbidity 2014–2016. Oxford: National Perinatal Epidemiology Unit, University of Oxford 2018.

Chapter 22

Gamete and Embryo Cryopreservation

Rachel Cutting

1 Introduction

Cryopreservation is a fundamental adjunct for any in vitro fertilisation (IVF) programme for both gametes and embryos. Sperm can be frozen for use in donor cycles, treatment cycles or to preserve fertility. After the first successful frozen-thawed embryo live birth was reported in 1983, embryo cryopreservation is routinely used to store supernumerary embryos, to improve cumulative pregnancy rates and to help effectively implement a single embryo transfer policy. However, oocyte cryopreservation has proved to be more challenging as the survival rates and pregnancy rates were initially low.

Improvements though in cryopreservation techniques for both oocytes and embryos have increased the effectiveness and efficiency and therefore widened the application of these techniques. For oocyte cryopreservation there has been a shift from it being classed as experimental to it being offered as a mainstream treatment option. The improvements to embryo cryopreservation and a greater understanding of endometrial receptivity have now changed the perception that fresh embryos have higher success rates than cryopreserved embryos. Further evidence shows that controlled ovarian stimulation cycles have poorer obstetric and perinatal outcomes [1] and that 'freeze all' cycles can reduce the complication of ovarian hyperstimulation syndrome (OHSS). Subsequently this may see a shift to performing more frozen embryo transfers than fresh embryo transfers. Centres therefore need to optimise their cryopreservation programmes to ensure the best outcomes for patients.

This chapter will review the current techniques and applications for cryopreservation.

2 Cryopreservation Methods

2.1 Use of Cryoprotectants

Although discovered by accident in 1949, the use of cryoprotectants for both gametes and embryos is essential to maximise survival and ensure viability is preserved. They reduce intracellular ice formation by facilitating dehydration of the cell to minimise intracellular water. Permeating cryoprotectants such as glycerol, propandiol (PROH), dimethyl sulphoxide (DMSO), or ethylene glycol (EG) enter into the cell to displace water. Non-permeating cryoprotectants (e.g. sucrose) do not permeate the cell but increase the extracellular osmolarity to enhance dehydration by generating an osmotic gradient across the cell membrane. Although used very successfully, caution needs to be exercised because if intracellular concentration of cryoprotectants becomes too high there may be a toxic effect.

2.2 Rapid Freezing

Rapid freezing is a simple method which is used for sperm cryopreservation where after drop-wise addition of cryoprotectants and equilibration, the straws are placed in direct contact with liquid nitrogen vapours before plunging into liquid nitrogen [2]. Although this method is routinely used, there is a lack of reproducibility and control of overcooling rates.

2.3 Slow Freezing

Slow freezing is a well-established method for cryopreservation. The first protocol for embryo cryopreservation was reported in 1985 [3] with more recent modifications only really being applied to the concentrations of cryoprotectant in the media. Slow dehydration is achieved by using programmable equipment set to initial cooling rates of -0.3 to -0.5 °C/min for embryos and -0.5 to -1 °C/min for sperm. This utilises relatively low concentrations of cryoprotectants; the concentration of the permeating cryoprotectants is approximately 1.5 M (usually PROH), and the concentration of non-permeating cryoprotectants is 0.1–0.3 M [4]. Dehydration is achieved by exposing the cells to hypertonic solutions of cryoprotectants at supra-zero temperatures followed by a progressive increase in solute concentration of the extracellular phase due to extracellular ice formation. Ice nucleation (seeding) which is induced at -5 to -8 °C controls ice formation and therefore prevents release of latent heat which could disrupt the cooling rate. During a slow rate freezing programme when dehydration of the cellular environment is almost complete (after -40 °C) the rate of cooling is increased and cells can be placed into liquid nitrogen [4]. The majority of embryo cryopreservation until more recently was carried out using this methodology with survival rates being in the region of 60–80%.

2.4 Vitrification

Boldt [5] describes vitrification as a process by which an aqueous solution is converted to a solid, glass-like amorphous substance by rapid changes in temperature of the solution. This process which is being increasingly used for oocytes, early cleavage embryos and blastocysts involves usually a 10–15 minute pre-equilibration period with low concentrations of cryoprotectants (1–2 mol/l) followed by a short exposure time to high permeating cryoprotectant concentrations (5–6 mol/l) and non-permeating cryoprotectants (0.5–1.0 mol/l). Rapid cooling is then induced (>20,000 °C/min). The high concentrations of cryoprotectant increase viscosity to prevent ice nucleation.

There are multiple commercially available devices for vitrification which can be classified as open or closed. Open systems have direct contact with liquid nitrogen during cooling and storage. Although successful, concerns have been raised regarding contamination risks from liquid nitrogen. Closed systems circumnavigate this problem but the disadvantage is that they cannot achieve a high cooling rate and may have the potential toxicity effects of longer exposure to high concentrations of cryoprotectants. However, studies have shown that closed systems are as equally effective as open systems [6].To ensure vitrification is a success, warming rates must also be considered to prevent ice nucleation.

Edgar and Gook [7] suggested in their critical appraisal of cryopreservation methods that vitrification shows higher survival rates than slow freezing and therefore should be the method of choice for oocytes and blastocysts, but either method can be used equally effectively for cleavage stage embryos.

3 Sperm Cryopreservation

Cryopreservation of human sperm was first described more than 50 years ago and is now used routinely for a range of clinical applications: treatments with donor sperm, fertility preservation and IVF treatment. More recently there has been an increase in the use of surgically retrieved sperm and having the ability to successfully store testicular sperm negates the need for further surgery. A meta-analysis [8] concluded that there was no difference between fertilisation rates and clinical pregnancy rates when using fresh versus cryopreserved-thawed testicular sperm which makes sperm cryopreservation for azoospermic patients an effective option.

However, it is notable in the laboratory that parameters such as motility, velocity and viability are altered after cryopreserved samples are thawed. However, more subtle changes may occur such as damage to the structure and function of sperm, which in turn may affect the fertilisation potential of the sperm.

A study [9] combined examining the ultrastructural changes with sperm parameters after cryopreservation. The group reported that viability significantly decreased which was thought to be related to the physical and chemical environment during the process including the high solute content of intracellular fluid following dehydration, toxic effects of cryoprotectants and damage to the membranes by rapid changes in osmolarity and temperature. Motility was also significantly affected with an increase in the percentage of immotile sperm after thawing. By using scanning and electron microscopy it was found that the percentage of normal morphological sperm decreased after thawing. Furthermore, after examining organelles it was found that the acrosome, which is vital for the process of fertilisation, was the most severely affected. This study found no differences relating to chromatin and nuclear content morphology. However, there is no consensus on this final point as cryopreservation was found to induce chromatin decondensation [10] and cause an increase in sperm DNA fragmentation [11].

There is still much work to do before the optimal method of human sperm cryopreservation is determined. The preferable technique may be to use methods which do not require cryoprotectants to reduce osmotic and toxic effects. Ozkavukcu [9] suggested that different methods may work best for different groups, for example, simple vapour freezing for donor sperm but more complex methods for sub/infertile men. There is evidence more recently that specific devices can be used effectively for very low sperm counts and individual sperm [12]. Small volume vitrification devices are also being developed which negate the need for permeating cryoprotectants [13].

Whilst sperm banking for post-pubertal men is routinely offered, preserving fertility for prepubertal boys who do not yet produce sperm cells has been impossible. However, advances in spermatogonial stem cell storage followed by transplantation in animal models may provide hope for a future solution [14].

4 Oocyte Cryopreservation

Renewed interest in oocyte cryopreservation, especially in countries where the creation of supernumerary embryos is forbidden, has led to improvements in survival and pregnancy rates such that now oocyte cryopreservation is considered a routine treatment option for medical, social and legal reasons.

Initially poor survival rates were attributed to the surface area/volume ratio and its relationship with the cell permeability due to the large size of the oocyte [15]. However, zygotes with almost identical surface/volume ratios can be successfully cryopreserved and therefore it is the differences in membrane permeability not surface/volume ratio which influence survival rates of oocytes. However, oocytes are susceptible to cryodamage and may be damaged due to chilling injury which could lead to ultrastructural damage. However, since the introduction of vitrification, spindle recovery has been shown to have improved; there is less cortical granule loss and vacuolisation and increased survival rates have been reported. Furthermore a systematic review and meta-analysis [16] concluded that there was no difference between vitrified and fresh oocytes in terms of fertilisation, cleavage and clinical pregnancy rates, although there was a reduced ongoing pregnancy rate in the cryopreserved group.

Further studies are required especially where the same end points are defined to ensure patients are provided with evidence-based statistics so they can make an informed choice, especially if they are choosing to delay childbirth for social reasons. However, for patients considering oocyte cryopreservation for fertility preservation reasons, it offers realistic hope and overcomes the ethical issues if embryos are frozen

and a partner withdraws consent for the embryos to be used in a treatment.

5 Embryo Cryopreservation

There is no consensus over the best way to cryopreserve embryos and there are differences in the selection criteria of embryos to cryopreserve with respect to quality and the method used. However, it has been reported that having strict morphological selection criteria may lead to better post-thaw recovery for both cleavage embryos and blastocysts [17].

Cryopreservation of pronuclear (PN) embryos, although selecting fertilised oocytes offers no information regarding developmental and morphological competence of the embryos and many centres may prefer freezing post embryo cleavage [7]. However, freezing at PN stage has routinely been used due to its reproducible survival rates and has been widely used when there is a risk of OHSS. Freezing at the cleavage stage does however help determine the embryo potential prior to storage and has the advantage that even if an embryo has partially survived the thaw process (some cells within the embryo may lyse leaving others viable) it may still have the potential to implant and result in a live birth. Clinic policy is usually to consider the embryo to have survived if 50% of the original blastomeres are intact.

Prolonged culture to the blastocyst stage aids embryo selection and assessment of embryo potential but until more recently cryopreservation of blastocysts has not been as successful as for cleavage stage embryos. Changes to methods used such as vitrification and refinements to the techniques, for example, artificially shrinking the blastocoeles prior to vitrification have been shown to improve survival rates [18]. Survival post thaw can be more difficult to assess in blastocysts than in cleavage stage embryos as it is difficult to assess an increase in cell number. However, a marker of survival can be taken as blastocelic re-expansion. Ahlostrom et al [19] assessed pre-freeze and post-thaw parameters of blastocyst quality to determine if it was possible to predict blastocysts with high potential. The study found that blastocoele expansion and trophectoderm cell quality were the most significant morphological pre-freeze predictors of a live birth and that the most predictive factor post thaw was degree of re-expansion. They concluded that re-expanding blastocysts assessed within

2–4 hours with >60% viability should be selected for transfer.

Slow freezing is still used for early cleavage stage embryo freezing, although more recently there seems to be a shift towards vitrification. This is supported in the literature as vitrification for both cleavage stage and blastocysts appears to be associated with a significantly higher post-thaw survival rate than slow freezing [20]. With improvements in outcomes from blastocyst cryopreservation and the requirement to reduce multiple birth rates, blastocyst transfer and cryopreservation are becoming more routine.

Further randomised trials which use the same criteria for post-thaw survival and defined outcome points, such as live birth rates per oocyte thawed, are required before one method can be recommended over another.

6 Cryopreservation Issues

6.1 Safety

The increase in success with both slow freezing and vitrification has meant that oocyte cryopreservation is now an accepted practice in ART. This has further been validated by Noyes et al. [21] who reported that more than 900 babies have been born following oocyte cryopreservation without any apparent increase in congenital anomalies.

Frozen embryo transfer is now a routine treatment in an IVF programme. The European Society of Human Reproduction and Embryology (ESHRE) reported a total of 114,593 frozen embryo replacement cycles (FER) from the 2010 register of data [22]. From this analysis of the 120,634 ART infants born, 94,609 (78.4%) were born after IVF/ICSI fresh cycles and 17,689 (14.7%) after FER treatments. Many studies have provided reassuring data on safety and efficacy of embryo cryopreservation with data suggesting better obstetric and perinatal outcomes from FER cycles [1].

6.2 Ethics

Any aspect of ART is not without ethical concerns and the cryopreservation of gametes and embryos is no exception. An increasing number of those diagnosed with cancer are surviving long term and the use of cryopreservation is increasing; however, posthumous use will always raise ethical concerns. Improvements to oocyte cryopreservation are of benefit to women suffering from cancer as it removes the risks of a partner withdrawing consent for use if embryos are stored. However, some may see storing oocytes for social reasons, for example, to delay motherhood as morally unacceptable. There is also the ethical dilemma of how to manage a storage bank in the absence of regulation. The Human Fertilisation and Embryology Authority (HFEA) imposes strict laws regarding storage periods (statutory storage period is 10 years with controls in place to only allow extension of storage in certain circumstances). Many patients find reaching a decision regarding their stored embryos difficult especially with respect to allowing embryos to perish. Therefore, other countries which have no regulations may have unwanted embryos remaining in storage indefinitely. There is also the ethical question of ownership of embryos after couples separate with several high profile court cases reaching the press in recent years.

In order to prevent problems, effective and adequate patient information, counselling and consent are required.

7 Conclusion

Gamete and embryo cryopreservation is an important component to any fertility programme and has widespread routine use. Further research is required with sperm, oocytes and embryos to understand the real effects of cryopreservation so that not only are cryosurvival rates maximised but the chance of achieving a live birth is also improved.

References

[1] Maheshwari A, Pandy S, Shetty A, Hamilton M, Bhattacharya S. Obstetric and perinatal outcomes in singleton pregnancies resulting from the transfer of frozen thawed versus fresh embryos generated through in vitro fertilization treatment: a systematic review and meta-analysis. *Fertil Steril.* 2012 Aug;98(2):368–77

[2] Di Santo M, Tarozzi N, Nadalini M, Borini A. Human sperm cryopreservation: update on techniques, effect on DNA integrity, and implications for ART. *Adv Urol.* 2012;2012:854837

[3] Lassalle B and Testart J. Human embryo features that influence the success of cryopreservation with the use of 1,2 propandiol. *Fertil Steril.* 1985;44:645–651

[4] Coticchio G, Bonu M, Borini A, Flamigni C. Oocyte cryopreservation: a biological perspective. *Eur J Obstet Gynecol Reprod Biol.* 2004;115:S2–S7

[5] Boldt J. Current results with slow freezing and vitrification of the human oocyte. *Reprod Biomed Online.* 2011;23:314–322

[6] Papatheodorou A, Vanderzwalmen P, Panagiotidis Y, Prapas N, Zikopoulos K, Georgiou I, Prapas Y. Open versus closed oocyte vitrification system: a prospective randomized sibling-oocyte study. *Reprod Biomed Online.* 2013 Jun;26(6):595–602

[7] Edgar and D Gook D. A critical appraisal of cryopreservation (slow cooling versus vitrification) of human oocytes and embryos. *Human Reprod Update.* 2012; 18(5):536–554

[8] Ohlander S, Hotaling J, Kirshenbaum E, Niederberger C, Eisenberg ML. Use of fresh versus cryopreserved sperm. *Fertil Steril.* 2014 Feb;101(2):e12

[9] Ozkavukcu S, Erdemli E, Isik A, Oztuna D, Karahuseyinoglu S. Effects of cryopreservation on sperm parameters and ultrastructural morphology of human spermatozoa. *J Assist Reprod Genet.* 2008 Aug; 25(8):403–11

[10] Fortunato A, Leo R, Liguori F. Effects of cryostorage on human sperm chromatin integrity. *Zygote.* 2012;8:1–7

[11] Gosálvez J, Núñez R, Fernández JL, López-Fernández C, Caballero P. Dynamics of sperm DNA damage in fresh versus frozen-thawed and gradient processed ejaculates in human donors. *Andrologia.* 2011;**43**:373–7

[12] Stein A[1], Shufaro Y, Hadar S, Fisch B, Pinkas H. Successful use of the Cryolock device for cryopreservation of scarce human ejaculate and testicular spermatozoa. *Andrology.* 2015 Mar;3(2):220–4

[13] Chen Y, Li L, Qian Y, Xu C, Zhu Y, Huang H, Jin F, Ye Y. Small-volume vitrification for human spermatozoa in the absence of cryoprotectants by using Cryotop. *Andrologia.* 2015 Aug;47(6):694–9

[14] Tournaye H, Dohle GR, Barratt CL. Fertility preservation in men with cancer. *Lancet.* 2014 Oct 4;384(9950):1295–301

[15] Leibo SP and Pool TB. The principal variables of cryopreservation: solutions, temperatures, and rate changes. *Fertil Steril.* 2011;96(2):269–76

[16] Potdar N, Gelbaya TA, Nardo LG. Oocyte vitrification in the 21st century and post-warming fertility outcomes: a systematic review and meta-analysis. *Reprod Biomed Online.* 2014 Aug;29(2):159–76

[17] Alpha Scientists in Reproductive Medicine and ESHRE Special Interest Group in Reproductive Medicine. The alpha consensus meeting on cryopreservation key performance indicators and benchmarks: proceedings of an expert meeting. *Reprod BioMed Online.* 2012;25:146–67

[18] Mukaida T, Oka C, Goto T, Takahashi K. Artificial shrinkage of blastocoeles using either a micro-needle or a laser pulse prior to the cooling steps of vitrification improves survival rate and pregnancy outcome of vitrified human blastocysts. *Hum Reprod.* 2006 Dec;21(12):3246–52.

[19] Ahlström A, Westin C, Wikland M, Hardarson T. Prediction of live birth in frozen-thawed single blastocyst transfer cycles by pre-freeze and post-thaw morphology. *Hum Reprod.* 2013 May;28 (5):1199–209

[20] Loutradi K, Kolibianakis E, Venetis C, Evangelos E, Pados G, Bontis I, Tarlatzis B. Cryopreservation of human embryos by vitrification or slow freezing: a systematic review and meta analysis. *Fertil Steril.* 2008; 90(1):186–93

[21] Noyes N, Porcu E, Borini A. Over 900 oocyte cryopreservation babies born with no apparent increase in congenital anomalies. *Reprod Biomed Online.* 2009; 18(6):769–76

[22] Kupka MS, Ferraretti AP, de Mouzon J, Erb K, D'Hooghe T, Castilla JA, alhaz-Jorge C, De Geyter C, Goossens V. The European IVF-Monitoring (EIM) Consortium, for the European Society of Human Reproduction and Embryology (ESHRE). Assisted reproductive technology in Europe, 2010: results generated from European registers by ESHRE. *Hum Reprod.* 2014; 29(10):2099–113

Chapter 23

Quality Management in Reproductive Medicine

Bryan Woodward
Linsey White

1 Introduction

For fertility clinics to be successful, quality must be a priority. Quality is not just about ticking boxes, it is about ensuring jobs are completed to the best standard possible. Quality is defined as:

> the degree to which a set of inherent characteristics fulfils requirements
>
> (ISO9000:2000)

Quality can be considered as consistent conformance to patient expectations, and has also been referred to as a 'journey where you never arrive', since maintaining quality is a continuous process:

> the race for quality has no finish line so technically it is more like a death march
>
> (www.despair.com)

Comparison to a death march is perhaps unfair! The process of achieving quality can be extremely rewarding, and is more like a 'eureka moment' when the people involved realise the benefits that quality brings to an organisation.

Achieving quality requires quality systems to be in place throughout the organisation. This enables troubleshooting via a cycle of continuous improvement, which enhances quality, leading to better patient satisfaction, alongside improved satisfaction of investors and staff.

1.1 Establishing a Quality Management System

The first step in achieving quality is to establish a quality management system (QMS). For the United Kingdom, the Human Fertilisation and Embryology Authority (HFEA) requires all licensed fertility clinics to have a QMS, stating:

The authors would like to thank Mrs Marcia McNicol from MCM Compliance Ltd. for offering advice on this chapter.

> The centre must put in place a QMS and implement this system to continually improve the quality and effectiveness of the service provided in accordance with the conditions of this licence and the guidance on good practice as set out in the HFEA's Code of Practice.
>
> (Guidance Note T32, HFEA Code of Practice, 2015)

The HFEA provides its own definition of a QMS as:

> The organisational structure, defined responsibilities, procedures, processes and resources for implementing quality management (i.e. the co-ordinated activities to direct and control an organisation with regard to quality), including all activities which contribute to quality, directly or indirectly
>
> (Section 23.1, HFEA Code of Practice, 2015)

The QMS requires regular review and needs to adapt to new legislation. For example, in 2004, the European Union Tissues and Cells Directive 2004/23/EC (EUTCD) established standards of quality and safety for the donation, procurement, testing, processing, preservation, storage and distribution of human cells and tissues. All HFEA-licensed fertility clinics had to revise their QMS to align themselves to the HFEA's interpretation of the EUTCD.

1.2 External Standards

Many clinics consult external standards to establish a QMS, such as the International Organization for Standardization (ISO; www.iso.org), which provide sets of standards for a specific level of quality.

ISO standards that relate to assisted conception include:

ISO 9000:2000. Quality Management Systems: Fundamentals and vocabulary

ISO 9001:2008. Quality Management Systems: Requirements

ISO 15189:2012. Medical Laboratories: Requirements for Quality and Competence

Other approaches to QMS development originate from successful care manufacturing companies, and

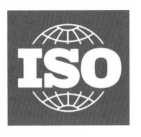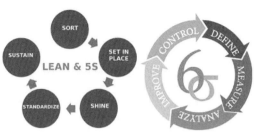

Fig. 23.1 Three popular external standards: ISO, Lean & 5S and Six Sigma

include 'Lean & 5S' and 'Six Sigma' (Figure 23.1). 'Lean & 5S' is an operating philosophy orginally developed by Toyota to help reduce costs and turnover time.

> A systematic approach to identify and eliminate waste through continuous improvement by flowing the product only when the customer needs it in pursuit of perfection
>
>> US Department of Commerce's National Institute of Standards & Technology Manufacturing Extension Partnership

Similarly, Motorola developed 'Six Sigma', a philosophy that reduces 'variability' to help solve problems. 'Six Sigma' solves all problems using a five-step DMAIC process: Define, Measure, Analyse, Improve, Control.

External standards tend to be short documents with wide-ranging statements to allow interpetation by different industries. For reproductive medicine, more specific organisations also need consideration, such as the HFEA, the Care Quality Commission, the NHS Litigation Agency and the UK Accreditation Service.

Whatever the approach, clinics with a well thought out QMS have the foundations for implementing effective quality management on a daily basis. All areas can be evaluated, from the way staff practice, to the actual treatment protocols and the results achieved.

The HFEA states:

> The centre should:
>
> a) identify the processes needed for quality management, for providing and managing resources and for assisted conception procedures, and
>
> b) ensure these processes, including the interaction between them, are effective and continually improved.
>
> (Section 23.2 and 23.3, HFEA Code of Practice, 2015)

In summary, the QMS provides a management framework to monitor and enhance performance. All activities that contribute to quality, either directly or indirectly, are considered. If quality is present, then the QMS ensures patients receive an agreed standard of care throughout their treatment, whilst the clinic works to continually improve the service delivered by achieving high standards and consistency throughout.

According to the HFEA, specific QMS documentation is needed:

> The following documentation must form part of the QMS:
>
> a. a quality manual
> b. standard operating procedures (SOPs) for all activities authorised by this licence and other activities carried out in the course of providing treatment services that do not require a licence
> c. guidelines
> d. training and reference manuals, and
> e. reporting forms.
>
> (Guidance Note T33, HFEA Code of Practice, 2015)

This chapter will introduce and discuss the key steps and accountabilities within a QMS. This will take into account the elements mentioned in Guidance Note T33.

1.3 The Quality Manual

The Quality Manual is the backbone of the QMS. This document should consist of easily digestible sections for ease of reference. The introduction should briefly describe the clinic's location, activities that take place and the legal entity. It is important to clarify the scope, to segregate any parts of the organisation excluded from the QMS, e.g. diagnostic hormone assays may be referred out to another organisation and therefore be beyond the clinic's scope.

The Quality Manual should reference documented policies and procedures, describe how documents are controlled, how audits are conducted and how non-conformances (NCs) are addressed. When the benefits of quality are appreciated, then the Quality Manual becomes the Bible for a fertility clinic (alongside the HFEA Code of Practice in the United Kingdom).

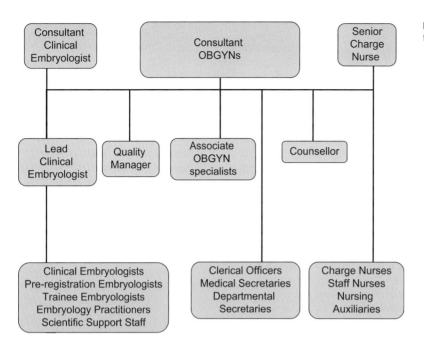

Fig. 23.2 An organisational chart for a fertility clinic

1.4 Organisational Structure, Management and Responsibility

A clinic should have enough staff in place of sufficient grade and experience to perform the treatments to a required level of quality. All staff should comply with ethical conduct, which is usually covered by the codes of conduct from respective professional bodies, e.g. the Royal College of Nursing (RCN), the Royal College of Obstetrics and Gynecologists (RCOG) and the Royal College of Pathologists (RCPath). Laboratory staff additionally sign up to codes from the Health and Care Professions Council (HCPC), the Association of Clinical Embryologists (ACE) and the Association of Biomedical Andrologists (ABA).

A designated individual, or 'Person Responsible' (PR), should have overall responsibility for all licensable activity taking place. In the United Kingdom, the PR has to be approved by the HFEA. The PR and senior management of the different areas (medical, nursing, scientific and administration) form the management team to direct the organisational structure by assigning clear roles and responsibilities to all staff and ensuring they have everything they need to fulfill these roles. Consideration should also be given to other individuals (from other departments, other clinics, diagnostic laboratories and suppliers), with the patients at the heart of the organisation's care.

The HFEA states that:

The centre must have an organisational chart which clearly defines accountability and reporting relationships (Guidance Note T11, HFEA Code of Practice, 2015)

The organisational chart (Figure 23.2) requires periodic and timely reviews to ensure its effectiveness in supporting the clinic's needs. For example, an increase in patient numbers may warrant an increase in the number of certain types of staff.

Each position within the organisation should be clearly defined by a job description specifying the requirements, e.g. appropriate education, skills, training and experience. Job descriptions can not only be used as part of the hiring process but also to develop staff to ensure they are sufficiently skilled to meet the clinic's objectives. If employees are engaged they feel more valued, and this in turn benefits the clinic. A training system can cover training needs, with individuals having a personal training file, which includes evaluation of performance and competence, and an annual appraisal report from their line manager. If quality is present, individuals will competently perform their designated tasks in line with the SOPs to benefit the clinic.

1.5 The Quality Manager

For quality management to work, a Quality Manager must be appointed. This person must have a deep understanding of all aspects of the QMS. The Quality Manager may have other responsibilities within the clinic, although increasingly this is becoming a full-time job.

The Quality Manager's role is vast, but includes the following:

i) ensuring resources are available for implementation and maintenance of the QMS, and that staff are aware of the associated tasks;

ii) monitoring of training compliance to ensure that employee knowledge, skills and attitude is of appropriate standard, and offer support and retraining where necessary;

iii) delegating the audits and identifying the need for changes and opportunities for improvement;

iv) establishing the quality policy and objectives.

1.6 The Quality Policy and Objectives

The Quality Policy is a written document that shows the clinic's intention to work towards key areas, e.g. achieving patient satisfaction, training staff and working with suppliers to achieve the best outcomes for patient treatment.

The HFEA defines a Quality Policy as:

the overall intentions and direction of an organisation related to quality as formally expressed by centre management. A quality policy statement defines or describes an organisation's intentions and commitment to quality and provides a framework for setting quality objectives and planning.

(Section 23.6, HFEA Code of Practice, 2015)

And

Centre management should ensure the quality policy includes a commitment to:

a) providing a service that meets its users' needs and requirements

b) meeting the provisions of this Code of Practice

c) continually improving the effectiveness of the quality management system

d) upholding good professional practice, and

e) ensuring the health, safety and welfare of all staff and visitors to the centre.

(Section 23.7, HFEA Code of Practice, 2015)

The Quality Policy should be approved by the PR and be available throughout the clinic, to both staff and patients. To ensure the quality objectives meet user's needs, they should be measurable and regularly reviewed such that the objectives are reached and maintained.

2 Document Control and Record Keeping

For quality to exist, all staff need to perform SOPs the same way, using the same recording methods to minimise variation between operators. To help this, all documents and records should be controlled through the QMS (Figure 23.3). This ensures that only current approved versions of documents and record sheets are available. If an SOP is changed, it is essential that all staff use and have access to all up-to-date documentation to ensure all processes are carried out as per the

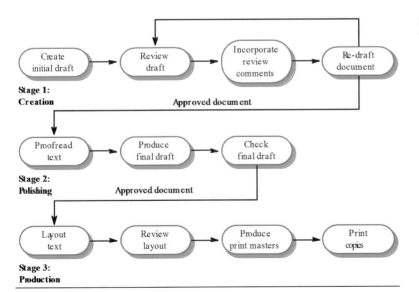

Fig. 23.3 The process of document control

Stage 1: Creation — Create initial draft → Review draft → Incorporate review comments → Re-draft document — Approved document

Stage 2: Polishing — Proofread text → Produce final draft → Check final draft — Approved document

Stage 3: Production — Layout text → Review layout → Produce print masters → Print copies

changed SOP. Adherence to older uncontrolled versions of SOPs could impact on the safety of patients, their gametes and/or embryos and also on staff.

Any deviations from agreed processes should be recorded as non-conformance reporting to ensure traceability of all events. Staff should be allowed the opportunity to justify deviations and update appropriate procedures if required. Whilst a deviation is a non-conformance to the SOP, it can occasionally lead to an improvement. This is what quality improvement is all about.

All documents and templates should abide by the following guidelines:

- All documents should be assigned unique IDs to allow them to be controlled and tracked e.g. SOP-XXX, FORM-YYY.
- Each document should have a numerical revision or version which should be updated each time the document is reviewed and changed (with previous versions archived for reference).
- Document changes should be carried out by someone with technical expertise of the process. The changed document should then be peer reviewed before approval for use. For traceability, a full justification of why changes were made should be recorded, assessing the possible impact of the change, including any changes to risk level and validation documented.
- Documents should be available at all times to operators completing the process and this should be in the format that cannot be amended or deleted.
- Documents should follow the same templates to allow consistency throughout
- Referencing other documents where applicable e.g. links to related worksheets (electronic hyperlinks are often used to make this simpler).
- Documents should be appropriately filed to allow traceability with a recommended retention of files for a specific period of time.

2.1 Quality Indicators, Audits and Quality Assurance

Quality indicators, often referred to as Key Performance Indicators (KPIs), allow for evaluation of clinic procedures.

Regarding KPIs, the HFEA states:

Required standards of quality and safety, in the form of quality indicators for all activities authorised by this licence and other activities carried out in the course of providing treatment services that do not require a licence, must be established.

(Guidance note T35, HFEA Code of Practice, 2015)

Examples of KPIs include: how many eggs are collected (clinicians) and how many oocytes fertilised (embryology). However, a word of warning: do not overdo KPIs; there should be enough to capture the essence, but any more than that dilutes the user's attention, drawing focus away from key measurements.

Alongside KPIs are audits: systematic, independent and documented processes for obtaining evidence and evaluating it objectively to determine the extent to which criteria are fulfilled. Audits establish whether all activities that affect quality are being carried out effectively. They can be used to measure compliance with policies, procedures or requirements (e.g. the HFEA Code of Practice).

The HFEA states that:

audits must be performed at least every two years, by trained and competent staff and in an independent way. Findings and corrective actions must be documented and implemented.

(Guidance Note T11, HFEA Code of Practice, 2015)

However, auditing is best performed as an iterative process (see Figure 23.4), with audits scheduled and completed in accordance with the audit schedule plan.

Audits can be performed internally (within the organisation) and externally (via external assessment, e.g. from the HFEA). External audits often provide a focus to get things done and are a good way of driving continuous improvement. Thus, HFEA inspections should be welcomed, as they give patients and staff a further degree of confidence in the clinic.

Table 23.1 The three types of audit

Audit Type	Description
Vertical	Assesses a complete process from start to finish, e.g. the patient pathway, from arrival, to treatment, to departure after treatment
Horizontal	Assesses one aspect of the system, e.g. the training records for all staff are examined
Examination (Witness)	Assesses one specific activity, e.g. observations of an egg collection procedure to ensure compliance with the SOP

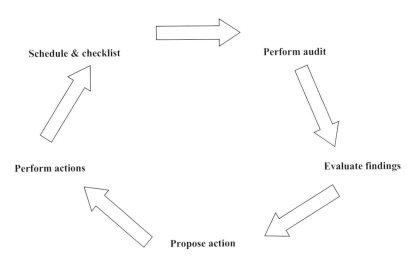

Fig. 23.4 The continuous audit loop

There are three main types of audit: vertical, horizontal and witness (see Table 23.1).

Both internal and external audits may uncover non-conformances to processes. These require an action plan with time frames for completion, as part of quality improvement, e.g. staff retraining.

Trends may be identified from on-going KPI monitoring. These should be investigated in order to identify and initiate actions to resolve root causes.

2.2 Non-Conformance (NC) Reporting and Corrective Action Preventative Action (CAPA)

It is important that all NCs in the clinic are investigated to assess potential impact and minimise any detrimental outcome. Things sometimes do not go according to plan. When NCs are investigated, a report should be generated to describe what went wrong, the immediate resolution implemented, the impact on the NC and the remediation needed to return to conformance. Problems with existing or potential quality issues need to be resolved in order to prevent their occurrence and recurrence. This involves corrective and preventive actions (CAPA).

Corrective actions (CA) identify problems and prevent their recurrence. CA are planned alongside reactive processes, with the latter being remedial action to immediately rectify an NC. One method of CA is the '5 whys' which is a problem-solving method carried out by asking 'why' no fewer than five times to drill down to the underlying cause of an issue.

Preventive actions (PA) are planned to prevent an undesirable event occurring. This is based on verifiable information that the clinic has been made aware of. If the PA are good, NCs are minimised. Clinic staff may not be aware that a smooth running organisation is often the result of PA! PAs are often identified at routine audits.

Risk management involves CAPA. However, CAPA is only effective if the information obtained is accurate and well-organised.

2.3 Risk Management

Risk management is the process of identifying and controlling all potential risks that the fertility service may pose. These could be risks to patients and their gametes or embryos, or risks to staff by any process.

Risk management should be integrated into all processes throughout the QMS to mitigate risk as much as possible. Through identification of all the potential hazards at an early stage, appropriate controls can be identified and incorporated into the service development to eliminate or reduce risks. This is a proactive process, and all staff should be engaged in risk management, and encouraged to identify potential risks.

There are three stages to risk analysis: defining the intended procedure, identifying the hazard, and estimating the risk level for each hazard. Actions can then be taken to either accept the risk (if it is considered small enough to do so) or reduce the risk (if it is considered unacceptable to allow to continue). Risk management is about reducing risks to an acceptable level, accepting that no clinic will ever eliminate all risks.

2.4 Patient Satisfaction and Complaints

The HFEA requires patient satisfaction surveys to be carried out to identify, assess and react to emerging issues and to identify opportunities for the continuous improvement of service.

Audits also help to ensure patient satisfaction:

The customer's perception of the degree to which the customer's requirements have been fulfilled.

(ISO 9000:2000)

Complaints are inevitable, and clinics should have a clear complaints procedure that is accessible to patients. Complaint data is valuable, as it makes clinics reassess whether they have the right controls in place. Complaints should never be ignored. They should be subsequently evaluated alongside the responses and any CA that were instigated. This allows any trends to be observed, so that quality can be improved.

If patients do not feel complaints have been resolved, they can contact the HFEA, provided the complaint is reported within six months of the event. However, the HFEA cannot intervene in disputes about funding and treatment costs and have a limited remit to intervene if a clinic refuses treatment.

3 Control of Equipment

3.1 Validation

Validation should be carried out on all critical equipment and processes to verify they are working as required, and thereby give confidence in the system.

Typically validation documents include the following:

- A Validation Master Plan (VMP): this is the starting point, defining the scope, planning and management of complete validation process. The VMP summarises details of the equipment and the strategy for the whole validation process.
- A User Requirement Specification (URS): this describes the needs and purpose of the equipment.
- The Qualifications: documents provided by the company supplying the equipment, including:
  - Installation Qualification (IQ): to verify installation of equipment.
  - Operation Qualification (OQ): to demonstrate the ability of the equipment or process to operate as specified in URS.
  - Process Qualification (PQ): to display satisfactory completion of the OQ, demonstrating outputs of process meets all specifications.

- A Validation Report (VR): to summarise all documents and verify that all the requirements of VMP have been met. The VR should also provide a timeline for revalidation depending on changes to processes and trends.

3.2 Calibration and Maintenance

All equipment requires maintenance and calibration, with the frequency defined by manufacturer specifications. Alternatively, a risk assessment should be carried out to assess frequency required based on usage, importance of equipment, breakdown and trends in error.

Where there is not foolproof verification that a process is working as intended, calibration and maintenance helps to highlight potential problems with equipment, before it goes wrong! Calibration and maintenance means you minimise 'down-time', which allows all patients to be treated to the same standard without glitches.

It is also important to keep records of unplanned maintenance, as this could signify suboptimal equipment. Most importantly, a malfunctioning item should be switched off and clearly labelled as 'not in use'. Larger items such as incubators may not easily be removed from an embryology lab, so it is essential the whole team is notified that the incubator should not be used (often it is the most used equipment that is likely to fail due to constant use).

3.3 Traceability and Identification

High level identification and traceability should be in place to allow verification, history and location of process chains for all equipment and consumables. Incoming consumables should be approved either by supplier or in-house testing as suitable for use, e.g. by CE-marking of the product.

Regarding CE-marking, the HFEA states

The centre should use only media and consumables that have been CE-marked at a classification suitable for their intended purpose. Modifying existing devices (for example, adding calcium ionophore to culture medium) or using them 'off label' for purposes not intended by the manufacturer (for example, using a medium for a different purpose from that specified) has safety implications. It may also count as manufacture of a new device under the Medical Devices Regulations.

(section 26.4, HFEA Code of Practice, 2015)

All consumables should be identified as 'approved for use' and receipted in such a way to prevent deterioration to quality. Fertility clinics need to confirm the equipment or supplies that they purchase comply with all legislative requirements.

Consumables should be batch controlled by logging the product identifier, batch number and expiry date. This allows ease of traceability and recall.

3.4 Third Party Agreements

Third party agreements (TPAs) should be established to describe the method for the acceptance of external services or incoming products. This allows approval and monitoring of the suppliers to ensure needs and expectations are met. TPAs are sometimes referred to as Service Level Agreements (SLAs), more often for services rather than products, although the two are often used to mean both.

The HFEA defines a TPA as

an agreement in writing between a person who holds a licence and another person which is made in accordance with any licence conditions imposed by the Authority for the purpose of securing compliance with the requirements of Article 24 of the first Directive (relations between tissue establishments and third parties) and under which the other person -

(a) procures, tests or processes gametes or embryos (or both), on behalf of the holder of the licence, or

(b) supplies to the holder of the licence any goods or services (including distribution services) which may affect the quality or safety of gametes or embryos

(Mandatory Requirement 2A, HFEA Code of Practice, 2015)

Controls should be implemented to establish a method for acceptance of services/incoming goods to ensure providers/suppliers are approved, monitored and evaluated on their ability to supply the service/product and also that the supplied service/product meets the quality requirements that are needed.

For culture media, the temperature is critical. TPAs with companies supplying culture media should stipulate that the 'cold chain' (temperature from the factory, throughout transit to the clinic) is not broken. This can be monitored by dataloggers that measure temperature throughout transit. This confirms that the quality of the media will be optimal for clinic use. If there is a change to the transport method without prior agreement from the clinic, then the TPA has not been adhered to (Figure 23.5).

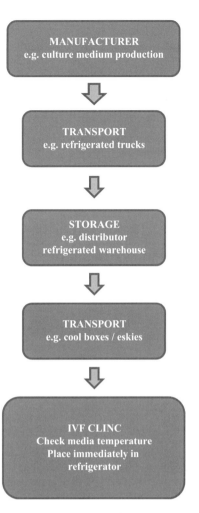

Fig. 23.5 The importance of maintaining a cold chain for transport of culture medium (and why third party agreements are important)

4 The Management Review Meeting (MRM)

All of the above are aspects of the continual process of quality management. It is important that the management team reviews quality matters annually to ensure the process continues to provide optimal quality. This meeting is termed the Management Review Meeting, and is not just a talking shop or a tick-box exercise. Rather the MRM is an opportunity to get a group of senior decision makers together to review the organisation's quality and to make improvements where necessary. As such, the MRM is one of the most important meetings that a fertility clinic has. It also makes good business sense!

5 Conclusion

This chapter has summarised some of the key aspects of how to set up and run a successful QMS for reproductive medicine. The aim was to offer an insight into the benefits that the pursuit of quality can bring to a clinic. It is hoped that with correct guidance, everyone will see the benefits of bringing quality to a clinic, from staff and service delivery and ultimately to our patients.

Chapter

24

Early Pregnancy

Maya Chetty
Janine Elson

1 Introduction

Early pregnancy problems are common and cause significant physical and psychological morbidity and mortality. Miscarriage is thought to affect one in five pregnancies and ectopic pregnancy to occur in 1 in 100 gestations though these rates are higher in pregnancies resulting from assisted reproductive techniques (ART) than in spontaneous pregnancies. According to the third annual report of the Confidential Enquiry into Maternal Deaths by MBRRACE-UK, in 2009–2014, 12 women died from early pregnancy-associated causes [1]. Nine of these women died as a direct result of an ectopic pregnancy and three women died following termination or attempted termination of pregnancy. In the triennium 2012–2014, the maternal mortality rate due to early pregnancy problems was 0.29 per 100,000 maternities.

2 Terminology

It is important that the terminology used in early pregnancy problems does not distress women further. For this reason the term 'abortion' should be avoided, and the term 'miscarriage' used instead to describe a non-viable intrauterine pregnancy. It is also important that terminology is used consistently to allow comparison of research data. The European Society of Human Reproduction and Embryology (ESHRE) early pregnancy special interest group published a consensus statement in 2015 advocating the use of terminology as in Table 24.1 [2].

3 Diagnosis of Ectopic Pregnancy and Miscarriage

Ultrasound in the early stages of pregnancy (up to 10 weeks of gestation) is important and necessary for many clinical reasons. A recent RCOG Scientific Impact Paper [3] reassures that ultrasound for clinical reasons is safe during the early stages of pregnancy

and the benefits outweigh any potential risks. During the first 10 weeks of pregnancy the fetus is most vulnerable because it is extremely small, the cells are dividing quickly and the placenta is not attached so there is limited blood flow. Certain types of ultrasound (colour and pulse waved Doppler) use a higher power output and should not be recommended at all during the early stages of pregnancy. Ultrasound for non-medical reasons is not recommended. It is important that healthcare professionals have a good knowledge of the safety principles of ultrasound.

Transvaginal ultrasound is more effective than transabdominal ultrasound for visualising the structures of the pelvis and should be the preferred approach for the assessment of an early pregnancy [4]. A transabdominal ultrasound scan should be considered for women with an enlarged uterus or other pelvic pathology, such as fibroids or a large ovarian cyst.

3.1 Pregnancy of Unknown Location

If a woman has a positive pregnancy test and no intrauterine or extrauterine pregnancy is visible on transvaginal ultrasound scan, this is termed a pregnancy of unknown location (PUL). PULs include complete miscarriages that have not been seen previously on ultrasound scan, viable intrauterine pregnancies that are too small to visualise and some ectopic pregnancies. Two measurements of human chorionic gonadotrophin (hCG) taken 48 hours apart can be used to determine subsequent management. A single progesterone measurement may also help to identify PULs that are likely to resolve spontaneously. It is important to remember that neither hCG nor progesterone concentrations can be used to identify the location of a pregnancy and that no method is validated in ART. When the serum hCG increases by more than 63% in 48 hours a transvaginal ultrasound should be performed 7–14 days later to determine the location of the pregnancy. An earlier repeat scan

Table 24.1 Terminology for classifying pregnancy failure prior to viability for research purposes [2]

Term	Description of pregnancy loss and clinical or ultrasound findings
Pregnancy loss	Spontaneous pregnancy demise
Early pregnancy loss	Spontaneous pregnancy demise before 10 weeks of gestational age (before 8th developmental week)
Non-visualised pregnancy loss	Spontaneous pregnancy demise based on decreasing serum or urinary β-hCG levels and non-localisation on ultrasound, if performed
Biochemical pregnancy loss	Spontaneous pregnany demise based on decreasing serum or urinary β-hCG levels, without an ultrasound evaluation
Resolved pregnancy loss of unknown location (resolved PUL)	Pregnancy demise not visualised on transvaginal ultrasound with resolution of serum β-hCG after expectant management
Treated pregnancy loss of unknown location (treated PUL)	Pregnancy demise not visualised on transvaginal ultrasound with resolution of serum β-hCG after medical management
Miscarriage	Intrauterine pregnancy demise confirmed by ultrasound or histology
Early miscarriage	Intrauterine pregnancy loss <10 weeks' size on ultrasound
Anembryonic (empty sac) miscarriage	Intrauterine pregnancy loss with a gestational sac but without a yolk sac or an embryo on ultrasound
Yolk sac miscarriage	Intrauterine pregnancy loss with a gestational sac and yolk sac, without an embryo on ultrasound
Embryonic miscarriage	Intrauterine pregnancy loss with an embryo without cardiac activity on ultrasound
Fetal miscarriage	Pregnancy loss ≥10 weeks' size with a fetus (≥33 mm) on ultrasound
Ectopic pregnancy	Ultrasonic or surgical visualisation of a pregnancy outside of the endometrial cavity

should be considered when the initial hCG is 1500 IU/ litre or more. When there is a decrease in serum hCG of more than 50% after 48 hours, a continuing pregnancy is unlikely and a urine pregnancy test should be done in 14 days. When the change in serum hCG concentration is between a 50% decline and 63% rise, the woman should be referred to the early pregnancy service within 24 hours [4].

3.2 Miscarriage

If on transvaginal ultrasound an intrauterine pregnancy is seen and the crown–rump length is less than 7 mm and there is no visible heartbeat, a second scan should be performed a minimum of 7 days after the first before making a diagnosis. Further scans may be needed before a diagnosis can be made. If on transvaginal ultrasound scan an intrauterine gestation sac is seen with a mean gestation sac diameter >/= 25 mm

(with no obvious fetal pole) or a fetal pole with crown rump length >/=7 mm (the latter without evidence of fetal heart activity), a second opinion and/or second scan a minimum of 7 days later should be performed. If there is no growth, this is suggestive of a diagnosis of miscarriage [4].

The presence of transvaginal bleeding or lower abdominal pain and ultrasound images showing heterogenous irregular echoes in the midline of the uterine cavity [5] suggest the diagnosis of an incomplete miscarriage. Retained products are usually seen as a well-defined area of hyperechoic tissue within the uterine cavity as opposed to blood clots, which are poorly outlined. Blood clots will be also seen sliding within the uterine cavity when pressure is applied on the uterus by a transvaginal probe [6]. If a measurable focus of hyperechoic tissue is seen, in 85% chorionic villi are identified on evacuation of retained products of conception (ERPC) [7].

3.2.1 Complete Miscarriage

The diagnosis of a complete miscarriage can only be made by ultrasound if an intrauterine pregnancy has been seen previously. If this is the case and on a transvaginal ultrasound scan the ET < 15 mm and there is no evidence of retained products of conception (RPOC) there is unlikely to be a significant amount of RPOC and so this can be labelled a complete miscarriage. It should be remembered, however, that even with a 2 mm ET, 57% may still have chorionic villi present. The cessation of pain and bleeding is also suggestive of a complete miscarriage.

3.2.2 Threatened Miscarriage

Women with vaginal bleeding and a confirmed viable intrauterine pregnancy should be reassessed if the bleeding becomes heavier or persists for more than 14 days. Whether or not the use of progesterone treatment for women who bleed in early pregnancy reduces the risk of miscarriage will hopefully be answered by the ongoing randomised controlled trial PRISM. In ART, luteal support with progesterone is conventionally continued until between 8 and 12 weeks gestation. There is, however, increasing evidence that early cessation of progesterone support does not increase miscarriage rates even in presence of bleeding [8].

3.2.3 Management of Miscarriage

Until recently the mainstay of treatment for the management of miscarriage has been surgical management, or the evacuation of RPOC, under general anaesthetic. Over the past decade, however, the focus has shifted from urgent surgical management to more individualised treatment and patient choice between expectant, medical and semi-elective surgical management.

It is currently recommended that expectant management should be used as first-line management in women with a confirmed diagnosis of miscarriage for the first 7–14 days. In situations where expectant management is not suitable, such as when there is an increased risk of haemorrhage or there is evidence of infection, or if expectant management is not acceptable to the woman, other management options should be explored [4]. Sufficient information and appropriate support should be provided regardless of the treatment method.

The success rate of expectant management varies widely. The type of miscarriage is significant with higher success rates seen in incomplete miscarriages

(80–94%) and lower success rates in early embryonic demise (28–76%) [9]. The chance of successful resolution also increases with the length of the follow-up. Women should be counselled to allow 2 weeks for expectant management and around 50% will resolve in this time. If there is no evidence of infection, women can continue with expectant management after this if they wish, and should be reviewed again at a minimum of 14 days. The infection rate with expectant management is 2% at 14 days and 3% at 8 weeks, and this is not significantly different from surgical management [10].

Medical management offers women the option of active treatment of miscarriage without the need for surgery and can be offered in the outpatient setting. The most commonly used drug is misoprostol, a prostaglandin analogue. This is licensed for oral use only but can be administered vaginally, sublingually or rectally. The antiprogesterone drug mifepristone should not be used to treat missed or incomplete miscarriage as it has not been shown to increase success rates compared to misoprostol alone. Current guidelines suggest a single vaginal dose of 800 micrograms of misoprostol for women with a missed miscarriage and 600 micrograms (or 800) for women with an incomplete miscarriage. Pain relief and antiemetics should also be offered. Women should be advised to seek help if bleeding has not started 24 hours after treatment and if the urine pregnancy test at 3 weeks after medical management is positive [4].

The success rate of medical management depends on the type of miscarriage, the drug regimen and the time allowed for products to be passed. Studies show success rates ranging from 70–96% for incomplete miscarriages and 52–92% for embryonic demise. For women diagnosed with incomplete miscarriages, medical management does not increase the rate of success over expectant management alone. Complications of medical management include the diarrhoea and vomiting associated with prostaglandin use and heavy bleeding requiring emergency evacuation in around 5% of cases [11].

Surgical management of miscarriage is the most successful option for the management of miscarriage, with a complete evacuation rate of 97% [12]. It is the most appropriate treatment for women who present with excessive bleeding, are haemodynamically unstable, have signs of infected RPOC or where there is a provisional diagnosis of gestational trophoblastic disease. Other women may prefer surgical intervention because it is quick and this may help with the grieving process. Suction curettage under general anaesthesia or manual vacuum aspiration under local anaesthetic in an outpatient setting can be used to remove RPOC. Cervical priming with misoprostol can be used to reduce the risk of uterine perforation. All at-risk women should be screened for *Chlamydia trachomatis*.

The MIST trial [10] looked at the incidence of infection in women managed surgically, medically and expectantly and no difference in the rate of infections was seen. Excessive bleeding is less likely to occur with surgical management than with expectant or medical management. Cervical damage and uterine perforation are uncommon complications of surgical management, with rates of 0.3% and 1.9% respectively. Intrauterine adhesions can form as a result of the trauma to the endometrium during surgical curettage in up to 8% of women. These can be a cause of subfertility and recurrent miscarriage. Fetomaternal haemorrhage can occur in surgical procedures and it is therefore recommended that non-sensitised RhD negative women who undergo evacuation should be given anti-D.

3.3 Ectopic Pregnancies

Any pregnancy implanted outside the uterine cavity is termed an ectopic pregnancy. More than 10,000 ectopic pregnancies are diagnosed annually in the United Kingdom with an incidence of around 11 per 1,000 pregnancies [1]. Ectopic pregnancy continues to be a cause of maternal death although the case fatality rate has fallen over recent years, most likely due to earlier diagnosis and treatment. Risk factors include tubal damage following surgery or infection, smoking and IVF, although the majority of women with an ectopic pregnancy do not have an identifiable risk factor. Ectopic pregnancies can be divided into those that are extrauterine (tubal, ovarian and abdominal) and those that are uterine (interstitial, cervical, caesarean scar and cornual). Around 95% of ectopic pregnancies occur within the fallopian tube, with the ampullary region of the tube being the most common site.

3.3.1 Tubal

Tubal ectopic pregnancies should be positively identified using transvaginal ultrasound. An inhomogenous or noncystic mass that moves separate to the ovary is most commonly seen, though an empty

extrauterine gestational sac or an extrauterine gestational sac containing a yolk sac and/or embryonic pole may be present [14]. Free fluid is also often seen on ultrasound and is not diagnostic of ectopic pregnancy though it can be the result of a tubal rupture or of blood leaking from the fimbrial end of a tube [15].

Tubal ectopic pregnancies can be treated surgically, medically or expectantly. The serum hCG level is not useful for making a diagnosis of ectopic pregnancy but is useful for determining the success of conservative management options. The National Institute for Health and Care Excellence (NICE) recommends that medical management with systemic methotrexate should be the first-line management for women who are able to return for follow-up and who meet the following criteria:

- no significant pain
- an unruptured ectopic pregnancy with a mass smaller than 35 mm with no visible heartbeat
- a serum hCG between 1500 and 5000 IU/litre
- no intrauterine pregnancy (as confirmed on ultrasound scan) [4].

Methotrexate should not be given at the first visit because of the chance that there is a viable intrauterine pregnancy.

For women who have minimal pain, have low (less than 1500 IU/litre) and declining hCG levels, and are willing and able to attend for follow-up, expectant management is a reasonable option. Success rates vary from 57 to 100% and depend upon case selection [16].

Women who have a tubal ectopic pregnancy and significant pain, an adnexal mass of 35 mm or larger, a visible fetal heartbeat on ultrasound scan, a serum hCG level of 5000 IU/litre or more or where treatment with methotrexate is not an acceptable option, should be offered surgery as first-line treatment. A laparoscopic approach is generally preferred to an open approach and in the presence of a healthy contralateral tube, salpingectomy should be performed rather than salpingotomy as there is a lower rate of persistent trophoblast. However, salpingotomy should be considered in women with a history of fertility-reducing factors (previous ectopic pregnancy, contralateral tubal damage, previous abdominal surgery or previous pelvic inflammatory disease) [13].

3.3.2 Cervical

A cervical pregnancy is a pregnancy that has implanted into the cervical mucosa, below the internal os. These

Box 24.1 Sonographic criteria for the diagnosis of cervical ectopic pregnancy

- Empty uterus
- Barrel shaped cervix
- Gestational sac below internal os (uterine arteries)
- Absence of sliding sign
- Blood flow around sac with Doppler

Box 24.2 Sonographic criteria for the diagnoses of caesarean scar implantation

- Empty uterine cavity
- Anterior location of gestation sac at level of internal os at site of previous caesarean section scar
- Thin or absent layer of myometrium between the gestational sac and the bladder
- Prominent trophoblastic/placental circulation on Doppler examination
- Empty endocervical canal

Box 24.3 Sonographic criteria for the diagnosis of interstitial pregnancy

- Empty uterine cavity
- Products of conception/gestational sac located laterally in the interstitial (intramural) part of the tube and surrounded by less than 5 mm of myometrium in all imaging planes.
- The 'interstitial line sign', which is a thin echogenic line extending from the central uterine cavity echo to the periphery of the interstitial sac.

are rare, occurring in 1 in 1,000–95,000 pregnancies. The sonographic criteria for the diagnosis of cervical pregnancy are listed in Box 24.1. The sliding sign distinguishes cervical ectopic pregnancies from miscarriages that are in the cervical canal. Pressure is applied to the cervix using the probe. In a miscarriage the gestational sac slides against the endocervical canal, whereas in a cervical ectopic it does not [17].

A single serum hCG level carried out at diagnosis is useful in deciding management options. An hCG level greater than 10,000 IU/litre is associated with a decreased chance of successful medical management with methotrexate [18].

Medical management with systemic or local injection of methotrexate has a 91% success rate. Surgical methods of management are associated with a high failure rate and high rates of excessive bleeding. They should therefore be reserved for women with life-threatening bleeding. Dilatation and curettage with additional measures to control haemorrhage is the traditionally used method, though successful hysteroscopic resection with uterine artery embolisation has more recently been described.

3.3.3 Caesarean Scar

Caesarean scar pregnancy is defined as implantation into the myometrial defect occurring at the site of a previous uterine incision. It occurs in 1 in 200 pregnancies and these pregnancies may be potentially viable pregnancies or miscarriages within the scar. Caesarean scar pregnancy is diagnosed primarily by transvaginal ultrasound but MRI can be a useful adjunct (Box 24.2).

Intervention should be considered in women with a first trimester caesarean scar pregnancy and a surgical approach is thought to be the most effective [13].

3.3.4 Interstitial

A pregnancy implanted in the interstitial part of the fallopian tube is an interstitial pregnancy. 3D ultrasound or MRI can be useful adjuncts to transvaginal ultrasound in the diagnosis of interstitial pregnancy (Box 24.3). A single serum hCG level should be carried out at diagnosis and a repeat at 48 hours may be useful in deciding further management. If hCG levels are low or falling, expectant management may be appropriate otherwise medical management with methotrexate or surgical management should be used. Surgical options include laparoscopic cornual resection, salpingotomy and hysteroscopic resection under laparoscopic or ultrasound guidance [13].

3.3.5 Ovarian

Ovarian pregnancies are rare, occurring in 0.0003% of all pregnancies. There are no agreed sonographic criteria though suggestive findings with an empty uterus are listed in Box 24.4. As the diagnosis of ovarian pregnancy can be difficult to make with certainty pre-operatively, the diagnosis is usually confirmed histopathologically after diagnostic laparoscopy and surgical treatment. Laparoscopic removal of the gestational products by enucleation or wedge resection is preferred [19]. Oophorectomy is only occasionally required. Medical management with methotrexate

> **Box 24.4** Sonographic findings suggestive of an ovarian pregnancy
>
> - Wide echogenic ring with internal echolucent area on surface of ovary
> - Negative sliding organ sign
> - Separate corpus luteum
> - Echogenicity of ring greater than ovary

> **Box 24.6** Sonographic criteria for the diagnosis of abdominal pregnancy
>
> - Absence of intrauterine gestation sac
> - Absence of dilated tube and complex adnexal mass
> - Gestational sac surrounded by bowel loops and separate to peritoneum
> - Mobility when subjected to pressure in posterior cul-de-sac

> **Box 24.5** Sonographic criteria for the diagnosis of cornual pregnancy [20]
>
> - Single interstitial portion of fallopian tube in main uterine body
> - Gestational sac, mobile and separate from uterus surrounded by myometrium
> - Vascular pedicle adjoining gestational sac to unicornuate uterus

may be considered where surgery is risky or where there is persistent trophoblast.

3.3.6 Cornual

A cornual pregnancy is a pregnancy implanted in the rudimentary horn of a unicornuate uterus (Box 24.5). Cornual pregnancies should be managed by excision of the rudimentary horn by laparoscopy or laparotomy. Urinary tract anomalies can be associated with unicornuate uteri and attention should be paid to this during surgery.

3.3.7 Abdominal

Abdominal pregnancy is a rare form of ectopic pregnancy with an incidence of around 1.3% of ectopic pregnancies. In advanced abdominal pregnancy MRI can be a useful diagnostic adjunct, and can help to plan the surgical approach (Box 24.6). An early abdominal pregnancy can be removed laparoscopically [21] or alternatively could possibly be managed medically with systemic methotrexate or with ultrasound-guided fetocide. Advanced abdominal pregnancy should be managed by laparotomy.

3.3.8 Heterotopic

A heterotopic pregnancy is a coexisting ectopic and intrauterine pregnancy. It should be considered following ART, where there is an intrauterine pregnancy and persistent pain, and where there is a persistently raised hCG post miscarriage or termination of pregnancy.

The intrauterine pregnancy should be considered in the management plan and methotrexate only given if the intrauterine pregnancy is non-viable or the woman does not wish to continue with the pregnancy. In clinically stable women, the ectopic pregnancy can be managed with local injection with potassium chloride or hyperosmolar glucose. If the woman is clinically unstable then surgical removal is the treatment method of choice. Where the ultrasound findings are of a non-viable pregnancy, expectant management is an option [13].

3.3.9 Anti-D

Rhesus negative women who undergo surgical management of ectopic pregnancy, or where bleeding is repeated, heavy or associated with abdominal pain should be offered anti-D prophylaxis [13]. Whether or not women who undergo expectant or medical management should be offered anti-D is controversial.

3.3.10 Fertility following Ectopic Pregnancy

In the absence of a history of subfertility or tubal pathology, there is no difference in the risk of future tubal ectopic pregnancy between the different management methods. Women who do have a previous history of subfertility should be advised that treatment of their tubal ectopic pregnancy with expectant or medical management is associated with improved reproductive outcomes compared with radical surgery. Women receiving methotrexate for management of tubal ectopic pregnancy can be advised that there is no effect on ovarian reserve and women undergoing treatment with uterine artery embolisation and systemic methotrexate for non-tubal ectopic pregnancies can be advised that live births have been reported in subsequent pregnancies. Women undergoing laparoscopic management of ovarian pregnancies can be reassured that they have good future fertility prospects [13].

3.4 Early Pregnancy Issues Specific to ART

Most ART pregnancies use progesterone supplementation and this will affect serum progesterone levels. There is evidence that hCG levels are altered both by ART and by multiple embryos which must be taken into account when interpreting results.

Initial studies show an increased rate of monozygotic twins with blastocyst transfers over cleavage stage embryos and over natural conception. This may also be increased with ICSI, extended culture and maternal age. However changes in culture media may affect the rate of monozygotic twins [22]. Clearly monozygotic twinning is associated with significant morbidity and mortality in both early pregnancy and in more advanced gestations.

3.5 Support and Counselling

Women should be provided with evidence-based information and support to allow informed decision-making. Emergency contact details should be given and information about how to access support and counselling services given. After an early pregnancy loss, women should be offered the option of a follow-up appointment.

Muscle relaxation training may reduce anxiety and improve quality of life in women undergoing treatment for ectopic pregnancy with methotrexate. After treatment with methotrexate, women should be advised to wait three months before trying to conceive due to a higher malformation rate, though conception in this time should not be considered an indication for termination [13].

4 Service and Training

Early pregnancy assessment services should provide dedicated services seven days a week for women with early pregnancy complications. Self-referrals from women with recurrent miscarriages, previous ectopic and molar pregnancies should be accepted as well as direct referrals from A+E, GPs etc. Ultrasound and assessment of serum hCG should be offered and diagnostic and therapeutic algorithms used (Box 24.7). Women should have access to all appropriate management options with clear referral pathways in place where required [4].

Box 24.7   NICE quality standards

- Statement 1. Women referred to early pregnancy assessment services are seen by the service at least within 24 hours of referral.
- Statement 2. Women who are referred with suspected ectopic pregnancy or miscarriage are offered a transvaginal ultrasound scan to identify the location and viability of the pregnancy.
- Statement 3. Women with a suspected miscarriage who have had an initial transvaginal ultrasound scan are offered a second assessment to confirm the diagnosis

---

Box 24.8   Practice points

- Medical management is appropriate for selected tubal, cervical and interstitial pregnancies
- Surgical management for cervical and caesarean scar pregnancies needs an available haemostatic technique
- Laparoscopic removal of rudimentary horn method of choice for cornual pregnancies
- Oophorectomy is only needed for advanced ovarian ectopics
- Primary abdominal pregnancies in first trimester can be managed laparoscopically
- Monitor MZ twin rates

    –Culture media/sequence

Clinicians undertaking ultrasound for the diagnosis of early pregnancy problems, medical management via ultrasound guided techniques and surgical management should be appropriately trained. Senior support should be available to allow the full range of surgical options to be offered. Virtual reality simulators can be a useful training tool for surgical procedures.

5 Conclusion

Miscarriage and ectopic pregnancy are sadly a common consequence of infertility treatment and have important physical and psychological consequences. Transvaginal ultrasound is the main diagnostic tool. Clinicians working in infertility should be familiar with the diagnosis and management of early pregnancy problems and have close links to early pregnancy services. Women should be treated with compassion and respect, and they should be supported in choosing the management method that best suits them. Non-tubal ectopic pregnancies still present a diagnostic challenge. Current guidelines exist to aid clinicians in the management of these relatively rare conditions (Box 24.8).

References

1. Knight M, Nair M, Tuffnell D, Kenyon S, Shakespeare J, Brocklehurst P, Kurinczuk JJ (Eds.) on behalf of MBRRACE-UK. *Saving Lives, Improving Mothers' Care – Surveillance of maternal deaths in the UK 2012–14 and lessons learned to inform maternity care from the UK and Ireland Confidential Enquiries into Maternal Deaths and Morbidity 2009–14.* Oxford: National Perinatal Epidemiology Unit, University of Oxford; 2016 [www.npeu.ox.ac.uk/mbrrace-uk].

2. Kolte AM, Bernardi LA, Christiansen OB, Quenby S, Farquharson RG, Goddijn M, Stephenson MD; ESHRE Special Interest Group. Early Pregnancy Terminology for pregnancy loss prior to viability: a consensus statement from the ESHRE early pregnancy special interest group. *Hum Reprod.* 2015 Mar; 30(3): 495–8. doi: 10.1093/humrep/deu299. Epub 2014 Nov 5.

3. RCOG. Ultrasound from conception to 10+0 weeks of gestation. Scientific Impact Paper No. 49. March 2015.

4. NICE. Ectopic pregnancy and miscarriage: diagnosis and initial management. Clinical Guideline 154. December 2012.

5. Luise C, Jermy K, Collons WP, Bourne TH. Expectant management of incomplete, spontaneous first-trimester miscarriage: outcome according to initial ultrasound criteria and value of follow-up visits. *Ultrasound Obstet Gynecol* 2002; 19: 580–2.

6. Elson J, Salim R, Tailor A, BAnerjee S, Zosmer N, Jurkovic D. Prediction of early pregnancy viability in the absence of an ultrasonically detectable embryo. *Ultrasound Obstet Gynecol* 2003; 21: 57–61.

7. Sawyer E, Ofusasia E, Ofili-Yebovi D, Helmy S, Gonzalez J, Jurkovic D. The value of measuring endometrial thickness and volume on transvaginal ultrasound scan for the diagnosis of incomplete miscarriage. *Ultrasound Obstet Gynecol* 2007; 23: 205–9.

8. Kohls G1, Ruiz F, Martínez M, Hauzman E, de la Fuente G, Pellicer A, Garcia-Velasco JA. Early progesterone cessation after in vitro fertilization/intracytoplasmic sperm injection: a randomized, controlled trial. *Fertil Steril* 2012; 98(4):858–62. doi: 10.1016/j.fertnstert.2012.05.046. Epub 2012 Jun 29.

9. Graziosi GC, Mol BW, Ankum WM, Bruinse HW. Management of early pregnancy loss. *Int J Gynecol Obstet* 2004; 86: 337–46.

10. Trinder J, Brocklehurst P, Porter R, Read M, Vyas S, Smith L. Management of miscarriage: expectant, medical, or surgical? Results of randomized controlled trial (miscarriage treatment (MIST) trial). *BMJ* 2006; 332: 1235–40.

11. Gronlund A, Gronlund L, Clevin L, Andersen B, Palmgren N, Lidegaard O. Management of missed abortion: comparison of medical treatment with either mifepristone + misoprostol or misoprostol alone with surgical evacuation. A multi-center trial in Copenhagen County, Denmark. *Acta Obstet Gynecol Scand* 2002; 81: 1060–5.

12. Sotiriadis A, Makrydimas G, Papatheodorou S, Ionnidis JP. Expectant, medical, or surgical management of first-trimester miscarriage: a meta-analysis. *Obstet Gynecol* 2005; 105: 1104–13.

13. RCOG. Diagnosis and management of ectopic pregnancy. Green-top guideline no. 21. November 2016.

14. Brown DL, Doubilet PM. Transvaginal sonography for diagnosing ectopic pregnancy: positivity criteria and performance characteristics. *J Ultrasound Med* 1994; 13: 259–66.

15. Nyberg DA, Hughes MP, Mack LA, Wang KY. Extrauterine findings of ectopic pregnancy of transvaginal US: importance of echogenic free fluid. *Radiology* 1991; 178: 823–6.

16. Craig LB, Khan S. Expectant management of ectopic pregnancy. *Clin Obstet Gynecol* 2012; 55: 461–70.

17. Jurkovic D, Hacket E, Campbell S. Diagnosis and treatment of early cervical pregnancy: a review and a report of two cases treated conservatively. *Ultrasound Obstet Gynecol* 1996: 8: 373–80.

18. Kung FT, Chang SY. Efficacy of methotrexate treatment in viable and nonviable cervical pregnancies. *Am J Obstet Gynecol* 1999; 181: 1438–44.

19. Joseph RJ, Irvine LM. Ovarian ectopic pregnancy: aetiology, diagnosis and challenges in surgical management. *J Obstet Gynecol* 2012; 32: 472–4.

20. Mavrelos D, Sawyer E, Helmy S, Holland TK, Ben-Nagi J, Jurkovic

D. Ultrasound diagnosis of ectopic pregnancy in the non-communicating horn of a unicornuate uterus (cornual pregnancy). *Ultrasound Obstet Gynecol* 2007; 30: 765–70.

21. Shaw SW, Hsu JJ, Chueh HY, Han CM, Chen FC, Chang YL et al. Management of primary abdominal pregnancy: twelve years of experience in a medical centre. *Acta Obstet Gynecol Scan* 2007; 86(9): 1058–62.

22. Moayeri SE, Behr B, Lathi RB, Westphal LM, Milki AA. Risk of monozygotic twinning with blastocyst transfer decreases over time: an 8-year experience. *Fertil Steril* 2007; 87: 1028–32.

Evaluation and Management of Recurrent Miscarriage

H. M. Bhandari

S. Tewary

M. K. Choudhary

RECURRENT MISCARRIAGE

1 Definition

The spontaneous loss of a pregnancy before the viable gestation is termed miscarriage. Miscarriage therefore includes all pregnancy losses from conception until 23 completed weeks of pregnancy. It remains the commonest adverse outcome of pregnancy and can either be sporadic or recurrent (RM). Currently, no consensus exists on the definition of RM. The Royal College of Obstetricians and Gynaecologists (RCOG) guideline defines RM as the loss of three or more consecutive pregnancies [1]. However, the American Society for Reproductive Medicine (ASRM) has adopted the definition of consecutive loss of two or more clinical pregnancies, documented either by ultrasonography or histopathological examination [2]. RM can be either 'primary' (no previous live birth) or 'secondary' (following a live birth).

2 Epidemiology

About 1% of the couples trying to conceive experience three or more consecutive miscarriages and about 5% of the couples have two or more consecutive miscarriages [3]. Nearly half (45%) of these women have secondary RM. In one in five women with secondary RM, the previous pregnancies are complicated by either prematurity or intrauterine growth restriction of the fetus [4]. Approximately one-third of couples (32%) with RM would have experienced conception delays and one in five (22%) late miscarriage [4].

3 Risk Factors for RM

The chance of having a subsequent successful live birth following RM is inversely related to the number of previous miscarriages and maternal age [5].

3.1 Maternal Age

Maternal age has been shown to be a strong, independent risk factor for miscarriage in a large prospective register linkage study [6]. The UK census data from 2011 reports that the standardised average age of mothers at first childbirth was 27.9 years, compared to 23.7 years in 1971. The report also found an increased percentage of births to mothers aged 35 years or more, which almost trebled from 7.5% in 1971 to 20% in 2011. The age-related risk of miscarriage in recognised pregnancies increases sharply after the age of 35 years, rising from 11% at 20–24 years to 93% at 45 years and older. In women aged 40 years or older, only 41.7% achieved live birth within 5 years as opposed to 81.3% of women aged 20–24 years [5]. Women aged 20 years with 2 previous miscarriages have a 92% chance of success in the next pregnancy compared with only a 60% chance of success in women aged 45 years [7].

3.2 Number of Previous Miscarriages

While around three quarters of women with 3 miscarriages achieve a live birth within 5 years, only about half have successful pregnancy following 6 or more previous miscarriages [5]. The risk of further miscarriage increases by 45% after 3 or more pregnancy losses [6].

3.3 Environmental Factors

A matched case control study by Lashen et al. [8] demonstrated significantly higher odds of RM in obese women (OR 3.51, 95% CI 1.03–12.01). In couples with RM, maternal obesity has been found to be an independent factor increasing the risk of miscarriage in a subsequent pregnancy.

Frequent and excessive maternal alcohol consumption, passive smoking and caffeine consumption in the peri-conceptual period have been associated with an increased risk of RM. However, there is no evidence from randomised controlled studies about lifestyle adaptations to improve reproductive outcome in women with otherwise unexplained RM.

4 Causes of RM

It has been widely accepted that RM is a heterogeneous condition. RM may be associated with several factors such as parental genetic and embryonic chromosomal conditions, maternal antiphospholipid syndrome, inherited thrombophilias, congenital and acquired uterine abnormalities, endocrine dysfunction, infectious diseases, endometrial abnormalities, immunological dysfunction and environmental factors. The common potentially associated causative factors for RM and their further management are discussed in this chapter.

4.1 Genetic Abnormalities

It is estimated that only 30% of the embryos are successful in resulting in a live birth. The remainder is either lost prior to implantation (30%) or post-implantation, 30% as early pregnancy loss (before 6 weeks' gestation) and 10% as clinical miscarriage [9]. The exceptionally high attrition rate of human embryos is attributed mainly to the high prevalence of chromosomal and genetic aberrations throughout all stages of pre-implantation embryo development. Chromosomal abnormalities account for about half of all the cases of sporadic miscarriages and amongst these abnormalities, about 50% are due to chromosomal segregation errors such as trisomy. The rest are non-trisomies, predominantly monosomy X and triploidy [10]. Although chromosomal segregation errors can lead to miscarriage, these have not been identified as risk factors for RM, but can provide useful information about the prognosis for future pregnancy.

Chromosomal translocations refer to chromosome abnormalities that are caused by the rearrangement of segments of DNA between non-homologous chromosomes. Translocations are of two types: reciprocal translocation in which there is an exchange of two terminal segments from different chromosomes, or Robertsonian translocation in which there is centric fusion of two acrocentric chromosomes with the loss of the short arms. In couples with two or more consecutive miscarriages, a carrier rate of 3–6% for either a Robertsonian or reciprocal translocation has been reported [11]. Carriers of a balanced reciprocal translocation themselves usually have no loss or gain

of genetic information and hence are usually phenotypically normal. However, 50–70% of their gametes may have an unbalanced chromosomal pattern at meiosis resulting in embryos inheriting an unbalanced translocation that is in turn associated with an increased risk of miscarriage. The miscarriage risk for couples where one is a carrier of a reciprocal translocation can be up to 72.4% [12]. Children born with unbalanced translocation generally have multiple congenital malformations and/or mental disability [4]. The importance of recognising the risk is not that it can be treated but that there may be an opportunity to avoid the birth of an affected child e.g. through antenatal screening and termination of the pregnancy after appropriate counselling or in selected cases through pre-implantation diagnosis.

4.2 Thrombophilias

Pregnancy is naturally a hypercoagulable state which is protective to the pregnant mother especially during the intra-partum and post-partum period. However, when this natural pivotal change in the pregnancy physiology is affected by a thrombophilic defect, early and late adverse pregnancy outcomes can occur. Thrombophilias, both inherited and acquired, are known to cause a predisposition to venous and arterial thrombosis. The thromboses in decidual vessels are thought to be related to intrauterine growth restriction, fetal death and recurrent miscarriage [4].

4.2.1 Acquired Thrombophilia or Antiphospholipid Syndrome (APS)

APS is the most important and treatable cause of RM [1, 4]. Diagnosis of APS is made when at least one clinical and one laboratory criterion is present (Table 25.1) [13].

Anti-phospholipid antibodies (APA) are present in 15% of women with RM [14] compared to a prevalence of less than 2% in the low risk obstetric population. APA are thought to contribute to RM by altering the extra-villous trophoblast function, initiating a local inflammatory response and by triggering thrombosis of the microvasculature of the placenta later in pregnancy. APS if left untreated can reduce the live birth rate to 10% [15].

4.2.2 Inherited or Hereditary Thrombophilias

The recognised inherited thrombophilias are listed in Box 25.1. Inherited thrombophilic mutations have

Table 25.1 Clinical and laboratory criteria to diagnose antiphospholipid syndrome. At least one clinical and one laboratory criteria should be present to diagnose antiphospholipid syndrome.

Clinical criteria	Laboratory criteria

Vascular (arterial/venous/small capillary) thrombosis History of adverse pregnancy outcome
  – Three or more consecutive miscarriages before 10 weeks gestation
  – One or more morphologically normal fetus/es lost after 10 weeks gestation
  – One or more preterm births before 34 weeks gestation owing to placental insufficiency or severe pre-eclampsia
	IgG and/or IgM ACA in medium or high titre on 2 or more occasions at least 12 weeks apart
	IgG and/or IgM anti-B2 glycoprotein1 antibodies (in the titre of >99th centile) on 2 or more occasions at least 12 weeks apart.
	LA present in plasma on 2 or more occasions at least 12 weeks apart.

Box 25.1   Inherited thrombophilias

Types of Inherited Thrombophilia

Activated protein C resistance (commonly due to Factor V Leiden mutation)

Prothrombin gene mutation (Factor II)

Protein S deficiency

Protein C deficiency

Anti-thrombin III deficiency

Methylenetetrahydrofolate reductase (MTHFR) mutation

---

been implicated as a possible cause of RM. However, prospective data on the outcome of untreated pregnancies in women with inherited thrombophilias are scarce. Their association with late pregnancy loss is stronger than with early pregnancy loss [1].

4.2.3 MTHFR Mutation

MTHFR is a key enzyme in one-carbon metabolism which catalyses the conversion of 5,10-methylenetetrahydrofolate into 5-methyltetrahydrofolate. MTHFR gene polymorphisms are commonly associated with hyperhomocysteinaemia, the milder forms of which have been identified as a risk factor for thrombosis. There is no convincing evidence to suggest hyperhomocysteinaemia is a risk factor for RM.

4.3 Structural Abnormalities – Uterine and Cervical

Congenital uterine abnormalities, depending on the type and degree of anatomical distortion, are thought to impair reproductive outcome. They are associated with an increased risk of spontaneous miscarriage and other pregnancy complications such as preterm labour, fetal malpresentation, low birth weight and increased perinatal mortality rates [16]. Although the exact aetio-pathophysiology remains uncertain, they are found to be significantly more prevalent in women with miscarriage than in the general population. The incidence of congenital uterine anomalies may range from 2.7% to 16.7% in the general population or in fertile women and from 1.8% to 37.6% in women with two or more consecutive miscarriages [17]. The prevalence of all congenital uterine anomalies in women with two or more miscarriages appears to be similar to those with three or more miscarriages.

Fibroids are common, benign tumours of the uterus occurring in up to 77% of women approaching the age of 50. The prevalence of fibroids in women with RM is reported as 8.2% [18]. Although cavity distorting sub-mucous and intramural fibroids and large non-cavity distorting intramural fibroids may interfere with implantation [19], their effect on the risk of RM remains poorly understood. An observational study found that mid-trimester miscarriages were significantly commoner in women experiencing RM with either cavity distorting or non-cavity distorting fibroids compared to women with otherwise unexplained RM [18]. In this study, resection of fibroids distorting the uterine cavity removed the risk of mid-trimester loss and increased live birth rate by twofold in subsequent pregnancies [18].

Intrauterine adhesions (Asherman's syndrome) have been thought to increase the risk of RM by endometrial fibrosis and inflammation and diminishing intrauterine volume [20]. The reported incidence of intrauterine adhesions on diagnostic hysteroscopy following three or more spontaneous miscarriages is around 10%, but a study found that 97.5% of women with three or more miscarriages have had two or more surgical management of miscarriage procedures [20]. However, there is no evidence from prospective studies to confirm the causal relationship of intrauterine adhesions to RM.

A diagnosis of cervical weakness is based on a history of recurrent mid-trimester miscarriages or recurrent preterm deliveries following painless cervical dilatation in the absence of contractions, bleeding or other causes of RM. The exact incidence of cervical weakness in women with RM is unknown and there are no objective tests that can reliably identify women with cervical weakness in the non-pregnant state [1].

4.4 Endometrial Causes

There is a growing body of evidence from in-vitro and animal studies to suggest that decidualising endometrial stromal cells serve as sensors of embryo quality upon implantation and that any perturbations in endometrial decidualisation may cause recurrent miscarriage [9]. It has also been suggested that in some women with RM the duration of uterine receptivity is prolonged, widening the implantation window. Decidualising stromal cells from women with RM may fail to discriminate between high and low quality embryos and thereby allow developmentally compromised embryos to implant resulting in miscarriage which may then be recurrent. There are no standardised investigations however, to assess endometrial dysfunction and the current treatments to improve endometrial function are empirical.

4.5 Endocrine Abnormalities

Uncontrolled diabetes mellitus is a known risk factor for miscarriages and congenital malformations, but well managed, diabetes alone is not found to be a risk factor for miscarriage and thus should not cause recurrent miscarriage.

Physiological changes of pregnancy demands increased thyroid hormone production which is adequately accommodated by a normal thyroid gland. An underactive thyroid gland may not be able to meet the demands of changes in pregnancy; however, there is no evidence to suggest that women with miscarriage or RM have more overt or subclinical hypothyroidism.

The role of anti-thyroid antibodies in RM is not completely established. The prevalence of thyroid peroxidase antibodies (TPO-Ab) in women with recurrent miscarriage is reported to be higher. In a systematic review, it was identified that the presence of thyroid antibodies was associated with an increased risk of RM (OR 2.3, 95% CI 1.5–3.5), when compared with the absence of thyroid antibodies [21].

The role of prolactin in RM is controversial. Prolactin is essential for female reproduction and high levels are associated with ovulatory dysfunction. Hyperprolactinaemia is thought to affect the hypothalamo-pituitary-ovarian axis, resulting in impaired folliculogenesis, oocyte maturation and/or a short luteal phase [2]. In one study bromocriptine-treated hyperprolactinaemic women with RM had a significantly higher percentage of successful pregnancies overall [22]. An observational study, however, identified that those women with RM and significantly lower serum prolactin levels were at an increased risk of miscarriage in subsequent pregnancy [23].

Polycystic ovarian syndrome (PCOS) is the most common endocrine condition in women of reproductive age. The reported prevalence of PCOS in women with RM ranges from 4.8% to 82%, and the wide range of apparent prevalence is the result of the huge variation in the diagnostic criteria used for PCOS before the establishment of the Rotterdam criteria [24]. PCOS has been associated with an increased risk of miscarriage, but the exact mechanism remains unclear. The markers of PCOS are not predictive of pregnancy loss following spontaneous conception amongst ovulatory women with RM. The increased risk of miscarriage in PCOS women may be due to hyperandrogenaemia, hyperinsulinaemia and insulin resistance. The prevalence of hyperandrogenaemia in RM women is 11% [25]. In RM women, increased follicular phase free androgen index is associated with an increased risk of miscarriage in subsequent pregnancy [25]. Insulin resistance is prevalent in 17–27% of women with RM [24]. Hyperinsulinaemia in PCOS is attributed to obesity as well as to insulin resistance independent of body weight. It is found to be an independent risk factor for miscarriage and is thought to play a key role in implantation failure by suppressing circulating levels of glycodelin and IGFBP-1. However, there is no strong association between hyperinsulinaemia and RM.

4.6 Infection

There is a paucity of evidence to suggest infections such as toxoplasmosis, rubella, cytomegalovirus, herpes, listeria and bacterial vaginosis cause first trimester RM. Therefore, routine screening for these infections as a part of RM evaluation is not recommended and neither is any routine use of antibiotics.

4.7 Immune Dysfunction

The survival of a genetically 'foreign' semi-allogenic fetus and the placenta requires significant regulation of the maternal immune system and this maternal tolerance is mediated by MHC proteins, endometrial leukocytes and the cytokines.

HLA class 1b alleles and polymorphisms (HLA –C, –E, -F and –G) seem to induce suppression of the maternal immune system, but their exact link to pregnancy complications such as RM has not been convincingly established [26].

Uterine natural killer (uNK) cells are the most abundant of all decidual leucocytes. They are a rich source of cytokines and growth factors and are thought to play a role in conferring immunotolerance towards paternal antigens, in decidualisation by regulating trophoblast invasion and vascular remodelling. There is no convincing evidence to suggest that uNK cell density is different in women with RM when compared to controls, and the uNK cell density does not appear to predict future pregnancy outcome.

Peripheral NK cells are phenotypically and functionally different from uNK cells and have no role in decidualisation, implantation and hence in RM.

4.8 Psychological

Miscarriage can be a distressing event and can induce obvious emotional responses, such as anxiety, depression, denial, anger, marital disruption, and a sense of loss and inadequacy [4].

4.9 Male Factor

Studies examining the role of sperm DNA damage in RM patients have shown mixed results. There is insufficient evidence to suggest that tests of DNA fragmentation have predictive value in the prospective identification of women at risk of RM. At present, sperm DNA testing is not recommended as a part of the clinical evaluation of RM.

4.10 Unexplained

Despite the range of available investigations, the aetiology of RM is unknown in 50% to 70% of couples [2]

and remains challenging and frustrating to both clinicians and couples. Although the majority of unexplained RM may occur by chance, a certain proportion of women will go on to have more miscarriages, which statistically would be unlikely to occur due to chance alone [27]. Older women with unexplained RM generally do not have any specific underlying pathology and the prognosis in these women remains good. However, in younger women who are less likely to suffer from RM, an unidentified aetiological factor may well be the reason for their unexplained RM [27].

5 Recommended Investigations for Couples with RM

The couple should be seen together at a dedicated recurrent miscarriage clinic and a detailed history should be obtained, taking into consideration the aetiological factors and family history, as discussed earlier. Though the RCOG defines RM as three or more consecutive miscarriages, it may be reasonable to undertake evaluation of a couple after two first trimester miscarriages, especially if they were diagnosed either by an ultrasonography or histopathological examination.

5.1 Karyotyping

If the karyotype of the products of conception (POC) is normal, then RM is less likely to have occurred as a consequence of chance [27]. Normal fetal karyotype in RM is associated with a poor prognosis for future pregnancies and with an increased number of further miscarriages, whereas RM associated with abnormal karyotype of the POC occurs as a result of chance [4] and carries good prognosis for future pregnancies. Hence, it is recommended that in the evaluation of RM, cytogenetic analysis of POC should be undertaken, where possible, at third and subsequent miscarriages [1].

Though balanced translocations are found in 3–6% of couples with RM, the risk of a subsequent pregnancy with an unbalanced translocation is less than 2%. The chances of these couples having a healthy baby in future pregnancy is 81%, which is not different from non-carriers (83%) [11]. Hence routine karyotype screening of all couples with RM is not cost-effective and is not recommended [1]. However, when an unbalanced chromosomal translocation is identified in the POC, evaluating parental karyotype for balanced translocation would be more appropriate [1].

5.2 Testing for Thrombophilias

Patients with a history of first trimester RM or one or more second trimester miscarriages should be screened for APA [1]. It is important to perform screening ideally in a non-pregnant state, preferably 12 weeks after an antecedent pregnancy episode to minimise false positive results. ACA and anti-B2 glycoprotein antibodies are detected using an enzyme linked immunosorbent assay [13]. Detection of LA specificity can be improved by dilute Russell's viper venom time test and one other test (either modified APTT or a dilute PT), but a confirmatory step (e.g. using a high phospholipid concentration, platelet neutralising reagent or LA-insensitive reagent) is needed to demonstrate phospholipid dependence [13]. If the initial test is positive it is important to repeat the test after a minimum of 12 weeks to confirm the diagnosis.

Patients with a history of second trimester miscarriage should be tested for inherited as well as acquired thrombophilia [1]. Testing for MTHFR mutation is not a part of recommended evaluation for RM.

5.3 Investigations for Structural Abnormalities

A transvaginal pelvic ultrasound scan should be used to screen all women with RM for structural abnormalities. Three-dimensional transvaginal pelvic ultrasound scans appear to be more promising in the diagnosis and classification of congenital uterine anomalies and in identification of other structural abnormalities such as sub-mucous fibroids or intra-uterine synechiae. Magnetic resonance imaging of the pelvis may be required for doubtful or complex cases, particularly for the assessment of associated abnormalities of cervix and vagina. Though considered 'gold standard', invasive surgical procedures such as combined diagnostic hysteroscopy and laparoscopy, should be reserved for a definitive diagnosis.

5.4 Hormonal Profile

The current evidence does not suggest routine screening for PCOS and thyroid function tests (including TPO-Ab), and prolactin and HbA1C are not imperative unless clinically indicated.

5.5 Immune Dysfunction

The exact role of immune dysfunction in RM has not been fully established. Routine testing for immune dysfunction is not currently recommended and these investigations should be reserved for research purposes.

There are no standardised investigations to assess endometrial dysfunction and further research is required before recommending endometrial assessment for evaluation of RM.

6 Treatment Options for Couples with RM

A recognised aetiology is identified in less than half of the couples investigated for RM. Couples with RM should be managed by a specialist clinic and the treatment depends upon whether there is an identifiable cause for RM (Figure 25.1).

6.1 Genetic Abnormalities

6.1.1 Parental Translocations

Referral to a clinical geneticist to discuss prognosis for future pregnancies should be undertaken for a structural genetic factor such as balanced translocation identified in parents. Options for these couples to have biological but unaffected offspring are a) prenatal diagnosis of the fetus by chorionic villous sampling or amniocentesis in early pregnancy following a natural conception or b) IVF/ICSI-PGD with transfer of unaffected embryos. The use of donor gametes for assisted conception and adoption are the other reproductive options.

The couples who have proven fertility should be made aware that IVF/ICSI-PGD may have physical, mental and/or financial implications for them. Overall LBR following IVF/ICSI-PGD for parental translocation carriers is between 20.6% and 29.4% per embryo transferred [28]. In couples with RM and carriers of reciprocal translocation, the cumulative LBR is 74% following natural conception and 35% following IVF/PGD [29], suggesting that IVF/PGD for these couples does not necessarily improve reproductive outcomes.

6.1.2 Embryo Aneuploidy Screening

IVF/ICSI-PGS is undertaken to screen embryos for aneuploidies, and selecting a euploid embryo for transfer is thought to result in improved LBR for couples with unexplained RM or those with advancing maternal age and repeated trisomic pregnancies. However, a retrospective study identified that in

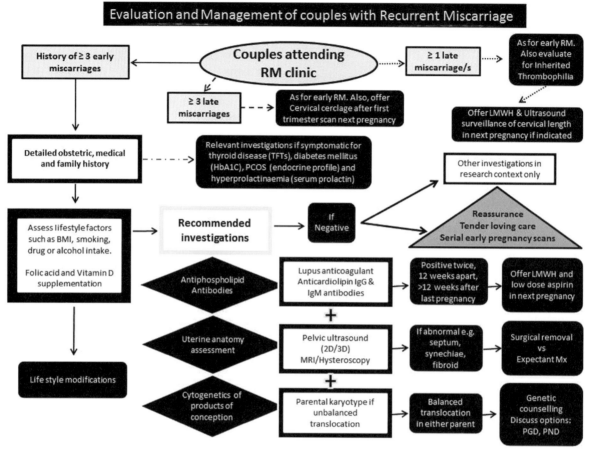

Fig. 25.1 Flow chart illustrating the evidence-based evaluation and management of couples with recurrent miscarriage. RM: recurrent miscarriage, LMWH: Low molecular weight heparin, BMI: Body mass index, TFTs: Thyroid function tests, HbA1C: Glycosylated haemoglobin, PCOS: Polycystic ovarian syndrome, 2D/3D: 2/3-Dimensional, MRI: Magnetic resonance imaging, PGD: Pre-implantation genetic diagnosis, PND: Prenatal diagnosis

women with RM, per attempt at IVF/ICSI PGS is not effective in improving LBR or decreasing miscarriage rate as compared with expectant management, except in those PGS cycles that complete transfer of a euploid embryo [30].

6.2 Anti-phospholipid Syndrome

The Cochrane Database Systematic Review identified that in women with RM and APS the only treatment which significantly improves pregnancy outcome is aspirin and unfractionated heparin [31]. Treatment improves the chances of achieving LBR in subsequent pregnancy by more than 70% and the miscarriage risk is decreased by 54% when compared to aspirin alone. LMWH appears to be as efficacious and as safe as unfractionated heparin and has an

advantage of being a once daily dose with reduced risk of osteoporosis and thrombocytopenia. These women should continue thromboprophylaxis until six weeks postnatally as they remain at risk of complications through their pregnancy, primarily of venous thromboembolism [1]. The dosage of LMWH is calculated according to the pre-pregnancy weight of the patient [32]. There is no consensus as to when the treatment should be initiated. However, the British Society of Haematology guidelines suggest that for women with APS with RM, antenatal administration of LMWH combined with low dose aspirin should begin as soon as pregnancy is confirmed [13].

Other treatment options such as corticosteroids and immunoglobulins have not been shown to improve birth rate in women with RM and APS [31].

6.3 Inherited Thrombophilia

While treatment options for women with RM and APS have been studied in RCTs, the optimal treatment options for women with RM and inherited thrombophilias remain a controversial topic due to a lack of good prospective data on the outcome of untreated pregnancies with inherited thrombophilias. The efficacy of anticoagulants for such patients has not yet been assessed in appropriate RCTs. Currently there is a multicentre RCT (ALIFE2) being conducted worldwide to assess the benefits of LMWH plus standard pregnancy surveillance versus standard surveillance alone in women with RM and inherited thrombophilia [33]. Treatment for inherited thrombophilia found in women with RM in the meantime should be offered only in research context. However, LMWH therapy may improve LBR in women with a history of second trimester miscarriage associated with inherited thrombophilia [1].

6.4 Structural Uterine Abnormalities

Hysteroscopic correction of uterine anomolies such as septate uterus, arcuate uterus and in some cases of partial bicornuate uterus can restore normal anatomy. Observational studies have provided evidence that surgical correction of septate uterus in women with RM may improve reproductive outcome [17, 34]. There is no evidence from RCTs assessing the benefits of surgical correction of uterine abnormalities on pregnancy outcome. The results of a multicentre randomised controlled trial assessing whether or not hysteroscopic septum resection improves reproductive outcome in women with a septate uterus are awaited (TRUST trial). NICE has found that the current evidence from non-randomised studies on efficacy of hysteroscopic metroplasty for women with RM to be adequate to support its use provided that the clinicians undertaking this procedure are appropriately trained and arrangements are in place for clinical governance, consent and audit [35].

The surgical management of RM women with Asherman's syndrome (intrauterine synechiae), uterine fibroids and uterine polyps is controversial, and there is no conclusive evidence that surgical treatment reduces the risk of further pregnancy loss. Hence, any surgical intervention should only be undertaken after careful counselling of the women informing them about lack of robust evidence to support this to improve reproductive outcome as well as the associated risks of a surgical approach.

History-indicated cervical cerclage should be offered to women with three or more previous preterm births and/or second trimester losses and an ultrasound-indicated cerclage is offered to women with one or more spontaneous mid-trimester losses or preterm births and with an evidence of cervical length of less than 25 mm on transvaginal ultrasonography [36]. For women with a history of second trimester miscarriage who have not undergone a history-indicated cervical cerclage, serial transvaginal ultrasound scans to assess cervical length would be useful in determining whether a cervical cerclage is required to prevent further mid-trimester miscarriage or preterm birth [1].

6.5 Other Treatments

Immune modulating therapies have been proposed as potential therapeutic strategies for women with unexplained RM. Progesterone acts as an immunomodulator, but the PROMISE trial provided good evidence that first trimester vaginal progesterone supplementation for women with unexplained RM does not improve reproductive outcomes [37].

Vaginal progesterone supplementation for high-risk women of preterm delivery has not been found to be beneficial in reducing the risk of preterm birth and adverse neonatal outcomes (OPPTIMUM) [38].

The authors of a Cochrane intervention review on 'hCG for preventing miscarriage' concluded that there was not enough evidence to support the use of hCG in RM women [39].

Paternal cell immunisation, third-party donor leukocytes, trophoblast membranes and intravenous immunoglobulin (IVIG) provide no significant beneficial effect over placebo in improving the live birth rate for women with unexplained RM [40]. Though an initial systematic review of RCTs showed that IVIG increased LBR in women with secondary RM, the largest RCT and an updated meta-analysis showed no significant effect of treatment with IVIG [41].

The results of a multicentred, randomised, double-blind, placebo-controlled trial assessing the effectiveness, safety and tolerability of NT100 (a variant of granulocyte colony-stimulating factor) in improving outcome in pregnant women with a history of unexplained RM are awaited (RESPONSE trial).

Results from a multicentred, randomised, double blind, placebo-controlled trial are awaited which would provide evidence on the outcome of levothyroxine treatment on LBR and pregnancy complications in women with RM and TPO-Ab (T4-LIFE study) [42].

Metformin, an insulin-sensitising agent when administered pre-pregnancy for women with PCOS and infertility showed that metformin has no effect on the sporadic miscarriage risk [43]. There is a lack of evidence from RCTs assessing the role of metformin in PCOS women with RM, and the use of metformin in these women is not recommended [1].

There is evidence to suggest a possible benefit of endometrial scratch in improving IVF outcome in women with previous two or more failed IVF treatment cycles, but not in preventing miscarriage in women with RM. Further research is being undertaken by the Tommy's Miscarriage research group (SiM trial) which will answer whether endometrial scratch will benefit RM women.

6.6 Unexplained RM

It is important to highlight to, and encourage, couples that they have more than 50–60% chances of a successful pregnancy without treatment, depending on maternal age and parity [5, 6]. Although the data to support role of psychological component in RM is inconclusive, there is some evidence from two non-randomised studies which have shown significant benefit in a subsequent pregnancy following close monitoring and support in a dedicated RM clinic.

Lifestyle modification and stress reduction should also be emphasised and that leading a healthier lifestyle, free from tobacco, alcohol, illicit drugs and undue stress may improve the couple's chances for a successful pregnancy.

It may be tempting to use empirical treatment with aspirin, LMWH, progesterone, steroids and immunomodulators in women with unexplained RM. However, some of these agents have been found to be non-beneficial and the others have not been tested in good quality studies. It is also important to consider that these treatments could potentially cause serious adverse effects. Clinical evaluation of future treatments for RM should be performed only in the context of sufficiently powered RCTs to determine their efficacy [1].

7 Conclusions

Recurrent miscarriage can be a distressing situation for the couples and a challenging one for clinicians. In spite of advances in genetics, imaging, reproductive endocrinology and immunology and better understanding of RM than ever before, the majority of cases of RM still do not have a clearly defined aetiology. Couples with unexplained RM have a good chance of a successful pregnancy with 'tender loving care' and clinicians should resist the use of empirical treatments for these couples which may be of no benefit, but might cause harm. The significance of appropriate training of staff dealing with RM sufferers cannot be underrated and should be incorporated in routine clinical practice.

Abbreviations

ACA:	Anti-cardiolipin antibodies
ALIFE2:	Anticoagulants for **li**ving **f**etuses in women with **r**ecurrent miscarriage and inherited thrombophilia
APA:	Anti-phospholipid antibodies
APTT:	Activated partial thromboplastin time
APS:	Anti-phospholipid syndrome
ASRM:	American Society for Reproductive Medicine
DNA:	Deoxyribose nucleic acid
ELISA:	Enzyme linked immunosorbent assay
HbA1C:	Glycosylated haemoglobulin
hCG:	Human chorionic gonadotrophin
HLA:	Human leucocyte antigen
ICSI:	Intracytoplasmic sperm injections
IGFBP-1:	Insulin like growth factor binding protein-1
IgG:	Immunoglobulin G
IgM:	Immunoglobulin M
IVF:	In-vitro fertilisation
IVIG:	Intravenous immunoglobulin
LA:	Lupus anticoagulant

LBR:	Live birth rate	PGS:	Pre-implantation genetic screening
LMWH:	Low molecular weight heparin	POC:	Products of conception
MHC:	Major histocompatibility complex	PROMISE:	**Pro**gesterone in recurrent **mis**carriage
MTHFR:	Methylenetetrahydrofolate reductase		
NICE:	National Institute for Health and Care Excellence	PT:	Prothrombin time
		RCOG:	Royal College of Obstetricians and Gynaecologists
OPPTIMUM:	**Do**es **p**rogesterone **p**rophylaxis **to** prevent preterm labour **im**prove **outcome?**	RCT:	Randomised controlled trial
		RM:	Recurrent miscarriage
PAI-1:	Plasminogen activator inhibitor-1	TPO-Ab:	Thyroid peroxidase antibodies
PCOS:	Polycystic ovarian syndrome	uNK cells:	Uterine natural killer cells
PGD:	Pre-implantation genetic diagnosis		

References

1. RCOG, The investigation and treatment of couples with recurrent first trimester and second trimester miscarriage. Green-top Guideline No.17. April 2011 [cited 2016 21 August]; Available from: www.rcog.org.uk/globalassets/documents/guidelines/gtg_17.pdf.

2. ASRM, Evaluation and treatment of recurrent pregnancy loss: a committee opinion. *Fertil Steril*, 2012. **98**(5): p. 1103–11.

3. Stirrat, G.M., Recurrent miscarriage. *Lancet*, 1990. **336**(8716): p. 673–5.

4. Rai, R. and L. Regan, Recurrent miscarriage. *Lancet*, 2006. **368** (9535): p. 601–11.

5. Lund, M., et al., Prognosis for live birth in women with recurrent miscarriage: what is the best measure of success? *Obstet Gynecol*, 2012. **119**(1): p. 37–43.

6. Nybo Andersen, A.M., et al., Maternal age and fetal loss: population-based register linkage study. *BMJ*, 2000. **320**(7251): p. 1708–12.

7. Brigham, S.A., C. Conlon, and R.G. Farquharson, A longitudinal study of pregnancy outcome following idiopathic recurrent miscarriage. *Hum Reprod*, 1999. **14**(11): p. 2868–71.

8. Lashen, H., K. Fear, and D.W. Sturdee, Obesity is associated with increased risk of first trimester and recurrent miscarriage: matched case-control study. *Hum Reprod*, 2004. **19**(7): p. 1644–6.

9. Teklenburg, G., et al., Natural selection of human embryos: decidualizing endometrial stromal cells serve as sensors of embryo quality upon implantation. *Plos One*, 2010. 5(4): e10258. DOI: 10.1371/journal.pone.0010258.

10. Koifman, A., D. Chityat, and A. Bashiri, *Genetics of Recurrent Pregnancy Loss*. 1st edn. Recurrent Pregnancy Loss: Evidence-Based Evaluation, Diagnosis and Treatment. 2016: Springer International Publishing. XV 208.

11. Franssen, M.T., et al., Reproductive outcome after chromosome analysis in couples with two or more miscarriages: index [corrected]-control study. *BMJ*, 2006. **332**(7544): p. 759–63.

12. Sugiura-Ogasawara, M., et al., Poor prognosis of recurrent aborters with either maternal or paternal reciprocal translocations. *Fertil Steril*, 2004. **81**(2): p. 367–73.

13. Keeling, D., et al., Guidelines on the investigation and management of antiphospholipid syndrome. *Br J Haematol*, 2012. **157**(1): p. 47–58.

14. Rai, R.S., et al., Antiphospholipid antibodies and beta 2-glycoprotein-I in 500 women with recurrent miscarriage: results of a comprehensive screening approach. *Hum Reprod*, 1995. **10**(8): p. 2001–5.

15. Rai, R.S., et al., High prospective fetal loss rate in untreated pregnancies of women with recurrent miscarriage and antiphospholipid antibodies. *Hum Reprod*, 1995. **10**(12): p. 3301–4.

16. Venetis, C.A., et al., Clinical implications of congenital uterine anomalies: a meta-analysis of comparative studies. *Reprod Biomed Online*, 2014. **29**(6): p. 665–83.

17. Grimbizis, G.F., et al., Clinical implications of uterine malformations and hysteroscopic treatment results. *Hum Reprod Update*, 2001. 7(2): p. 161–74.

18. Saravelos, S.H., et al., The prevalence and impact of fibroids

and their treatment on the outcome of pregnancy in women with recurrent miscarriage. *Hum Reprod*, 2011. **26**(12): p. 3274–9.

19. Sunkara, S.K., et al., The effect of intramural fibroids without uterine cavity involvement on the outcome of IVF treatment: a systematic review and meta-analysis. *Hum Reprod*, 2010. **25**(2): p. 418–29.

20. Cogendez, E., et al., Post-abortion hysteroscopy: a method for early diagnosis of congenital and acquired intrauterine causes of abortions. *Eur J Obstet Gynecol Reprod Biol*, 2011. **156**(1): p. 101–4.

21. van den Boogaard, E., et al., Significance of (sub)clinical thyroid dysfunction and thyroid autoimmunity before conception and in early pregnancy: a systematic review. *Hum Reprod Update*, 2011. **17**(5): p. 605–19.

22. Hirahara, F., et al., Hyperprolactinemic recurrent miscarriage and results of randomized bromocriptine treatment trials. *Fertil Steril*, 1998. **70**(2): p. 246–52.

23. Li, W., et al., The relationship between serum prolactin concentration and pregnancy outcome in women with unexplained recurrent miscarriage. *J Obstet Gynaecol*, 2013. **33**(3): p. 285–8.

24. Cocksedge, K.A., et al., A reappraisal of the role of polycystic ovary syndrome in recurrent miscarriage. *Reprod Biomed Online*, 2008. **17**(1): p. 151–60.

25. Cocksedge, K.A., et al., Does free androgen index predict subsequent pregnancy outcome in women with recurrent miscarriage? *Hum Reprod*, 2008. **23**(4): p. 797–802.

26. Dahl, M. and T.V. Hviid, Human leucocyte antigen class Ib molecules in pregnancy success and early pregnancy loss. *Hum Reprod Update*, 2012. **18**(1): p. 92–109.

27. Saravelos, S.H. and T.C. Li, Unexplained recurrent miscarriage: how can we explain it? *Hum Reprod*, 2012. **27**(7): p. 1882–6.

28. De Rycke, M., et al., ESHRE PGD Consortium data collection XIII: cycles from January to December 2010 with pregnancy follow-up to October 2011. *Hum Reprod*, 2015. **30**(8): p. 1763–89.

29. Hirshfeld-Cytron, J., M. Sugiura-Ogasawara, and M.D. Stephenson, Management of recurrent pregnancy loss associated with a parental carrier of a reciprocal translocation: a systematic review. *Semin Reprod Med*, 2011. **29**(6): p. 470–81.

30. Murugappan, G., et al., Intent to treat analysis of in vitro fertilization and preimplantation genetic screening versus expectant management in patients with recurrent pregnancy loss. *Hum Reprod*, 2016. **31**(8): p. 1668–74.

31. Empson, M., et al., Prevention of recurrent miscarriage for women with antiphospholipid antibody or lupus anticoagulant. *Cochrane Database Syst Rev*, 2005. Issue 2. Art. No.: CD002859. DOI: 10.1002/14651858.CD002859.pub2.

32. RCOG, Reducing the risk of venous thromboembolism during pregnancy and the puerperium. Green-top Guideline No 37a. April 2015 [cited 2016 21 August]; Available from: www.rcog.org.uk/globalassets/documents/guidelines/gtg-37a.pdf.

33. de Jong, P.G., et al., ALIFE2 study: low-molecular-weight heparin for women with recurrent miscarriage and inherited thrombophilia: study protocol for a randomized controlled trial. *Trials*, 2015. **16**: p. 208.

34. Sugiura-Ogasawara, M., et al., Does surgery improve live birth rates in patients with recurrent miscarriage caused by uterine anomalies? *J Obstet Gynaecol*, 2015. **35**(2): p. 155–8.

35. NICE, Hysteroscopic Metroplasty of a Uterine Septum for Recurrent Miscarriage. IPG 510 January 2015 [cited 2016 21 August]; Available from: www.nice.org.uk/guidance/ipg510.

36. RCOG, Cervical cerclage. Green-top Guideline No 60. May 2011 [cited 2016 21 August]; Available from: www.rcog.org.uk/globalassets/documents/guidelines/gtg_60.pd.

37. Coomarasamy, A., et al., PROMISE: first-trimester progesterone therapy in women with a history of unexplained recurrent miscarriages: a randomised, double-blind, placebo-controlled, international multicentre trial and economic evaluation. *Health Technol Assess*, 2016. **20**(41): p. 1–92.

38. Norman, J.E., et al., Vaginal progesterone prophylaxis for preterm birth (the OPPTIMUM study): a multicentred, randomised, double-blind trial. *Lancet*, 2016. **387**(10033): p. 2106–16.

39. Morley, L.C., N. Simpson, and T. Tang, Human chorionic gonadotrophin (hCG) for preventing miscarriage. *Cochrane Database Syst Rev*, 2013. Issue 1: Art. No.: CD008611. DOI: 10.1002/14651858.CD008611.pub2.

40. Porter, T.F., Y. LaCoursiere, and J.R. Scott, Immunotherapy for recurrent miscarriage. *Cochrane Database Syst Rev*, 2006. Issue 2. Art. No.: CD000112. DOI: 10.1002/14651858.CD000112.pub2.

41. Stephenson, M.D., et al., Intravenous immunoglobulin and idiopathic secondary recurrent miscarriage: a multicentered randomized placebo-controlled trial. *Hum Reprod*, 2010. **25**(9): p. 2203–9.

42. Vissenberg, R., et al., Effect of levothyroxine on live birth rate in euthyroid women with recurrent miscarriage and TPO antibodies (T4-LIFE study). *Contemp Clin Trials*, 2015.

43. Palomba, S., et al., Effect of preconceptional metformin on abortion risk in polycystic ovary syndrome: a systematic review and meta-analysis of randomized controlled trials. *Fertil Steril*, 2009. **92**(5): p. 1646–58.

Sperm Retrieval
The Practical Procedures

Kevin McEleny

1 Why Perform Sperm Retrieval?

Surgical sperm retrieval (SSR) is used in situations where sperm suitable for fertility treatment cannot be obtained by other means, principally from the ejaculate. Even sperm obtained from cryptozoospermic samples can be used for intracytoplasmic sperm injection (ICSI) and the major indication is therefore azoospermia. On occasion, sperm suitable for treatment cannot be recovered due to problems with ejaculation and if techniques like penile vibratory stimulation or electro-ejaculation fail in men with conditions such as spinal cord injuries, or if sperm suitable for ICSI cannot be recovered from the post-orgasm urine in men with retrograde ejaculation, then SSR may be needed. A rare indication would be an 'emergency' retrieval procedure where a patient cannot for psychological reasons, produce a sperm sample on the day of oocyte retrieval and there are therefore no sperm available to proceed to treatment. As an alternative to cancelling the cycle, some authors have reported success by utilising SSR, although oocyte cryopreservation would be an appropriate alternative approach. In cases of obstructive azoospermia (OA), reconstructive male genital tract surgery where applicable, should be considered. Some authors describe excellent outcomes for vaso-vasostomy particularly in situations where the interval between vasectomy and reversal is short and the female partner is young with no fertility issues [1].

Some studies have suggested that there may also be occasional situations where SSR techniques may be indicated where sperm is available in the ejaculate. The Cornell group examined their outcomes in patients with cryptozoospermia where the couples had had at least one round of ICSI treatment using ejaculated sperm and one round of treatment using sperm recovered by microdissection testicular sperm extraction (MicroTESE). In an understandably small

number of cases examined in this retrospective analysis, by comparing the two approaches that were performed closest (temporally) to each other, a significantly higher fertilisation rate was identified in the MicroTESE group. Furthermore, a higher pregnancy rate was found when more than six sperm were seen in the ejaculate, following the post-preparation spin down examination of the samples. Due perhaps to the small sample size, no other significant findings were identified [2].

A multicentre study from Europe recruited couples who had experienced recurrent treatment failure using ICSI, in cases where the male partner had a high percentage of DNA fragmentation in his sperm. Sperm taken by testicular biopsy in this group showed a significantly lower percentage of sperm DNA fragmentation and also a significant number of clinical pregnancies. Although other studies have now shown similar results, as with the Cornell study, it is perhaps difficult to apply the results of this work to more general andrological practice. However, it is important to remember that SSR can be considered in situations other than azoospermia [3].

2 The Development of Surgical Sperm Retrieval

The introduction of ICSI and the first reported pregnancies using this technique [4] has revolutionised the care of couples with male factor subfertility. It paved the way then for sperm to be recovered surgically from the testes and to be used to treat couples affected by male factor subfertility. Prior to this, the only options available for couples were male genital tract reconstructive surgery in situations where it was an option (ie vaso-vasostomy, vaso-epididymostomy, or in the rare occasion of ejaculatory duct obstruction, trans-urethral resection of the ejaculatory ducts) or using donor sperm. It is worth mentioning that despite the rise of assisted reproductive techniques, these procedures are still valuable (and indeed cost-effective) in appropriate cases.

The mechanism of the azoospermia indicates what type of procedure can be employed to recover sperm for ICSI. Techniques to recover sperm from men with OA are nearly always successful, and so the techniques used to recover sperm from such cases are usually minimally invasive. It is more difficult to recover sperm surgically from men with sperm-production problems that have resulted in non-obstructive azoospermia (NOA) and the chance therefore of achieving biological paternity is much lower. The introduction of the MicroTESE technique, which utilises optical magnification to directly inspect the testicular parenchyma, by Schlegal and co-workers in Cornell University [5], has significantly increased the chance of recovering sperm from men with NOA. This modern technique is considered the gold standard in terms of recovering sperm in this particularly difficult-to-treat category of couples, when compared to single-site or multi-site TESE. Indeed, as sperm can be recovered in approximately half of non-obstructive cases where single site TESE failed to recover sperm and a third of cases where multi-site TESE has failed, the case for performing these less effective procedures in such men is seriously weakened [6]. A further study examined the outcomes in men undergoing MicroTESE SSR with those undergoing multi-site biopsy. This study showed that the recovery rate in the MicroTESE arm was significantly higher than in the multi-site TESE arm [7].

3 Investigating the Azoospermic Man prior to SSR

The detailed assessment of male fertility is covered elsewhere in this book (Chapter 3), but a few key points should be reiterated. The history and examination findings can explain the mechanism or even, on occasions, the precise cause of the problem. It is unfortunately not uncommon to encounter patients who have never been examined before, to then find relevant abnormalities like absent vasa deferens, large varicoceles or low volume testes, which can explain the problem. Occasionally scrotal examination may reveal suspicious lumps. Testes cancer is the commonest solid malignancy in young men. Men with fertility problems are at an increased risk of developing it, (possibly due to the shared aetiology of Testicular Dysgenesis Syndrome) a fact that should

be explained in the clinic, along with instructions regarding testicular self-examination [8]. It is mandatory to examine the genitalia of men who have significant male fertility problems and those who are to undergo SSR, to ensure that there are no surprises on the day of the procedure in terms of the patient's anatomy and to ensure that the patient is suitable for such a procedure. It is not unheard of in patients admitted for sperm retrieval who have not been examined before, to be found unexpectedly to have cryptorchidism when they are on the operating table. This situation should never arise. Furthermore, a patient who cannot tolerate his testes being examined is unlikely to tolerate a local anaesthetic procedure well either, and finding this out in advance could prevent a procedure being abandoned on the day.

A clear explanation for the problem is of great significance to the patient. A high FSH will confirm a sperm-production problem and in an azoospermic male, indicates a non-obstructive aetiology. The reverse however is not necessarily true as a significant number of men with a normal FSH and azoospermia can also have a non-obstructive aetiology (late maturation arrest). In this situation, the FSH level is within the normal range as the biological trigger for inhibin B release is the pachytene stage of meiosis, not the production of mature sperm, meaning that the patient could have a normal FSH (and normal-sized testes) with no sperm production.

The testosterone level of patients should be recorded pre-procedure as patients with a sperm-production problem not uncommonly have a low testosterone. This should never be corrected in advance of the procedure with testosterone replacement therapy, which can, by interfering with the hypothalamo-pituitary-gonadal axis, inhibit endogenous testosterone production and thus interfere with any spermatogenesis that may be occurring. Some clinicians use HCG, FSH or clomifene to boost sperm production, but this is controversial [9]. Whilst karyotype or (where indicated) cystic fibrosis testing can provide useful aetiological information, it is helpful also to perform Y microdeletion testing prior to attempting SSR, in situations where the underlying reason for the azoospermia is not known. This is to exclude the Y microdeletion patterns AZFa and b, which are believed to be incompatible with successful sperm retrieval as they result in complete Sertoli cell–only syndrome and complete maturation arrest respectively, in affected males. (Those men who bear the more common defect AZFc have hypospermato-genesis and do therefore have a chance of undergoing successful SSR, although the couple should be aware that such a defect would be passed on to any male children that they may have through ART).

Appropriate assessment of the azoospermic man allows him to be put into (in most cases) a mechanistic category, which will then determine what the most appropriate surgical sperm retrieval procedure would be, assuming of course that the couple wish to undergo ICSI treatment. Some couples in whom a genetic problem is identified decline SSR and furthermore, some couples prefer to opt for donor sperm treatment even when SSR is a possibility. The clinician's role is to provide the couple with appropriate information within a supportive environment, which will enable them to make what is the right choice for them. Some couples require more information and support and although men are sometimes reluctant to seek it, should be offered counselling.

4 Consent and Aftercare for Surgical Sperm Retrieval

Men undergoing SSR should be aware of the complications that can occur, namely bleeding and infection as well as the chance of success. It is possible that a significant bleed or infection could lead to shrinkage or loss of a testicle, although this is extremely unlikely. Furthermore, there is also a chance that the patient could be rendered hypogonadal by the procedure, particularly if procedures like multi-site TESE or MicroTESE are used. It is helpful therefore to document the testicular size and (morning) testosterone level both before and after the procedure. To allow for the standard storage of gametes it is necessary that the patients undergo a screen for blood-borne viruses and are therefore routinely tested for HIV, Hepatitis B and Hepatitis C. It is also a requirement that the patient and his partner complete the appropriate documentation that is a requirement of HFEA-licensed fertility centres.

Most procedures for OA can be performed under local anaesthetic, which is safer and cheaper than general anaesthetic, but as above, it is important to ensure that it is something that the patient will tolerate. After a procedure such as percutaneous epididymal sperm aspiration (PESA), testicular sperm aspiration (TESA) and/or single-site biopsies, the wound can be covered with a non-adherent dressing

and padding and the patient will be fitted with a scrotal support that can be removed after 24 hours. The patient should very quickly be able to return to their usual activities. For more invasive procedures such as MicroTESE, the scrotal support should remain on a little longer and the patient should avoid strenuous activity for a slightly longer period of time post-procedure. In terms of analgesia, patients who have undergone minimally invasive procedures need only simple analgesia. In the more invasive cases, a generous injection of local anaesthetic into the spermatic cord and wound edges will minimise discomfort post-operatively and enable the patients to be discharged the same day. Patients in significant pain may require strong opiates, which can cause drowsiness and nausea, which may in turn delay discharge. In addition to local anaesthetic that can be administered at the end of the GA cases, simple analgesia such as a non-steroidal anti-inflammatory drug along with paracetamol and perhaps codeine for breakthrough pain prove sufficient in the majority of cases.

5 Procedures for Recovering Sperm from Men with Obstructive Azoospermia

The choices here lie between an aspiration-type procedure and testicular biopsy.

Sperm can be recovered from the epididymides of the majority of men who have OA. A small number of men will have an intratesticular obstruction and such an approach may then be unsuccessful. In this case testicular sperm extraction (TESE) or aspiration (TESA) could be used.

In terms of the epididymal procedures, PESA is the most commonly performed procedure. It is a quick and technically straightforward percutaneous procedure. It can be performed under local anaesthesia by means of a spermatic cord block combined with local skin infiltration. The epididymis is immobilised between the index finger and thumb of the operator's non-dominant hand. A fine butterfly is then passed into the epididymis and the fluid aspirated. Fluid aspirated from the epididymis is examined under a light microscope by a technologist for the presence of sperm and if motile sperm are not seen, the operator can proceed directly to TESE or TESA. PESA is particularly effective in patients with distended epididymides, such as vasectomised men or men with absent vasa.

An alternative to PESA is microsurgical epididymal sperm aspiration (MESA). This procedure involves surgical exposure of the epididymides via a scrotal incision, which can then be examined under the operating microscope. In this way an epididymal tubule can be precisely cannulated (PESA is a 'blind' procedure, whilst MESA is performed under direct vision). The aspirated epididymal fluid can be examined under a light microscope, as with PESA, to look for the presence of motile sperm. Some work has suggested that MESA may give better fertility outcomes than PESA, but the quality of some of this data is not strong. Some work has also suggested that a MESA procedure may provide sperm for more ICSI treatment cycles than a PESA procedure [10].

One other potential advantage of MESA is that on occasion, simultaneous reconstructive procedures, such as vaso-epididymostomy can be considered and the fact that the testes are exposed also facilitates multi-site TESE if required. MESA is usually performed under general anaesthetic as a day-case procedure and takes longer to perform than PESA. It is therefore a more expensive intervention.

As an alternative, a testicular source of sperm can be sought primarily, without an attempt to obtain it from the epididymis. TESA is a simple procedure to perform and is carried out under local anaesthetic. It involves passing a fine needle connected to a syringe (as with PESA) into the testes, to aspirate fluid. The sperm recovery rate according to some sources can be lower than with biopsy techniques and also it is not possible to send a sample for histological assessment, meaning that problems that can on occasion be observed histologically, such as intra-tubular germ cell neoplasia, can be missed. Like PESA it is a 'blind' technique and can therefore, in the testis, be associated with bleeding or haematoma formation. It can be used in conjunction with mapping techniques as advocated by some experts [11].

TESE can be unilateral or bilateral, single (one biopsy) or multi-site (more than one biopsy per testis) and can be performed under local or general anaesthetic as a closed technique, where the tunica albuginea is exposed via a small skin incision (suitable for single site biopsies only), or as an open technique where the testes are delivered via a raphe incision. What is performed depends on the preferences of the clinician and patient, as well as on the available facilities. Generally single-site biopsies are performed as a closed technique, whilst multi-site biopsies are performed as an open technique under general anaesthetic, but individual practices vary. Most patients for

surgical sperm retrieval are fit young men with few if any co-morbidities and the procedures are usually carried out on a day-case basis. Testicular biopsy techniques also have the advantage of providing the opportunity for a small piece of testicular parenchyma to be sent off separately in Bouin's medium for histological assessment. This will allow concomitant problems that may be of importance, such as intratubular germ cell neoplasia (carcinoma in situ-CIS) to be identified. The specimens for sperm extraction should be placed directly into warmed, buffered culture medium (e.g., G-MOPS), before transfer to the lab. After incising the tunica albuginea, the testicular parenchyma can be exposed and a representative sample removed for sperm retrieval. After achieving haemostasis, the tunica albuginea, dartos and skin are then closed using an absorbable suture. The wound is covered with a non-adherent dressing and the patient provided with a scrotal support and padding.

Ideally the operator will retrieve sperm of sufficient number and quality to permit storage for future ICSI attempts. It is disappointing for the couple if sperm deemed less than ideal for ICSI purposes is recovered, meaning that the male partner may need to go through another procedure before the couple can proceed to ICSI. Surgical sperm retrieval procedures should only take place where facilities are available for cryopreservation. Diagnostic biopsies for histology only (i.e., where sperm retrieval is not planned) should be strongly discouraged. The reason for this is that the absence of sperm on diagnostic biopsy does not mean that sperm cannot be recovered by more invasive means, as sperm production can be patchy within the testicle in cases of NOA and it is not therefore difficult to fail to find an area of active spermatogenesis in a testis by using a single-site biopsy. There is no evidence that the fertility outcomes obtained by using frozen sperm obtained from men with OA are any worse than those obtained by using fresh sperm. Separating the sperm retrieval procedure from the female treatment cycle makes things easier in terms of both decision-making and logistics.

'Offsite' procedures where the procedure is not performed in the fertility unit require robust standard operating policies to ensure that the recovered material is transported safely to the fertility unit, possibly in a transport incubator, which will maintain the temperature of the sperm. Such offsite sperm procurement techniques are still bound by HFEA regulations in the United Kingdom.

6 Procedures for Recovering Sperm from Men with Non-obstructive Azoospermia

Men with NOA represent some of the most challenging cases in terms of their ability to achieve biological paternity and it is important that all options for family formation are discussed including the use of donor gametes and adoption. Not all couples wish to proceed to SSR and ICSI and it is important that the couple are given time to reflect on their available choices. In terms of what procedures are used for recovering sperm in such cases, a literature review will show that a variety of techniques have been employed to recover sperm from men with this problem, including the testicular procedures described earlier. One important observation has been that the testes in men who have NOA can contain foci of normal spermatogenesis and this can be determined by parenchymal examination under magnification. Such foci may be located deep within the testes and may not be accessible by conventional open biopsy techniques. This concept led to the development of the MicroTESE procedure, which many centres now believe is the new gold standard for sperm recovery in such cases. MicroTESE is usually performed under general anaesthesia as a day-case procedure. The testes are delivered via a scrotal incision and the tunica albuginea incised to expose the testicular parenchyma. Most surgeons do this via an equatorial incision, as the sub-albugineal veins runs transversely across the testes and this approach allows them to be avoided. The parenchyma is then everted through the incision to expose the testicular lobules. Some experts advocate a longitudinal incision, with minimal eversion of the testicular parenchyma as an alternative approach. Through use of either approach, the lobules are then examined under an operating microscope with the aim of identifying individual seminiferous tubules that are relatively dilated and opalescent in appearance. These areas are then selected for sperm retrieval, as tubules are more likely to be sperm-bearing and this precise targeting means that small scattered areas of spermatogenesis can be located. Although numerous biopsies are often taken, the more precise method of selection means that the individual biopsies are very small and the total volume taken is less than with multi-site TESE. MicroTESE takes longer to perform but the post-operative recovery and other potential side effects are the same.

7 Patient Selection and Prognosis

Unfortunately, other than the identification of men with AZFa and b, there are no other reliable prognostic factors that would lead to exclusion of men with NOA, in terms of their suitability for sperm retrieval. Testis volume and FSH, two of the most widely used parameters have not been demonstrated to be of prognostic use in the majority of studies and there is a clear requirement for future scientific discovery to enable us to better pick men in whom SSR will be unsuccessful.

8 Conclusion

A range of techniques for the surgical retrieval of sperm are available. The underlying mechanism of azoospermia (or significant hypospermia) along with operator preference and scientific team experience will determine which technique is most suitable for a given situation. In general terms, a range of procedures can be successfully employed for cases of obstructive azoospermia, due to the high overall success rate, although there may be quantifiable differences between the methods in terms of the amount of sperm recovered. Non-obstructive azoospermia is however best addressed with the more advanced techniques such as MicroTESE, which have given hope to many couples seeking to achieve biological paternity.

References

1. Goldstein M, Shihua PL, and Matthews GJ. Microsurgical vasovasostomy: the microdot technique of precision suture placement. *J Urol* 1998; **159**: 188–90

2. Bendikson K, Neri Q, Takeuchi T et al. The outcome of intracytoplasmic sperm injection using occasional spermatozoa in the ejaculate of men with spermatogenic failure. *J Urol* 2008; **180**: 1060–64

3. Greco E, Scarselli F, Iacobelli M et al. Efficient treatment of infertility due to sperm DNA damage by ICSI with testicular spermatozoa. *Hum Reprod* 2004; **20**: 226–30

4. Palermo G, Joris H, Devroey P et al. Pregnancies after intracytoplasmic injection of single spermatozoon into an oocyte. *Lancet* 1992; **340**: 17–8

5. Schlegel PN. Testicular sperm extraction: microdissection

improves sperm yield with minimal tissue excision. *Hum Reprod* 1999; **14**: 131–5

6. Ramasamy R and Schlegel PN. Microdissection testicular sperm extraction: effect of prior biopsy on success of sperm retrieval. *J Urol* 2007; **177**: 1447–9

7. Tsujimura A, Matsumiya K, Miyagawa Y et al. Conventional multiple or microdissection testicular sperm extraction: a comparative study. *Hum Reprod* 2002; **17**: 2924–9

8. Jacobsen R, Bostofte E, Gerda Engholm G et al. Risk of testicular cancer in men with abnormal semen characteristics: cohort study. *BMJ* 2000; **321**: 789–92

9. Shiraishi K, Ishikawa T, Watanabe N et al. *Int J Urology* 2016; **23**: 496–500

10. Schroeder-Printzen I, Zumbé J, Bispink L et al. Microsurgical epididymal sperm aspiration: aspirate analysis and straws available after cryopreservation in patients with non-reconstructable obstructive azoospermia. *Hum Reprod* 2000; **15**: 2531–5

11. Beliveau M and Turek P. The value of testicular 'mapping' in men with non-obstructive azoospermia. *Asian J Andrology* 2011; **13**: 225–30

Preimplantation Genetic Testing

Joyce C. Harper
Sioban B. SenGupta

1 Introduction

In 2017, the World Health Organization published new nomenclature for preimplantation genetic diagnosis (PGD). They renamed the procedure preimplantation genetic testing (PGT), with PGT-M for monogenic diseases and PGT-SR for structural rearrangements. Preimplantation genetic screening (PGS) was renamed PGT-A (aneuploidy). In this chapter, PGT-M and PGT-SR will be referred to as PGT.

PGT is performed for couples who are at risk of transmitting a specific inherited disorder. The reproductive options for these couples are to remain childless, have no genetic testing on any pregnancy (reproductive chance), undergo prenatal or preimplantation genetic diagnosis, have gamete donation or adopt. The couples who opt for PGT have already been diagnosed with their disorder. They may have had an affected child, have a known family history or been diagnosed as an adult. There are a growing number of people who have had direct to consumer genetic testing or preconception genetic risk screening and have identified that they are at risk of transmitting a genetic disease to their children [1]. Most couples going through PGT are fertile, and may have been through prenatal diagnosis and termination of an affected pregnancy. PGT is not an easy option as the couple has to go through in vitro fertilization (IVF); it is expensive and the success rates are only comparable to routine IVF patients. The added problem is that there are cases where all of the embryos are affected as can be seen from the ESHRE PGD Consortium data where for all indications there are a number of cycles that reached PGT but do not have a transfer procedure [2].

PGT was first performed in 1989 in a series of couples who were at risk of transmitting a sex-linked disease to their children [3]. The biopsy was performed by removing one cell from cleavage stage embryos. A polymerase chain reaction (PCR) method was used which was able to detect a segment of the Y chromosome. Soon after this, other centres around the world successfully applied PGT for a variety of single gene and chromosomal disorders [4].

Biopsy has been performed to remove polar bodies or embryonic cells from cleavage or blastocyst stage embryos. The diagnosis has been performed using fluorescent in situ hybridization (FISH), PCR and more recently by array comparative genomic hybridization (a-CGH), next generation sequencing (NGS) and single nucleotide polymorphism arrays.

The technology in PGT has been applied as an adjunct to embryo selection methods used in IVF to select the chromosomally 'best' embryo for transfer; PGT-A [5]. PGT-A has been applied to patients of advanced maternal age, repeated implantation failure, repeated miscarriages, severe male factor infertility and more recently, good prognosis (Table 27.1).

2 Embryo Biopsy

For two decades, the prevalent method of embryo biopsy has been cleavage stage biopsy where usually one blastomere is biopsied from the cleavage stage embryo on day 3 of development [3]. The initial method used acid Tyrodes to drill a hole in the zona pellucida and aspiration to remove the blastomeres. To date, there is only one study examining the effects of biopsy but it is generally thought that the technique may have a negative effect on implantation and development.

For many years this method remained unchanged. It was only in the ESHRE PGD Consortium data collection for cycles performed in 2004 that the laser was used more often than acid Tyrodes. The other change was the introduction of $Ca^{2+}Mg^{2+}$ free biopsy media that reduced the junctions between blastomeres and made the biopsy easier [6].

Table 27.1 Differences between PGT-M/PGT-SR and PGT-A

	PGT-M and PGT-SR	PGT-A
Aims	Identify genetically normal embryos Achieve a genetically normal pregnancy/birth	Increase in IVF delivery rate
Indication	Monogenic disorder X-linked disease Known chromosome abnormality	Advanced maternal age Repeated implantation failure Repeated miscarriage Severe male factor Good prognosis
Fertility	Often fertile	Infertile or subfertile or recurrent pregnancy loss
Undiagnosed or inconclusive results	Never transfer these embryos	Can transfer these embryos
Prenatal Diagnosis	Indicated	Indicated for the same risk factors as natural conceptions

Adapted from [10]

The main issue with cleavage stage biopsy is that high levels of chromosomal mosaicism are seen at this stage [7]. Chromosomal mosaicism within the preimplantation embryo makes PGT highly problematic as the blastomere removed may not be representative of the rest of the embryo. This biological phenomenon has to be taken into account, especially in diagnosis examining chromosomes as it could lead to false positive and negative results.

Polar body biopsy was first reported by Verlinsky and colleagues where they originally biopsied only the first polar body (pre-conception diagnosis) [8]. It was soon realized that both the first and second polar body were required for an accurate diagnosis. The main limitation of polar body biopsy is that it only allows identification of the maternal genes and chromosomes. Therefore it cannot be applied if the male is carrying a chromosome abnormality or dominant single gene disorder. Polar body biopsy has been used in countries whose laws forbid 'embryo' biopsy, such as Germany and more recently Italy. The polar bodies can be removed simultaneously or sequentially; both procedures having advantages and disadvantages. Simultaneous removal requires fewer manipulations, but it may be difficult to distinguish between the first and second polar body (which might be necessary for some diagnoses) and the first polar body may degenerate. Sequential biopsy requires two biopsy stages but has the advantage of knowing which polar body is removed.

Blastocyst biopsy is now the most common method of embryo biopsy [2]. Following pioneering work from Muggleton Harris and others, it was

applied clinically ten years ago. Blastocyst biopsy can be performed in two ways. A hole can be drilled on day 3 and the embryos left in culture so that some of the trophectoderm cells herniate, which can be biopsied on day 5. The problem with this method is that inner cell mass may herniate instead of trophectoderm. In the second method, the hole is drilled on the morning of day 5, away from the inner cell mass to ensure that only trophectoderm cells herniate. The blastocyst can be returned to culture for a few hours to allow herniation and if required, trophectoderm can be gently aspirated. The cells are cut from the embryo using a laser. The blastocyst will collapse but usually rapidly reforms, sealing the hole in the trophectoderm where the cells have been removed.

One of the problems with blastocyst biopsy is that it gives a relatively short time for the diagnosis as transfer has to occur by day 6, giving just 24 hours for the diagnosis compared to 48–60 hours after cleavage biopsy. The introduction of vitrification as a method to cryopreserve blastocysts, and the reported high survival rates even after blastocyst biopsy has resulted in a shift to blastocyst biopsy and vitrification, allowing an unlimited amount of time for the diagnosis and batching of samples, consequently making the diagnosis cheaper.

Mosaicism is also seen at the blastocyst stage but at a much lower level [9]. Detection of mosaicism and its clinical significance is still being studied (see PGT-A section).

Blastocyst biopsy usually gives five cells that are analysed together which makes diagnosis easier and reduces the misdiagnosis rate. Since only approximately 50–60% of embryos reach the blastocyst stage, biopsy at this time results in fewer embryos to process which is more time and cost effective. This is especially relevant in comparison to polar body biopsy where at least 2–4 times the number of samples will have to be analysed.

Biopsy is an invasive procedure. In the case of blastocyst biopsy it removes some of the embryo or cells that will goonto make the placenta. Biopsy of the blastocoelic fluid and the use of spent culture media are being studied [10,11]. Whether there are two polar bodies, 1–2 blastomeres or 5 trophectoderm cells, the major advances in PGT over recent years have been the methods of diagnosis.

3 Diagnosis

3.1 Molecular Diagnosis

The polymerase chain reaction (PCR) is designed to enrich a DNA sample for one specific fragment, amplifying it to a level at which it can be visualized and subjected to further genetic analysis. It has become one of the most important methods in genetic testing and refinement of the PCR protocol for single cell analysis has proven highly successful. The sensitivity of PCR with fluorescently labelled primers is suitable for single cell analysis, allows multiple targets to be amplified simultaneously, and has reduced the problems of contamination and the time taken for the genetic analysis to be performed.

Allele dropout (ADO), the phenomenon where only one of the two alleles present in a cell is amplified to a detectable level, generally affects 5–20% of single cell amplifications (although in some instances the frequency is higher) and is a problem that is yet to be fully understood. This is an important consideration in the diagnosis of dominant disorders or recessive diseases where only one mutation can be detected. Multiple ADO events may appear to have occurred in cells that are monosomic for the chromosome being tested by PCR. Similarly contamination of DNA from cumulus cells, sperm or external sources will confound diagnosis.

A growing number of genes have been analysed by PCR–PGT and a variety of mutation detection strategies employed. Minisequencing [12] and real-time PCR assay with fluorescence resonance energy transfer (FRET) hybridization probes followed by melting curve analysis [13] are the most common methods used. The best protocols take into consideration the principal problems; amplification efficiency, contamination and allele dropout. It is now understood that an absence of amplification (PCR failure) should never be taken as an indication that an embryo is free of a mutation; amplification is unsuccessful in approximately 10% of isolated blastomeres regardless of their genotype.

In a multiplex PCR reaction, several loci can be investigated at once if the primers are labelled with different fluorescent tags and by designing primers to give PCR products of different size ranges. In all cases of molecular diagnosis, multiplex PCR of the mutation locus together with flanking linked polymorphic markers provides an additional means of determining the genotype of the embryo hence reducing the risk of misdiagnosis due to ADO.

Protocols based solely on the analysis of multiple microsatellite markers linked to and flanking the mutation site provide an indirect method for diagnosis by the identification of alleles in phase with the mutation. These protocols require the availability of DNA from at least two individuals in the family with the mutation so that the phase alleles can be identified by linkage analysis. Linkage based strategies without mutation detection are the most commonly used approach when reference samples for phase determination are available. In the case of *de novo* mutations, phase alleles can be identified using a combination of mutation detection and haplotyping of linked STR (short tandem repeat) markers by single sperm or polar body multiplex PCR [14].

There are a variety of methods aimed at non-specific amplification of the entire genome (whole genome amplification – WGA) [15]. Using these techniques a single genome can be amplified numerous times, thus providing sufficient DNA templates for many independent PCR amplifications including mutation detection and polymorphic markers that could test for ADO and contamination. WGA is required for a-CGH, SNP arrays and NGS. Methods include multiple displacement amplification (MDA) which is a non-PCR isothermal, strand-displacing amplification method. Other strategies involve fragmentation of DNA and ligation to linkers followed by PCR (PicoPLEX) or limited MDA followed by PCR for multiple annealing and looping-based amplification cycles (MALBAC).

PGT for mutations in the mitochondrial genome is complex due to random genetic drift during oogenesis resulting in heteroplasmy, where primary oocytes have a mixture of mitochondria with and without the inherited mutation. A bottleneck that operates at oogenesis determines the mutational load in primary oocytes. The size of the bottleneck appears to vary for different mitochondrial mutations and also between individuals. Determining a suitable threshold value for mutational load in embryos is difficult as the mutational load is also subject to random genetic drift in somatic tissue during development which will affect embryo survival and overall phenotype. PGT for mitochondrial mutations can be considered to be risk reducing rather than complete removal of the mutation, and couples need to be carefully counselled about the limitations of PGT for these disorders. PCR with restriction enzyme analysis has been used for the detection of specific mitochondrial mutations showing skewed meiotic segregation and the selection of embryos with a low mutational load. PGT for mutations in the mitochondrial genome requires extensive workup to allow semi-quantitative assessment of mutational load in single cells. Transplantation of nuclear DNA into enucleated donor oocytes or fertilized eggs may be clinically available in the future as a reproductive treatment option for females with mitochondrial mutations. The assessment of the mutational load by PGT is likely to still be needed to determine the extent of carry over of mitochondria during nuclear DNA transfer.

3.2 Examining Chromosomes

Fluorescent in situ hybridization (FISH) uses fluorescently tagged DNA probes that bind to their complementary sequence and can be visualized under a fluorescent microscope. The first chromosome analysis for PGT used FISH to identify the X and Y chromosomes. This method was rapidly applied to detect inherited chromosome abnormalities, such as translocations and non-inherited chromosome abnormalities for PGT-A.

The biopsied cells are spread, usually using HCl/Tween or methanol:acetic acid and FISH performed using appropriate probes. Early studies showed that the more probes used, the less efficient the procedure becomes. Today it is not advised to use FISH for PGT/PGT-A as more efficient techniques are available, such as a-CGH and NGS.

3.3 Array Comparative Genomic Hybridization

Comparative genomic hybridization is a technique that bridges the gap between molecular genetics and cytogenetics. In array-CGH, DNA from the test sample and DNA from a normal control DNA are amplified separately using WGA (Figure 27.1). The amplified DNA is differentially labelled with one of two fluorochromes, for example red for the test DNA

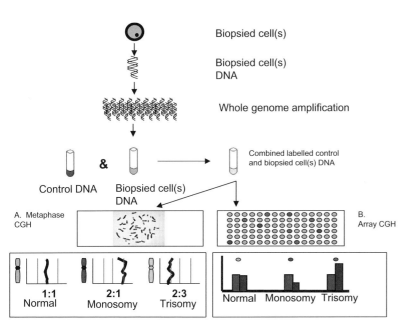

Fig. 27.1 Comparative genomic hybridization. First the biopsied material undergoes whole genome amplification and the embryonic DNA is labelled in green fluorescence. A control sample is labelled in red fluorescence. The samples are then co-hybridized onto an array platform and a computer analyses the ratio of red to green fluorescence. Adapted from [17].

and green for the control DNA. Following labelling, both DNAs are mixed together in equal proportions and are allowed to compete to hybridize onto an array platform containing clones of each chromosome (a-CGH) (Figure 27.1).

A number of studies were conducted to validate a-CGH. The method is robust and efficient compared to FISH and so, along with NGS, is the method of choice for PGT-SR and for PGT-A.

Since the analysis is fully automated, the whole procedure can be performed within 24 hours. For day-3 biopsy, it is possible to perform the embryo transfer on day 5 of embryo development in a fresh cycle [16]. However, for some groups, especially those performing blastocyst biopsy and/or transport PGT (where the diagnosis is done in a specialist PGT centre at a different location to the IVF unit), it is usually preferable to vitrify the biopsied embryos whilst the diagnosis and analysis is performed [17]. Also this is cost effective as the samples can be batched.

When arrays are applied to translocations, it is important that the smallest region of imbalance that may arise in embryos can be detected on the array. Therefore the number of clones present on the array in the region that is telomeric to each breakpoint should be checked to ensure that the region is sufficiently represented on the array to detect an imbalance. Couples need to be counselled so that they are aware that chromosomal aneuploidies other than those involved in the translocation will be detected on the array. This will be an ongoing issue for PGT as new technology detects more than just the abnormality being diagnosed.

There are some shortfalls of using a-CGH; it cannot detect polyploidies, such as triploidies as there is no imbalance in the total DNA content, it cannot detect balanced translocations or inversions as the total amount of DNA in the sample is the same as in the control sample and it cannot detect changes in DNA sequences (point mutations, intragenic insertions or deletions, triplet repeat expansion, etc.) or gains or losses in regions of the genome not covered by the array. a-CGH can pick up segmental abnormalities in preimplantation embryos but the clinical significance of this is not known.

3.4 Single Nucleotide Polymorphism Arrays

SNP arrays make use of the 10 million SNPs across the genome but a limitation has been the discovery of over 1,000 copy number variants (CNVs) with unknown clinical significance. SNP-based arrays offer other options for testing that are not available on a-CGH based systems. SNP-based arrays allow for simultaneous testing of specific genetic diseases by linkage analysis and the detection of aneuploidies of meiotic origin in each embryo. This will allow for the selective transfer of genetically and chromosomally euploid embryos for patients undergoing IVF with PGT-M. For SNP arrays the couple and appropriate relatives with the familial mutation(s), have to be tested to determine their haplotypes for linkage analysis. Karyomapping includes software to interpret the phasing of the SNP calls for linkage analysis [18].

The amount of information obtained is immense, and potentially it can also detect predispositions to common diseases, and late onset disorders if causative variants are included on the array. There are three problems when using SNP arrays; the relevance of some CNVs is unknown, parental DNA with familial reference samples need to be tested for linkage analysis and incidental large deletions leading to late onset disorders such as cancer predispositions may be identified in parents and their embryos.

3.5 Next Generation Sequencing

NGS has mainly been tested and applied in PGT-A for the detection of chromosomal imbalances in patients with translocations and has shown improved results compared to a-CGH [19]. Some groups have begun to use this technology in PGT-M with simultaneous aneuploidy screening. For NGS, WGA is required, and PCR-based whole genome amplification methods or MALBAC give better results compared to MDA on NGS platforms.

For PGT-A, only 0.1–2 x depth of read is required whereas monogenic disorders also require target enrichment of the WGA product by PCR. Diagnosis can be achieved by detection of the mutated allele together with the haplotype of linked SNPs. Alleles in phase with the mutation at the linked SNPs can be determined by haplotype analysis of family members with known genetic status similar to the analysis used for SNP arrays. Refinement in the analysis of genome wide data from WGA products is ongoing as exclusion of WGA artefacts improves the accuracy of diagnosis.

4 Preimplantation Genetic Screening

In 1995, two teams in the United States used PGT technology to detect chromosome abnormalities in polar bodies for patients going through IVF as an additional means of embryo selection, and this was applied to embryos by Munne et al. The technique was performed in patients with advanced maternal age, repeated implantation failure and repeated miscarriage with normal karyotypes in the parents. The technique was called a number of things, including preimplantation genetic diagnosis for aneuploidy screening (PGD-AS), PGS and now PGT-A.

Currently PGT-A is totally different to PGT-M and PGT-SR and its use more controversial. The patients are infertile or subfertile and the main aim is to aid current selection methods used in IVF [1]. In this situation, PGT-A has to be shown to improve delivery rates compared to other IVF selection methods. The only way this can reliably be achieved is through randomized controlled trials (RCT) [5].

This history of PGT-A can be separated into two versions. Up to 2010 we had version 1 which involved examination of just a few chromosomes by FISH. In 2004, the first RCT on PGT-A was reported and was followed by a study by Mastenbroek et al. Both studies were heavily criticized and were followed by eight more RCTs at the cleavage stage and one at the blastocyst stage all using FISH to examine a varying number of chromosomes, but none showed an increase in delivery rates (some showed a significant decrease in delivery rates).

The majority of PGT-A centres no longer perform PGT-A using FISH as it is felt that the method is not suitable for the accurate diagnosis of 1–2 cells. Additionally, after the ten RCTs using cleavage stage biopsy, it was felt that biopsy at this time may not be the most appropriate because the embryo is highly chromosomally mosaic. Therefore diagnosis at cleavage stage is based on the analysis of one cell that may not be representative of the rest of the embryo. In 2010, the ESHRE PGD Consortium wrote a position statement which stated that 'until results of RCTs using a different biopsy stage and arrays can demonstrate a significant increase in delivery rates, there is no evidence that routine PGT-A is beneficial for patients with advanced maternal age'.

In PGT-A version 2 centres stopped using FISH and tried a number of different methods, mainly a-CGH and NGS but also quantitative PCR to look at all of the chromosomes. In PGT-A v2, as well as applying the technique to poor prognosis patients, such as patients of advanced maternal age and repeated IVF failure, good prognosis patients were included. Most

PGT centres moved away from cleavage stage biopsy to avoid post zygotic mosaicism and concentrated on polar body and blastocyst biopsy.

ESHRE has embarked on a multi-centre RCT for patients with advanced maternal age using polar body biopsy and a-CGH. Polar body biopsy using a-CGH is an expensive technique as both polar bodies need to be analysed. But the technique will not be confused by post zygotic mosaicism which may be an advantage or disadvantage.

The only RCTs currently published for PGT-A version 2 are three pilot RCTs which used trophectoderm biopsy on good prognosis patients and one study on cleavage stage biopsy for advanced maternal age, but their limited sample size makes it impossible to draw conclusions. Lee et al. concluded that 'high-quality experimental studies using intention-to-treat analysis and cumulative live birth rates including the comparative outcomes from remaining cryopreserved embryos are needed to evaluate the overall role of PGT-A in the clinical setting'. Larger, well-designed RCTs using a-CGH on trophectoderm cells are about to be published.

A recent study reported that embryos that had low levels of chromosomal mosaicism after blastocyst biopsy for PGT-A went on to a successful delivery [20]. Other groups who are undertaking PGT for specific chromosome abnormalities are blinding the data for the other chromosomes and decoding the full chromosome complement at birth. Deliveries have been successful with embryos that would not have been transferred if the chromosome makeup was known before transfer (Khalaf, personal communication).

If poor prognosis patients are undergoing PGT-A, such as those of advanced maternal age who by definition produce few embryos, a trend in many IVF units is to bank embryos by vitrifying all the embryos from several cycles of IVF before warming all the embryos and performing the biopsy and diagnosis. In some US centres it is routine for patients to go through four egg collections before PGT-A is applied. From this cohort, there is an increased chance that a 'normal' embryo will be found, leading to increased pregnancy rates per embryo transfer procedure but very low pregnancy rates per egg collection.

But the world of IVF loves new technology, even unproven technology [5]. PGT-A accounts for more than all the other indications for PGT added together, according to the US data and the ESHRE PGD Consortium Data [2]. Kushnir et al. reanalysed the

SART data and concluded that PGT-A decreased the chances of live birth and that the improvements reported were likely to be as a consequence of patient selection. There are already IVF clinics in the United States that apply PGT-A to every embryo of every patient. It is highly probable that at some point in the near future, all IVF embryos will undergo genetic testing using NGS to determine which embryos are the 'best' from the cohort produced. Whatever the outcome of the PGT-A RCTs, patients may decide that it is beneficial to know the genetic make up of their embryos [114] and PGT-A will merge as the same technique will determine aneuploidy and genetic abnormalities.

5 Conclusion

PGT has been offered for 30 years. Blastocyst biopsy has increased in popularity and since vitrification shows excellent survival rates it is now possible to freeze all the embryos post biopsy giving more time to perform the diagnosis. For the diagnosis, FISH has been replaced by array-CGH, SNP arrays and NGS. These improvements have resulted in an increase in the number of diseases that can be diagnosed by PGT but also more controversial uses of this technology. PGT-A cycles have increased over the years and account for more cycles than all other indications added together.

The number of PGT cycles for monogenic disorders have been slowly increasing in number and it is predicted that this increase will continue [2].

It is key that diagnostic labs have appropriate training programmes for PGT clinical scientists and that PGT laboratories are accredited to ISO 15189 or equivalent. Embryologists need to perform the embryology and clinical scientists need to perform the genetic analysis. PGT centres should participate in external assessment schemes and are accredited to ensure that they meet international standards.

Whole genome scanning technology will bring challenges and opportunities, including ethical implications. Array CGH, SNP arrays and NGS sexes embryos which brings into discussion the issues surrounding social sex selection which is illegal in the EU. PGT for HLA matching and late onset disorders has resulted in much ethical debate.

The discussions will be ongoing as it is possible to diagnose non-disease causing traits. But current methods of PGT still require patients to go through expensive and time-consuming IVF procedures, with a relatively low success rate. For the majority of patients, this technique will only be used for serious conditions. For PGT-A, data from the RCTs using comprehensive chromosome analysis will be welcome to determine if this procedure has any benefit for infertile patients.

References

1. Harper JC, Aittomäki K, Borry P, Cornel MC, De Wert G, Dondorp W, Geraedts J, Gianaroli L, Ketterson K, Liebaers I, Lundin K, Mertes H, Morris M, Pennings G, Sermon K, Spits C, Soini S, Van Montfoort APA, Veiga A, Vermeesch JR, Viville S, Macek Jr. M. (2017) Recent developments in genetics and medically-assisted reproduction: from research to clinical application. *Human Reproduction Open* (in press)

2. De Rycke M, Belva F, Goossens V, Moutou C, SenGupta SB, Traeger-Synodinos J, Coonen E. (2015) ESHRE PGD Consortium data collection XIII: cycles from January to December 2010 with pregnancy follow-up to October 2011. *Hum Reprod.* Aug;

30(8):1763–89. doi: 10.1093/humrep/dev122. Epub 2015 Jun 12. PubMed PMID:26071418.

3. Handyside AH, Kontogianni EH, Hardy K, Winston RM. (1990) Pregnancies from biopsied human preimplantation embryos sexed by Y-specific DNA amplification. *Nature.* 19;344(6268):768–70. PubMed PMID: 2330030.

4. Harper JC, Handyside AH. (1994) The current status of preimplantation diagnosis. *Current Obs and Gynae.* 4:143–9.

5. Harper J, Jackson E, Sermon K, Aitken RJ, Harbottle S, Mocanu E, Hardarson T, Mathur R, Viville S, Vail A, Lundin K. (2017) Adjuncts in the IVF laboratory: where is the evidence for 'add-on' interventions? *Hum Reprod.*

2(3):485–91. doi: 10.1093/humrep/dex004.

6. Dumoulin JC, Bras M, Coonen E, Dreesen J, Geraedts JP, Evers JL. (1998) Effect of Ca^{2+}/Mg^{2+}-free medium on the biopsy procedure for preimplantation genetic diagnosis and further development of human embryos. *Hum Reprod.* 13(10):2880–3.

7. Harper JC, Coonen E, Handyside AH, Winston RML, Hopman AHN, Delhanty JDA. (1995) Mosaicism of autosomes and sex chromosomes in morphologically normal, monospermic, preimplantation human embryos. *Prenat Diagn.* 15:41–9.

8. Verlinsky Y, Rechitsky S, Evsikov S, White M, Cieslak J, Lifchez A, Valle J, Moise J, Strom CM. (1992) Preconception and

preimplantation diagnosis for cystic fibrosis. *Prenat Diagn.* 12(2):103–10. PubMed PMID: 1553355.

9. Fragouli E, Wells D. (2011) Aneuploidy in the human blastocyst. *Cytogenet Genome Res.* 133: 149–59.

10. Magli MC, Pomante A., Cafueri G, Valerio M, Crippa, A, Ferraretti AP, Gianaroli L. (2016) Preimplantation genetic testing: polar bodies, blastomeres, trophectoderm cells, or blastocoelic fluid? *Fertil Steril* Mar;105(3):676–83.e5. doi: 10.1016/j.fertnstert.2015.11.018. Epub 2015 Dec 1.

11. Feichtinger M, Vaccari E, Carli L, Wallner E, Mädel U, Figl K, Palini S, Feichtinger W. (2017) Non-invasive preimplantation genetic screening using array comparative genomic hybridization on spent culture media: a proof-of-concept pilot study. *Reprod Biomed Online.* Jun;34(6):583–9. doi: 10.1016/j.rbmo.2017.03.015. Epub 2017 Mar 28.

12. Fiorentino F, Biricik A, Nuccitelli A, De Palma R, Kahraman S, Iacobelli M, Trengia V, Caserta D, Bonu MA, Borini A, Baldi M. (2006) Strategies and clinical

outcome of 250 cycles of Preimplantation Genetic Diagnosis for single gene disorders. *Hum Reprod.* 21(3): 670–84. Epub 2005 Nov 25. PubMed PMID: 16311287.

13. Vrettou C, Traeger-Synodinos J, Tzetis M, Palmer G, Sofocleous C, Kanavakis E. (2004) Real-time PCR for single-cell genotyping in sickle cell and thalassemia syndromes as a rapid, accurate, reliable, and widely applicable protocol for preimplantation genetic diagnosis. *Hum Mutat.* 23(5):513–21.

14. Rechitsky S, Pomerantseva E, Pakhalchuk T, Pauling D, Verlinsky O, Kuliev A. (2011) First systematic experience of preimplantation genetic diagnosis for de novo mutations. *Reprod Biomed Online.* 22(4):350–61. Epub 2011 Jan 20.

15. Hughes S, Arneson N, Done S, Squire J. (2005) The use of whole genome amplification in the study of human disease. *Prog Biophys Mol Biol.* 88(1):173–89. Review.

16. Hellani A, Coskun S, Tbakhi A, Al-Hassan S. (2005) Clinical application of multiple displacement amplification in preimplantation genetic diagnosis.

Reprod Biomed Online. 10(3):376–80.

17. Harper JC, Harton G. (2010) The use of arrays in preimplantation genetic diagnosis and screening. *Fertil Steril.* 94(4):1173–7. Epub 2010 Jun 25. Review

18. Handyside AH, Harton GL, Mariani B, Thornhill AR, Affara N, Shaw MA, Griffin DK. (2010) Karyomapping: a universal method for genome wide analysis of genetic disease based on mapping crossovers between parental haplotypes. *J Med Genet.* 47(10):651–8. Epub 2009 Oct 25.

19. Yang, Z, Lin, J, Zhang, J, Fong, WI, Zhao R, Liu X, Podevin W, Kuang, Y, Liu J. (2015) Randomized comparison of next-generation sequencing and array comparative genomic hybridization for preimplantation genetic screening: a pilot study. *BMC Med Genomics* Jun 23;8:30. doi: 10.1186/s12920-015-0110-4.

20. Greco E, Minasi MG, and Fiorentino F. (2015) Healthy babies after intrauterine transfer of mosaic aneuploid blastocysts. *N Engl J Med.* Nov 19;373(21): 2089–90. doi: 10.1056/ NEJMc1500421.

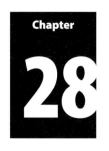

Chapter 28

Adjuvant Treatment and Alternative Therapies to Improve Fertility

Narmada Katakam
Luciano Nardo
Gavin Sacks

1 Adjuvant Treatment for the Uterus

With initial attempts of failed IVF, and also after miscarriages, it is quite common for women to assume and become convinced that there is a problem in the uterus or their body leading to the "rejection" of the embryos. This may be true for some women, but it is difficult to detect and predict which women this applies to. In fact, chromosomal errors in the embryos are probably the main underlying reason behind all reproductive failures, but uterine factors may have a role [1]. A recent analysis of more than 15,000 high grade blastocysts showed 30–90% were aneuploid, increasing significantly with a woman's age [2]. Sometimes preimplantation genetic screening (PGS) is useful either prior to or in conjunction with adjuvant treatment to assess the necessity and limit the number of embryo transfer cycles and repeated use of adjuvant treatments.

While the respective contributions of embryo and endometrium towards reproductive success should be individualised as much as possible, an estimate may be that about 20% of implantation problems are due to the uterus. Women should also be strongly counselled about the known embryo genetic contribution, and it is often helpful to turn around their perception, to illustrate that it is possible that they are highly receptive and not enough selective to embryo implantation, and it is simply that they are unable to detect which embryos to 'reject' [1].

2 Endometrial Receptivity Testing: Protein Expression

Endometrial receptor testing is still in experimental stage; this is done at a molecular level analysing the

expression of a group of genes related to endometrial receptivity. The testing is done by an endometrial biopsy in the luteal phase of the menstrual cycle and the endometrium is classified as receptive or non-receptive by a computational predictor, which suggests the window of implantation. Rescue of non-receptive endometrium by tailored embryo transfers in a displaced window of implantation resulted in higher pregnancy rate (51.7%) and implantation rate (33.9%) compared to the controls [3].

3 Endometrial Receptivity Testing: Immune Testing

Immune testing has a long and chequered history. With the exception of antiphospholipid antibodies and thyroid antibodies, few tests are widely available in routine clinical practice. The most well-known immune test is for natural killer (NK) cells. The purpose of NK testing is to attempt to be more discerning with immune therapy, so as to only target those who are possibly more likely to benefit from it.

Uterine NK (uNK) cells are rather specialised immune cells in the uterine mucosa participating in implantation, and are likely to play a significant role in ensuring its success [4]. Testing for uNK cells has, so far, primarily been done by immunohistochemistry, which is unable to detect subtypes or function. The enormous increase in numbers during the menstrual cycle (from 5% to more than 40% of all stromal cells) also makes reliable testing extremely difficult [5]. These technical issues explain why studies have been contradictory and, outside of research centres, this kind of testing should, in our opinion, be used with caution.

Peripheral blood NK (pbNK) cells testing has sometimes been dismissed as irrelevant in view of the functional differences of the majority of pbNK cells compared with uNK cells [4]. However, not only is there some evidence of correlation between pbNK

Declaration of interest: The authors report no declarations of interest. The authors alone are responsible for the content and writing of the paper.

and uNK numbers [5] but also pbNK testing can be an independent marker of systemic immune dysfunction. As with uNK testing, technical issues are critical and often underappreciated. However, there is evidence showing higher levels of activated pbNK cells in women with recurrent miscarriage and repeated IVF failure, and hence activated cells may be predictive of IVF success [5].

4 Immune Therapy

There is no evidence that immune therapy is beneficial when applied to all IVF cycles or all women with recurrent miscarriage. But, there is increasing evidence of benefit when given to women selected on basis of both their history and known immune dysfunction [6].

4.1 Corticosteroids

Reproductive failure and lower IVF success rates were noted in women with immune dysfunction. Immune-suppressive activity of corticosteroids was, therefore, expected to improve pregnancy outcome by reducing endometrial pro-inflammatory cytokines production and uNK cell activity [7]. The authors found that corticosteroids did not improve the clinical pregnancy rate in the study population, but subgroup analysis revealed a significantly higher pregnancy rate in the IVF, rather than ICSI group.

In a systematic review [6], there was a higher clinical pregnancy rate noted in the prednisolone group. However, data heterogeneity was substantial, thus suggesting a cautious interpretation of the results.

From various studies, significantly higher pregnancy and implantation rates were noted in women undergoing IVF, with high anticardiolipin antibody (ACA) when treated with methylprednisolone and low-dose aspirin. In presence of antithyroid antibodies (ATA) higher implantation and clinical pregnancy rates were seen in women treated with corticosteroids, aspirin and levothyroxine. In women with high uNK cells and unexplained recurrent miscarriage, live birth rates were higher in the prednisolone-treated group [8].

A number of investigators looking in to the use of steroids alone or in conjunction with other adjuvant treatments in women with positive antinuclear antibody (ANA) undergoing IVF have reported contradictory outcomes. The Cochrane review by Boomsma and colleagues (2012) [9] showed no evidence of improved clinical outcome with pre-implantation administration of glucocorticoids.

This clearly explains that steroids, in isolation or combination, are beneficial when used in targeted groups with immune dysfunction, high ACA, ATA or high uNK cells. Steroids are obviously cheap, easy to administer, widely available and have a fairly extensive history of use. The only known potential caution is the weak association with cleft palate; a threefold increase in oral clefts among offspring of women who received oral corticosteroids during pregnancy, which should be explained to the couple [10].

4.2 Intravenous Immunoglobulin (IVIg)

IVIg is a pooled blood product from numerous donors. Complications or side effects are seen in up to 35% of cases and are often related to the rate of infusion, total dose and brand of IVIg infused. Mild and transient side effects include flushing, headache, itching, low backache, nausea and fatigue. Serious and rare side effects include aseptic meningitis, severe anaphylactic reaction, acute renal failure and thrombotic events. We have previously argued that women should be provided with clear information of these side effects before embarking on the treatment [8].

Polanski et al. (2014) [6] reviewed 217 studies with high pbNK cells and identified only 3 eligible studies for analysis. The findings suggested that immune therapy for women with high pbNK cells is beneficial. Other authors found that, in women with high uNK cells and unexplained recurrent miscarriage, live birth rates were higher when IVIg was used [11]. A systematic review [12] showed significantly lower miscarriage rate, higher implantation rate, clinical pregnancy rate and live birth rate after IVIg treatment. However, the review noted numerous methodological flaws in the studies included, such as poor design, lack of randomisation, heterogeneous population, use of multiple adjuvant interventions, different doses and regimes of IVIg and lack of cost effective analysis.

4.3 Intralipid Infusion

Intralipid infusion therapy has been used for decades to correct fatty acid and calorie deficiency among those who are unable to feed orally. The intralipid infusion is an emulsion of soya bean oil, egg yolk, phospholipids, glycerin and water.

Intralipids function as immune-modulators by inhibiting pro-inflammatory factors such as TH1 cytokines [13]. It was shown that intralipid infusion could effectively suppress NK cells activity in patients with abnormal NK cytolytic activity. It is postulated that the fatty acids within the emulsion serve as ligands to activate peroxisome proliferator-activated receptors expressed by the NK cells, which would reduce NK cytotoxic activity resulting in enhanced implantation and maintenance of pregnancy [14].

A non-randomised trial showed a 46% clinical pregnancy rate with the use of 20% intralipid fat emulsion in women with recurrent implantation failure and elevated TH1 cytokine response on NK cell assay. It was noted that TH1:TH2 activity ratio decreased following treatment and this alteration in cytokine activity was deemed to be responsible for the outcome [15].

The first randomised controlled trial (RCT) with intralipid was recently presented at the ASRM Annual Meeting in Baltimore [16]. Women with repeated IVF failure and abnormal immune testing were randomised to receive intralipid or nothing. With over 100 in each group, the intralipid infusion group had significantly higher live birth rates (32%) than those who did not (12%). Given the relatively low cost and maternal-fetal safety, this type of immune therapy is likely to become more prevalent. However, caution is still necessary, not least because of the potential infection at the cannula site which has led recently to reported death [17].

4.4 Anti-tumour Necrosis Factor-Alpha

TNF-α antagonists suppress inflammatory response to tumor necrosis factor (TNF) and have been used in various autoimmune and immune-mediated conditions such as rheumatoid arthritis, ankylosing spondylitis, inflammatory bowel disease and psoriasis. Prolonged use of TNF inhibitors is associated with serious side effects such as lymphoma, demyelinating disease, congestive heart failure, induction of auto-antibodies and lupus-like syndrome [18]. Direct correlation between circulating TNF-α levels and IVF outcome has yet not been fully established [8], but its use has so far been directed at women with abnormal T cell activation.

An exaggerated TH1 response is harmful to the process of embryo implantation resulting in infertility. Anti-TNF-α agents, such as Entanercept (Enbrel),

Adalimumab (Humira) and Infliximab (Remicaid) were studied in infertile patients with raised TH1:TH2 cytokines ratio undergoing IVF, and a higher live birth rate was noted [19]. This treatment is however expensive and not used widely outside specialised centres.

5 Hormone Therapy: Metformin

Metformin is an insulin-sensitising agent. In women with polycystic ovary syndrome (PCOS), metformin appears to act as a brake on the response of polycystic ovaries to exogenous gonadotrophin stimulation minimising the risk of ovarian hyperstimulation syndrome (OHSS). Side effects, mainly gastrointestinal symptoms, occur in approximately 10% of patients on metformin. There is no evidence of teratogenicity.

An RCT comparing metformin with placebo in women with PCOS undergoing IVF treatment [20] demonstrated a significant increase in the clinical pregnancy rate beyond 12 weeks and a clinically significant reduction in the occurrence of severe OHSS. The Cochrane review [21] showed similar findings in terms of prevention of OHSS. A recent meta-analysis of metformin administration in women with PCOS undergoing ovulation induction with gonadotrophins found increased pregnancy and live birth rates in the treatment group [22]. Interestingly, Brewer and colleagues (2010) [23] concluded that women who took metformin in the fresh cycle of IVF treatment had a significantly higher live birth rate in the subsequent frozen embryo transfer cycle.

6 Improving Uterine Blood Flow

6.1 Aspirin

Aspirin (Acetylsalicyclic acid) is a non-steroidal anti-inflammatory agent (NSAID). Daily administration of low-dose aspirin results in vasodilation and increase in the peripheral blood flow by inducing a shift from thromboxane A2 to prostacyclin [24]. Aspirin was also shown to increase uterine blood flow [25], which in turn enhances the endometrial receptivity resulting in higher embryo implantation rates. However, these findings were not shown to translate into clinical use.

Aspirin was shown to be beneficial in women with recurrent miscarriage and antiphospholipid antibody syndrome (APS) as well as in prevention of early onset pre-eclampsia (CLASP Study). The Cochrane review [26] confirmed that administration of aspirin in IVF does not improve pregnancy rates. There was no significant difference noted between aspirin and control group for the live birth rate, clinical pregnancy rate or miscarriage rate.

6.2 Heparin

Heparin is an anticoagulant. It improves implantation by regulating the endometrial receptivity and decidualisation of endometrial stromal cells by several means.

In women with thrombophilia, impaired trophoblastic invasion of maternal vessels by the syncytiotrophoblast is noted due to micro-thrombi at the site of implantation [27]. In this group of women, heparin could improve implantation, however, published studies showed contradictory findings. Significant differences in pregnancy rates were noted in women with thrombophilia receiving heparin treatment with or without low-dose aspirin and no improvement in pregnancy rates when unfractionated heparin and low-dose aspirin were used [8]. A Cochrane systematic review [28] showed a 77% increase in live birth rate, 73% in implantation rate and a 78% reduction in miscarriage rate. The same review also found a 79% increase in live birth rate in women with history of three recurrent implantation failures (RIF). Interestingly, a similar improvement was not seen when studies included only unexplained RIF.

6.3 Vasodilators

Endometrial development plays a pivotal role in successful embryo implantation. Increased endometrial blood flow and thickness are likely to improve implantation and IVF success rates. Several agents have been tried to improve sub-endometrial blood flow and increase endometrial performance during IVF treatment.

6.3.1 Vasodilators: Nitric oxide (NO) and Nitroglycerine (NTG)

Nitric oxide is a vasodilator and regulates the smooth muscle of blood vessels. NO plays a significant role in decidualisation and implantation. NO production inhibitor in the post-ovulatory phase has been associated with pregnancy failure. Nitroglycerine (NTG) is an NO donor, and has been investigated to assess the efficacy in inducing uterine vasodilation and thereby endometrial receptivity. It was recently summarised that there was no significant difference in the implantation and pregnancy rates or the uterine artery Doppler between the placebo and the NTG groups [8].

Vasodilators: Sildenafil Citrate

Sildenafil citrate (Viagra) potentiates the effect of NO on vascular smooth muscle. Sildenafil improved radial artery resistance index, reduced uterine artery pulsatility index (PI) and endometrial thickness, and enhanced pregnancy rates in some studies, but similar findings in women undergoing either fresh IVF cycles or frozen embryo transfers were not noted [8].

7 Uterine Relaxants

The uterine smooth muscle contractility varies throughout the course of the normal menstrual cycle. The uterine activity in the IVF cycles is higher compared with the natural cycle conception, a phenomenon which is attributed to various factors including mechanical stimulation with the speculum, embryo transfer catheter stimulating the uterine wall, transfer in the early luteal phase and supraphysiological hormonal milieu. Increased contractility can result in an ectopic pregnancy. Various uterine smooth muscle relaxants are studied in an attempt to optimise IVF success rates and improve success [8].

7.1 Nitroglycerine (NTG)

NTG is an NO donor. It acts as a vasodilator and relaxes the smooth muscle of the uterus. However, use of NTG three minutes before embryo transfer did not show any significant difference in the ease of transfer or the pregnancy rates [29].

7.2 β2-Adrenergic Antagonists

Selective β2-adrenergic blockers (Ritodrine, Terbutaline and Salbutamol) are known uterine smooth muscle relaxants used in obstetrics for management of pre-term labour and before external cephalic version. Administration of these agents regularly for two weeks in the luteal phase, following oocyte retrieval did not show any improvement in the implantation and pregnancy rates [30], whilst resulting in adverse side effects such as hypotension and tachycardia.

8 Egg Quality

8.1 Dehydroepiandrostenedione (DHEA)

DHEA is an androgen produced primarily in the adrenal glands, gonads and brain. It is a precursor of androstenedione, testosterone and oestradiol. It has been suggested that the DHEA improves ovarian response by various methods: (a) via the androgen receptors in the ovary; (b) increasing the IGF-1 concentration and (c) regulating the LH-stimulated androgen and oestrogen production in the follicle [31].

There are few studies which report benefits of DHEA in this context. Initial observational studies showed improved ovarian response, increased number of oocytes retrieved and higher clinical pregnancy rates. However, an RCT [32] reviewing addition of DHEA to IVF protocols failed to reveal any significant difference between the treatment and the non-treatment groups in the number of live birth rates.

Potential side effects of long-term androgen supplementation in women seeking fertility have not been widely addressed. DHEA is unlicensed for prescription in Europe, and it is categorised as a food product in the United States. According to IVF Worldwide Survey, 2010, [33] there has been widespread use of various online preparations of DHEA targeted at the female fertility market. It is relatively cheap and widely available, and now commonly used as adjuvant therapy for poor responders in IVF, although evidence for benefit is poor.

8.2 Growth Hormone (GH)

Growth hormone plays a crucial role in growth and metabolism. It is essential to attain puberty and continues to play a role in ovarian function to include follicular development, oestrogen synthesis and oocyte maturation [33].

There was an unusual resurgence of interest on the use of growth hormone in assisted conception at the end of the first decade of the millennium. In a critical analysis by Homburg and colleagues, relevant studies in the last 25 years were reviewed and noted that GH was used in varied groups of patients including poor ovarian responders, PCOS and hypogonadotrophic-hypogonadism. GH appeared to be beneficial in relatively GH-deficient patients, for example hypogonadotrophic-hypogonadism. There was no convincing evidence in other therapeutic areas [34].

The Cochrane review [35] showed no significant difference in the number of live births when comparing GH-treated women with non-treated. However, there was considerable heterogeneity in the definitions, protocols and outcomes, and the number of subjects included in the studies was very small. In a recent RCT, when GH was added to the gonadotrophin-releasing hormone (GnRH) antagonist

protocol in poor responders, there was no difference in both clinical pregnancy rate and live birth rate [36].

There is not enough evidence to prove that supplementing GH in IVF cycles routinely is of benefit. There is positive effect noted in its use in poor responders, but given the size of the studies, the evidence is poor. Properly designed RCTs are needed if the findings are to be confirmed.

9 Antioxidants

In healthy individuals, reactive oxygen species (ROS) and antioxidants maintain a balance. Oxidative stress leading to rapid cellular damage occurs when this balance is disrupted. High levels of ROS and sperm DNA damage are detected in the semen of up to 25% of subfertile men as well as in cases of RM and IVF failure [37].

In women, the damage affects oocyte maturation, ovulation, embryo cleavage, blastocyst formation and implantation [38] Empirical oral antioxidants (combination of multivitamins and chelated amino acids) have not shown to improve oocyte quality and pregnancy rates [39]. However, they appeared to improve sperm parameters and oxidative stress.

10 Conclusion and Summary of Recommendations

Since pregnancy and childbirth form an anticipated trajectory of normal pathway of life, fertility problems and pregnancy loss can sometimes have a devastating effect and cause significant impact on the couple and wider family.

Even though most adjuvants have no evidence base, couples with poor prognosis are desperate, disheartened and are willing to try any additional option which might increase their chances ever so slightly. The selection of adjuvants should be carefully considered and clear explanation given to these vulnerable couples regarding efficacy and safety profile of these adjuvants to make an informed choice.

Absence of evidence at this moment of time does not mean evidence of absence of benefits of adjuvants in IVF. Empirical prescriptions of adjuvants could one day become a thing of the past; but for those recommending an adjuvant empirically now, caution is advised.

Here is the summary of available evidence. Undoubtedly, there is a need for large well-designed studies before recommending most of these adjuvants for routine use.

1. Corticosteroids: Steroids, in isolation or combination, are beneficial when used in targeted groups such as immune dysfunction, high ACA, ATA, high uNK cells. In presence of high NK cells activity and steroid use, a significantly higher pregnancy rate was noted in the IVF, rather than ICSI group.

2. IVIg treatment: Is beneficial for women with high pbNK cells, high uNK cells and unexplained recurrent miscarriage. There is significantly lower miscarriage rate, higher implantation rate, clinical pregnancy rate and live birth rate after IVIg treatment.

3. Intralipid infusion: Significantly higher live birth rates were noted when used in those with RIF and elevated TH1 cytokine response/ abnormal immune testing.

4. Anti-TNF-α agents: Higher live birth rate was noted in infertile patients with raised TH1:TH2 cytokines ratio. However, treatment is expensive and should be restricted to specialised centres.

5. Metformin: Administration in women with PCOS undergoing ovulation induction with gonadotrophins found increased pregnancy and live birth rates and a significantly higher live birth rate in the subsequent frozen embryo transfer cycle.

6. Aspirin: Beneficial in women with recurrent miscarriage and antiphospholipid antibody syndrome (APS).

7. Heparin: Significant difference in pregnancy rates were noted in women with thrombophilia, 78% reduction in miscarriage rate, 73% increase in implantation rate and 77% increase in live birth rate.

8. Vasodilators (Nitric oxide, Nitroglycerine and Sildenafil): No significant difference in the implantation and pregnancy rates was noted.

9. Uterine relaxants (Nitroglycerine and β2-Adrenergic antagonists): No significant difference in the implantation and pregnancy rates was noted.

10. Dehydroepiandrostenedione (DHEA): No significant difference noted in live birth rates.

11. Growth Hormone (GH): No significant difference noted in clinical pregnancy rate and live birth rates.

12. Antioxidants: Not shown to improve oocyte quality and pregnancy rates but appeared to improve sperm parameters and oxidative stress.

References

1. Teklenburg G, Salker M, Heijnen C, Macklon NS, Brosens JJ. The molecular basis of recurrent pregnancy loss: impaired natural embryo selection. *Mol Hum Reprod.* 2010;**16**(12):886–95.

2. Franasiak JM, Forman EJ, Hong KH, Werner MD, Upham KM, Treff NR, Scott RT Jr. The nature of aneuploidy with increasing age of the female partner: a review of 15,169 consecutive trophectoderm biopsies evaluated with comprehensive chromosomal screening. *Fertil Steril.* 2014 Mar;**101**(3):656–63.e1. doi: 10.1016/j.fertnstert.2013.11.004. Epub 2013 Dec 17. Review.

3. Ruiz-Alonso M, Blesa D, Díaz-Gimeno P, Gómez E, Fernandez-Sanchez M, Carranza F, Carrera J, Vilella F, Pellicer A, Simon C. The endometrial receptivity array for diagnosis and personalized embryo transfer as a treatment for patients with repeated implantation failure. *Fertil Steril.* 2013 Sep;**100**(3): 818–24.

4. Moffett A, Shreeve N. First do no harm: uterine natural killer (NK) cells in assisted reproduction. *Hum Reprod.* 2015;**30**(7): 1519–25.

5. Sacks G. Enough! Stop the arguments and get on with the science of natural killer cell testing. *Hum Reprod.* 2015; **30**(7):1526–31.

6. Polanski LT, Barbosa MA, Martins WP, Baumgarten MN, Campbell B, Brosens J, Quenby S, Raine-Fenning N. Interventions to improve reproductive outcomes in women with elevated natural killer cells undergoing assisted reproduction techniques: a systematic review of literature. *Hum Reprod.* 2014;**29**:65–75.

7. Boomsma CM, Macklon NS. Does glucocorticoid therapy in the peri-implantation period have an impact on IVF outcomes? *Curr Opin Obstet Gynecol.* 2008; **20**:249–56.

8. Nardo L, El-Toukhy T, Stewart J, Balen A, Potdar N. British Fertility Society Policy and Practice Committee: Adjuvants in IVF: Evidence for good clinical practice. *Hum Fertil.* 2015;**18**(1):2–15.

9. Boomsma CM, Keay SD, Macklon NS. Periimplantation glucocorticoid administration for assisted reproductive technology cycles. *Cochrane Database Syst*

Rev. 2012;Issue 6: Art. No.: CD005996. doi: 10.1002/ 14651858.CD005996.pub3.

10. Park-Wyllie L, Mazzotta P, Pastuszak A, Moretti ME, Beique L, Hunnisett L, et al. Birth defects after maternal exposure to corticosteroids: prospective cohort study and meta-analysis of epidemiological studies. *Teratology* 2000;**62**:385–92.

11. Moraru M, Carbone J, Alecsandru D, Castillo-Rama M, García-Segovia A, Gil J, et al. Intravenous immunoglobulin treatment increased live birth rate in a Spanish cohort of women with recurrent reproductive failure and expanded CD56 (+) cells. *Am J Reprod Immunol.* 2012;**68**:75–84.

12. Li J, Chen Y, Liu C, Hu Y, Li L. Intravenous immunoglobulin treatment for repeated IVF/ICSI failure and unexplained infertility: a systematic review and a meta-analysis. *Am J Reprod Immunol.* 2013;**70**:434–47.

13. Granato D, Blum S, Rössle C, Le Boucher J, Malnoë A, Dutot G. Effects of parenteral lipid emulsions with different fatty acid composition on immune cell functions in vitro. *JPEN J Parenter Enteral Nutr.* 2000;**24**:113–18.

14. Roussev RG, Acacio B, Ng SC, Coulam CB. Duration of intralipid's suppressive effect on NK cell's functional activity. *Am J Reprod Immunol.* 2008;**60**:258–63.

15. Ndukwe G. Recurrent embryo implantation failure after in vitro fertilisation: improved outcome following intralipid infusion in women with elevated T Helper 1 response. *Hum Fertil.* 2011; **14**(2):21–2.

16. El-khayat W, El Sadek M. Intralipid for repeated implantation failure (RIF): a randomized controlled trial, ASRM abstracts. *Fertil Steril.* 2015 Sep;**104**(3). doi: https://doi.org/ 10.1016/j.fertnstert.2015.07.080.

17. Royal College of Obstetricians & Gynaecologists, The administration of intralipid infusion and a recent Supreme Court ruling. Letter from President, April 2015.

18. Scheinfeld N. A comprehensive review and evaluation of the side effects of the tumor necrosis factor blockers etanercept, infliximab and adalimumab. *J Dermatolog Treat.* 2004; **15**(5):280–94. doi: 10.1080/ 09546630410017275. PMID 15370396.

19. Winger EE, Reed JL, Ashoush S, El-Toukhy T, Ahuja S, Taranissi M. Elevated preconception CD56+ 16+ and/or Th1:Th2 levels predict benefit from IVIG therapy in subfertile women undergoing IVF. *Am J Reprod Immunol.* 2011;**66**:394–403.

20. Tang T, Glanville J, Orsi N, Barth JH, Balen AH. The use of metformin for women with PCOS undergoing IVF treatment. *Hum Reprod.* 2006;**21**:1416–25.

21. Tso LO, Costello MF, Albuquerque LE, Andriolo RB, Freitas V. Metformin treatment before and during IVF or ICSI in women with polycystic ovary syndrome. *Cochrane Database Syst Rev.* 2009;Issue 2: Art. No.: CD006105. doi: 10.1002/ 14651858.CD006105.pub2.

22. Palomba S, Falbo A, La Sala G. Metformin and gonadotropins for ovulation induction in patients with polycystic ovary syndrome: a systematic review with meta-analysis of randomized controlled trials. *Reprod Biol Endocrinol.* 2014;**12**:3.

23. Brewer C, Acharya S, Thake F, Tang T, Balen A. Effect of metformin taken in the 'fresh' in vitro fertilization/ intracytoplasmic sperm injection cycle upon subsequent frozen embryo replacement in women with polycystic ovary syndrome. *Hum Fertil.* 2010;**13**:134–42.

24. Patrono C, García Rodríguez LA, Landolfi R, Baigent C. Low-dose aspirin for the prevention of atherothrombosis. *N Engl J Med.* 2005;**353**:2373–83.

25. Wada I, Hsu CC, Williams G, Macnamee MC, Brinsden PR. The benefits of low-dose aspirin therapy in women with impaired uterine perfusion during assisted conception. *Hum Reprod.* 1994;**9**:1954–7.

26. Siristatidis CS, Dodd SR, Drakeley AJ. Aspirin for in vitro fertilisation. *Cochrane Database Syst Rev.* 2011;Issue 8: Art. No.: CD004832.

27. Azem F, Many A, Ben Ami I, Yovel I, Amit A, Lessing JB, Kupferminc MJ. Increased rates of thrombophilia in women with repeated IVF failures. *Hum Reprod.* 2004;**19**:368–70.

28. Akhtar MA, Sur S, Raine-Fenning N, Jayaprakasan K, Thornton JG, Quenby, S. Heparin for assisted reproduction. *Cochrane Database Syst Rev.* 2013;Issue 8: Art. No.: CD009452. doi: 10.1002/ 14651858.CD009452.pub2.

29. Shaker AG, Fleming R, Jamieson ME, Yates RW, Coutts JR. Assessments of embryo transfer after in-vitro fertilization: effects of glyceryl trinitrate. *Hum Reprod.* 1993;**8**:1426–8.

30. Pinheiro OL, Cavagna M, Baruffi RL, Mauri AL, Petersen C, Franco JG Jr. Administration of beta2-adrenergic agonists during the peri-implantation period does not improve implantation or pregnancy rates in intracytoplasmic sperm injection (ICSI) cycles. *J Assist Reprod Genet.* 2003;**20**:513–16.

31. Nielsen ME, Rasmussen IA, Kristensen SG, Christensen ST, Møllgård K, Wreford Andersen E, et al. In human granulosa cells from small antral follicles, androgen receptor mRNA and androgen levels in follicular fluid correlate with FSH receptor

mRNA. *Mol Hum Reprod.* 2011;**17**:63–70.

32. Wiser A, Gonen O, Ghetler Y, Shavit T, Berkovitz A, Shulman A. Addition of dehydroepiandrosterone (DHEA) for poor-responder patients before and during IVF treatment improves the pregnancy rate: a randomized prospective study. *Hum Reprod.* 2010;**25**:2496–500.

33. Kucuk T, Kozinoglu H, Kaba A. Growth hormone co-treatment within a GnRH agonist long protocol in patients with poor ovarian response: a prospective, randomized, clinical trial. *Journal of Assisted Reproduction and Genetics.* 2008;**25**:123–7.

34. Homburg R, Singh A, Bhide P, Shah A, Gudi A. Growth hormone in fertility treatment - The

re-growth of growth hormone in fertility treatment: a critical review. *Hum Fertil.* 2012; **15(4)**:190–3.

35. Duffy JMN, Ahmad G, Mohiyiddeen L, Nardo LG, Watson A, Growth hormone for in vitro fertilization. *Cochrane Database Syst Rev.* 2010;Issue 4: Art. No.: CD000099. doi: 10.1002/14651858.CD000099.pub2.

36. Eftekhar M, Aflatoonian A, Mohammadian F, Eftekhar, T. Adjuvant growth hormone therapy in antagonist protocol in poor responders undergoing assisted reproductive technology. *Arch Gynecol Obstet.* 2013;**287**:1017–21.

37. Leach M, Aitken RJ, Sacks, G. Sperm DNA fragmentation abnormalities in men from

couples with a history of recurrent miscarriage. *Aust N Z J Obstet Gynaecol.* 2015;**55**:379–83.

38. Suzuki T, Sugino N, Fukaya T, Sugiyama S, Uda T, Takaya R, et al. Superoxide dismutase in normal cycling human ovaries: immunohistochemical localization and characterization. *Fertil Steril.* 1999;**72**:720–6.

39. Youssef MA, Abdelmoty HI, Elashmwi HA, Abduljawad EM, Elghamary N, Magdy A, Mohesen MN, Abdella RM, Bar MA, Gouda HM, Ali AM, Raslan AN, Youssef D, Sherif NA, Ismail AI. Oral antioxidants supplementation for women with unexplained infertility undergoing ICSI/IVF: Randomized controlled trial. *Hum Fertil.* 2015;**18(1)**:38–42.

Chapter 29

Male Fertility Preservation

Allan A. Pacey

1 Introduction

It is generally agreed that sperm banking should be routinely offered prior to the administration of any anti-neoplastic treatment to post-pubertal males following a diagnosis of cancer. It may also be required following a number of other diagnoses (e.g. some renal or rheumatoid conditions) as well as prior to some pelvic surgery or in cases of gender dysphoria. However, since there are over 5,000 new diagnoses of cancer in the United Kingdom each year in males of reproductive age (up to the age of about 44 years old), the majority of men banking their sperm will be following referral from an oncologist. This has led to the development of specific oncofertility pathways for men (and women) who need to preserve their fertility and these represent a number of significant challenges for health professionals in sperm banks and assisted conception units if a timely and effective service is to be provided. This chapter will review the latest thinking on how to provide an effective and efficient service, as well as consider the management of sperm banks in the longer term.

2 Referring Men for Sperm Banking

UK Clinical guidelines [1,2], and those from elsewhere in the world [3,4], each recommend that sperm banking should be a routine part of the care of all post-pubertal males prior to any anti-neoplastic treatment associated with a diagnosis of cancer. However, even with these guidelines in place, the evidence suggests that only a minority of men (<30%) actually bank sperm (although there are significant country-to-country differences in this as table II of reference [5]). There are two main reasons to explain this low uptake.

The first relates to the behaviour of oncologists themselves. For example, there are several studies showing that even with comprehensive guidelines in place, some oncologists simply do not raise the subject of fertility or make the patient aware that sperm banking is available and might be a good idea. This is for a number of different reasons which include the following: (i) difficulties in communication or embarrassment felt by the oncologist in raising the topic; (ii) lack of awareness about the local sperm banking facilities available and the pathway by which men might be referred; (iii) assumptions about the man's needs based on a perception of his family structure, his age or his sexual orientation and (iv) the need to start treatment quickly and a view that saving a man's life is preferable to preserving his fertility if by arranging sperm banking there will be a delay in him starting cancer treatment.

The second relates to the behaviour of men themselves when presented with a choice between starting treatment immediately or delaying treatment by a few days in order to bank sperm. There is no doubt that for some men this will be a difficult decision and in a prospective study of 91 newly diagnosed men who were offered the opportunity to bank sperm by their oncologist, the decision to decline the offer was specifically related to their quality of life scores [6] regardless of diagnosis and stage of disease. This suggests that some men may miss out the opportunity to bank sperm, because at the time of diagnosis they are feeling unwell. In this context, interview data [7] has shown that men's decisions to bank sperm need to be seen in the context of their experience *prior* to diagnosis and the fact that many had been to their General Practitioner many times before their symptoms had been taken seriously. Many men reported that at diagnosis they had been overwhelmed by the amount of information they had received and all emphasised the role of the oncologist in organising sperm banking and making it just part of the cancer journey, alongside other routine appointments such as blood tests, chest X-Rays and CT scans.

Whilst the literature says that some oncologists can be seen as barriers to sperm banking, others show that they are essential to facilitate the process.

Therefore, in running an effective fertility preservation service for men, it is recommended that strong links are developed between reproductive medicine specialists and key oncologists in the local area to make sure everyone is clear about the services available and the optimum methods of referral [8]. It is suggested that named link nurses be identified who can help to cross the boundary between the two specialties and who can help with the coordination of specific patients or serve as a conduit of information when protocols change.

3 Sample Procurement and Storage

Once a patient is identified who wishes to bank sperm, the next challenge is how to obtain a suitable specimen for cryopreservation. A common concern of health professionals is whether in oncology patients there will be sufficient sperm to bank because (i) the patient is very young, (ii) their disease may have compromised testicular function or (iii) they are too unwell to become sufficiently sexually aroused to produce an ejaculate by masturbation.

With regard to the first of these concerns (male age) the evidence is clear that sperm production is a relatively early event in puberty, with spermatogenesis commencing at an average of 13.4 years of age (range 11.7–15.3) [9]. This means that only a brief assessment of pubertal development is required before a referral can be considered. What is more problematic is whether young males of this age are sufficiently sexually mature to understand what is required of them in terms of giving the necessary consent and also the need for them to masturbate in a medical environment. The issue of providing a safe space for sample production and the provision of erotic material to facilitate sexual arousal is discussed in more detail in this chapter, but needless to say a young age is not necessarily a barrier to sperm banking once puberty has started.

Second is the issue of to what extent the patient's disease may have compromised his testicular function, thereby limiting the number or quality of sperm that can be recovered from an ejaculate and frozen. Whilst there is some evidence to suggest that the incidence of azoospermia in men attending for sperm banking is higher than is seen in the general population, there is on average sufficient sperm in the majority of men for use in assisted conception at a later date. For example, a recent study of 3,062 men banking sperm at the Hammersmith Hospital (London, UK) found that up to 11% had cryptozoospermia (where sperm were only seen in the centrifuged pellet) [10].

Finally, for those males who are unable (or unwilling) to produce a semen sample by masturbation (or where an ejaculate proves to be azoospermic), techniques of surgical sperm retrieval can be used if there is sufficient time to do so before the start of antineoplastic treatment and the male is well enough to undergo the procedure. Sometimes, sperm recovery can be undertaken at the time of other surgical procedures (e.g. orchidectomy) to avoid unnecessary delays and minimise the number of surgical procedures and outpatient visits.

However, the majority of males (>90%) are able to successfully produce ejaculates for sperm banking by masturbation and so consideration should be given to the clinical environment and other logistical arrangements which can be put in place for them to achieve this. For example, since men banking sperm at the time of diagnosis have a relatively poor understanding of the process and are doing it as part of a package of care being organised by their oncologist [7], to suggest that they are dealt with like all other male patients attending an assisted conception unit may not be ideal. Whilst some sperm banks are run as stand-alone services, others are inevitably linked to an in vitro fertilisation (IVF) unit and so consideration should be given to the fact that men with cancer do not necessarily identify as fertility patients at this stage, as well as the fact that they may not be in a serious relationship and may wish to attend alone, or with a friend, a healthcare professional, parent or guardian. Therefore a separate waiting area may be preferable, as might a separate consultation style and separate information sheets specifically tailored to sperm banking as part of oncology treatment.

A common area for discussion among health professionals is the provision of a suitable space for the collection of masturbatory ejaculates and whether or not the provision of erotic material is a good idea or not. With regard to the former, very little has been written about the needs of oncology patients and it is suggested that this is developed by understanding the needs of users through normal service evaluation activities (e.g. focus groups and/or questionnaires). However, with regard to the provision of suitable erotic material, several papers have been written to suggest it is a useful thing to provide [11]. Not only does it seem to improve ejaculate quality but it also increases the probability of obtaining a sample. However, those providing sperm banking services in the United Kingdom should be aware that it may be unlawful to provide erotica for use by males under the age of 18 years, although evidence suggests that minors would prefer to bring their own material with them [12]. Those working outside the United Kingdom should check their local laws with regard to the minimum age for the provision of erotic material (if it is allowed at all).

Finally, once an ejaculate is obtained, there are a fairly standard series of protocols for sperm cryopreservation (although it is likely that each laboratory will have its preferred method). Unfortunately, there is often significant loss of sperm viability during the freezing process [13], although for most men sufficient numbers of viable sperm do remain to allow sperm to be utilised during intracytoplasmic sperm injection (ICSI). However, sperm banks should monitor their ongoing sperm freezing rates by conducting regular post-thaw analysis of samples. Moreover, this information should ultimately be given to each patient so that they can know what to reasonably expect should they need to use their samples in treatment. This information can be revisited during post-treatment follow-up consultations as part of the suite of information which is discussed and revisited several times during the years that sperm is kept in storage.

4 Post-treatment Fertility Monitoring

Once anti-neoplastic treatment has ended, all men with banked sperm should be offered the opportunity to undergo regular semen analysis so that any long-term effects can be established and they can make their decisions about family planning and contraception appropriately. However, the literature suggests that men are often reluctant to engage with fertility monitoring programmes provided by sperm banks and often do so only when establishing a new relationship or planning to start a family [7]. Moreover, data from interviews suggest that a common deterrent to attending for semen analysis was men's anxiety about the result, with most preferring not to know if their semen quality was poor. Yet, ironically, information about recovered fertility is welcomed, even in men who did not want any more children, because it contributes to restored feelings of masculinity. Other reasons for non-attendance for post-treatment semen

analysis have been investigated [14] and include the following: (i) the lack of treatment side effects such as sickness and diarrhoea; (ii) a bad experience of the sperm banking process and (iii) having negative attitudes to disposal of the banked samples. These data suggest that there are complex physiological reasons why men might not accept invitations for semen analysis and a lack of response from them should not be taken as indicating that they are not interested in their banked sperm.

5 Natural Fertility of Cancer Survivors

Perhaps surprisingly, follow-up studies suggest that in many men spermatogenesis resumes (or remains unaffected) after anti-neoplastic treatment has ended. For example, in a cohort of 178 men treated for testicular cancer, approximately 60% had normal spermatogenesis five or more years after treatment and a further 20% had some sperm in their ejaculates [15]. Therefore, it is perhaps of no surprise that compared to men in the general population, many men remain fertile and go on to conceive without the need for assisted conception. For example, a follow-up study of 463 male cancer survivors with a mean age at diagnosis of 22 years found that 63% had become a father by the age of 35 years old, in comparison to 64% for men in the general population [16]. In addition, most studies suggest that those children fathered naturally have comparable health to those fathered by men without a cancer diagnosis; for example, there is no increased incidence of congenital anomalies [17] or the risk of developing cancer [18] in the children of cancer survivors.

6 Assisted Conception

Most studies suggest that only about 10% of men who bank sperm prior to cancer treatment ever return to use it in assisted conception (see table III of reference [5]). For some professionals who are in charge of sperm banks this might be seen as a failure but given the relatively high frequency of natural fertility in men after cancer treatment, this is perhaps to be expected. The challenge for sperm banks is how to maintain contact with men over an extended period of time and make sure their consent to storage and use remains up to date. If assisted conception using banked sperm is ultimately required, then there are relatively few studies to suggest whether any one technique is better than another. Live births using sperm banked over 20+ years have been seen with ICSI [19] as well as intrauterine insemination (IUI) [20] – the choice of treatment probably reflecting the quality of the sperm initially stored. In their UK guidelines, NICE give no specific recommendations in this regard, except to say that where infertility is already suspected, couples should not be forced to undergo 12 months of unprotected intercourse in order to demonstrate subfertility [2].

7 Long-Term Issues

For those involved in the provision of sperm banking services to men diagnosed with cancer, there are a number of specific long-term challenges. The most significant is how the sperm bank maintains long-term contact with men over what could amount to many decades (at the time of writing, UK law allows men to keep their frozen sperm for a total of 55 years). This may be significantly longer than men are in follow-up for their oncology (e.g. men with testicular cancer are typically discharged after five years). There are few studies to guide how this might be best achieved, although the recommendations of the HFEA Code of Practice [21] suggests that sperm banks should conduct regular audits of their stored material and should have a 'bring forward' system that alerts them to when consent may be about to expire or needs to be reviewed. We know that men do find it difficult to make the decision to dispose of banked samples, even when their fertility has recovered and their family is complete [7]. In a study of 19 men who requested elective disposal in two UK sperm banks [22], this decision was independently related to the following: (i) confidence about their fertility recovery; (ii) a view that fertility monitoring by post-treatment semen analysis was less important to them; (iii) a more positive attitude to disposal generally; (iv) less desire for future children and

(v) more likely to have experienced side effects during their cancer treatment. However, we know there is a 'hard-core' of men with banked sperm who simply do not respond to letters about their stored samples [23] and this seemed to be related to a complex interplay between past, present and future perspectives about their fertility and their banked sperm. The challenge for sperm banks is probably to devise invitation letters that address men's concerns whilst offering them tangible benefits and peace of mind. However, in this context, it is clear that information sources and resources produced about sperm banking are often pitched inappropriately and may actually hinder men's understanding of the issues. For example, an analysis of 66 online resources (such as patient information leaflets and websites) about sperm banking found that only a minority included information about the importance of long-term contact (18.2%) or discussed the issue of disposal when samples were no longer needed (10.6%) [24]. Moreover, for the most part, the readability of these resources (the reading age) was on average much higher than that of the general population, perhaps suggesting they were poorly understood by many men.

8 Conclusion

In conclusion, the evidence suggests that banking sperm for men with cancer is a much more complex aspect of reproductive medicine than might first appear. It is more involved than simply obtaining a sample of sperm and placing it in liquid nitrogen alongside samples from other men attending the clinic. If sperm banking services are to be offered wisely and effectively, then they need to take account of men's needs and aspects of their decision-making both at the time of cancer diagnosis and in the longer term.

References

1. Royal College of Physicians. *The Effects of Cancer Treatment on Reproductive Functions. Guidance on Management.* London: Royal College of Physicians, 2007.

2. National Institute for Health and Clinical Excellence. Fertility – Assessment and treatment for people with fertility problems. Nice Clinical Guideline 156, 2013. (accessed at www.nice.org.uk/guidance/cg156 on 1st November 2015)

3. European Society for Human Reproduction and Embryology Taskforce 7: Ethical considerations for the cryopreservation of gametes and reproductive tissues

for self-use. *Human Reproduction* 2004; **19**: 460–462.

4. Loren AW, Mangu PB, Beck LN, Brennan L, Magdalinski AJ, Partridge AH, Quinn G, Wallace WH & Oktay K. Fertility preservation for patients with cancer: American Society of Clinical Oncology Clinical Practice Guideline Update *Journal*

of Clinical Oncology 2013; **31**: 2500–2510.

5. Pacey AA & Eiser C. Banking sperm is only the first of many decisions for men: what healthcare professionals and men need to know. *Human Fertility* 2011; **14**: 208–217.

6. Pacey AA, Merrick H, Arden-Close E, Morris K, Rowe R, Stark D & Eiser C. Implications of sperm banking for health-related quality of life up to 1 year after cancer diagnosis. *British Journal of Cancer* 2013; **108**: 1004–1011.

7. Eiser C, Arden-Close E, Morris K & Pacey AA. The legacy of sperm banking: how fertility monitoring and disposal are linked with views of cancer treatment. *Human Reproduction* 2011; **26**: 2791–2798.

8. Pacey AA. Referring patients for sperm banking. In: A.A. Pacey and M.J. Tomlinson (Eds) *Sperm Banking – Theory and Practice.* Cambridge: Cambridge University Press, 2009; 110–128.

9. Nielsen CT, Skakkebaek NE, Richardson DW, Darling JA, Hunter WM, Jorgensen M, Nielsen A, Ingersley O, Keiding N & Muller J. Onset of the release of spermatozoa (spermarche) in boys in relation to age, testicular growth, pubic hair, and height. *Journal of Clinical Endocrinology Metabolism* 1986; **62**: 532–535.

10. Dearing C, Breen D, Bradshaw A, Ramsay J & Lindsay K. Trends and usage in a London National Health Service Sperm Bank for cancer patients. *Human Fertility* 2014; **17**: 289–296.

11. Wylie K & Pacey AA. Using erotica in government-funded health service clinics. *Journal of Sexual Medicine* 2011; **8**: 1261–1265.

12. Crawshaw MA, Glaser AW & Pacey AA. The use of pornographic materials by adolescent male cancer patients when banking sperm in the UK: Legal and ethical dilemmas. *Human Fertility* 2007; **10**: 159–163.

13. Nijs M & Ombelet W. Cryopreservation of human sperm. *Human Fertility* 2001; **4**: 158–163.

14. Pacey AA, Merrick H, Arden-Close E, Morris K, Barton LC, Crook AJ, Tomlinson MJ, Wright E, Rowe R & Eiser C. Monitoring fertility (semen analysis) by cancer survivors who banked sperm prior to cancer treatment. *Human Reproduction* 2012; **27**: 3132–3139.

15. Lampe H, Horwich A, Norman A, Nicholls J & Dearnaley DP. Fertility after chemotherapy for testicular germ cell cancers. *Journal of Clinical Oncology* 1997; **15**: 239–245.

16. Magelssen H, Melve KK, Skjaerven R & Fosså SD. Parenthood probability and pregnancy outcome in patients with a cancer diagnosis during adolescence and young adulthood *Human Reproduction* 2008; 23: 178–186.

17. Signorello LB, Mulvihill JJ, Green DM, Munro HM, Stovall M, Weathers RE, Mertens AC, Whitton JA, Robison LL & Boice JD Jr. Congenital anomalies in the children of cancer survivors: a report from the childhood cancer survivor study. *Journal of Clinical Oncology* 2012; 30: 239–245.

18. Sankila R, Olsen JH, Anderson H, Garwicz S, Glattre E, Hertz H, Langmark F, Lanning M, Møller T & Tulinius H. Risk of cancer among offspring of childhood-cancer survivors. Association of the Nordic Cancer Registries and the Nordic Society of Paediatric Haematology and Oncology. *New England Journal of Medicine* 1998; **338**: 1339–1344.

19. Horne G, Atkinson AD, Pease EH, Logue JP, Brison DR & Lieberman BA. Live birth with sperm cryopreserved for 21 years prior to cancer treatment: case report. *Human Reproduction* 2004; **19**: 1448–1449.

20. Feldschuh J, Brassel J, Durso N & Levine A. Successful sperm storage for 28 years. *Fertility and Sterility* 2005; **84**: 1017.

21. Human Fertilisation and Embryology Authority. *Code of Practice.* 8th Edition. London: HFEA, 2009.

22. Pacey AA, Merrick H, Arden-Close E, Morris K, Tomlinson MJ, Rowe R & Eiser C. How do men in the United Kingdom decide to dispose of banked sperm following cancer treatment? *Human Fertility* 2014; **17**: 285–288.

23. Eiser C, Merrick H, Arden-Close E, Morris K, Rowe R & Pacey AA. Why don't some men with banked sperm respond to letters about their stored samples? *Human Fertility* 2014; **17**: 278–284.

24. Merrick H, Wright E, Pacey AA & Eiser C. Finding out about sperm banking: what information is available online for men diagnosed with cancer? *Human Fertility* 2012; **15**: 121–128.

Chapter 30

Female Fertility Preservation

Nikoletta Panagiotopoulou

1 Introduction

Fertility preservation, which is defined by the National Center for Biotechnology Information as 'a method of providing future reproductive opportunities before a medical treatment with known risk of loss of fertility' (1), aims to mitigate the long-term effects of gonadotoxic treatment. Current evidence shows that timely fertility preservation counselling allows patients to better cope with the long-term effects of gonadotoxic treatment, including the potential for infertility (2). This chapter, thus, discusses the present status of fertility preservation in women and explores new developments in the field.

2 Establishing the Need for Fertility Preservation in Women Exposed to Gonadotoxic Treatment

Gonadotoxic treatments, such as radiotherapy, chemotherapy or surgery to reproductive organs, have been successfully used to treat cancer with considerably improved survival rates for young people diagnosed with cancer in the United Kingdom. As of 2010, there were more than 75,000 cancer survivors of reproductive age in the United Kingdom who were aged between 0 and 24 at the time of diagnosis (3), and the number is expected to further increase. In addition to cancer diagnoses, gonadotoxic treatment has been used for the management of non-oncological systemic diseases, such as autoimmune or haematological diseases (4). Therefore, fertility preservation should also be utilized in non-cancer conditions increasing the number of women who could benefit from it.

Evidence has shown that the reproductive capacity of women exposed to gonadotoxic treatment is reduced (5). Female reproductive capacity is dependent on effective ovarian function for ovulation, patency of fallopian tubes for fertilization and a suitable endometrial environment for implantation and in-utero development to term. Ovarian follicles are sensitive to the effects of agents that cause DNA damage such as radiotherapy and chemotherapy. Radiotherapy and chemotherapy destroy ovarian follicles and, therefore, reduce the ovarian reserve in a dose-dependent manner. Indeed, ovarian primordial follicles are particularly sensitive to radiation, with an estimated lethal dose required to destroy 50% of non-growing follicles (LD_{50}) of about 2 Gy (6). Effective sterilizing dose (ESD) is age dependent and it is estimated to be 20.3 Gy at birth but only 14.3 Gy at 30 years of age (7, 8). As a result, more than 97% of females treated with total body irradiation (20–30 Gy) during childhood will experience premature ovarian insufficiency (9). Moreover, the risk of premature ovarian insufficiency further increases if radiotherapy is combined with chemotherapy. Chemotherapy has two separate effects on ovarian function; an immediate effect induced by the growing follicle loss that is often reversible, and a delayed effect induced by primordial follicle pool depletion. If this reduction in the primordial follicle pool is almost complete, premature ovarian insufficiency may occur immediately after treatment. In addition to radiation-related ovarian damage, the uterus may be damaged by radiation to a field that includes the pelvis. A large retrospective cohort study showed that survivors who received pelvic irradiation are at increased risk of preterm delivery and low birth weight among their children (10). Moreover, pelvic irradiation has been associated with an increased risk of miscarriage and second trimester loss (11).

3 Estimating Fertility Prognosis after Gonadotoxic Treatment

The risk of gonadotoxic treatment to fertility cannot be assessed accurately and, therefore, fertility preservation counselling should be offered to all patients receiving gonadotoxic treatment. Natural progression of a disease means that fertility prognosis could change with the risk of premature ovarian insufficiency being dependent on the planned treatment rather than the disease itself.

Traditionally chronological age and the presence of menses have been used to predict reproductive performance (12). However, this relationship is not absolute (13) and hence there was a need for other markers of fertility potential. Endocrine profiles as well as the use of transvaginal ovarian sonography in the early follicular phase of the menstrual cycle are commonly used as markers of ovarian reserve for cancer survivors (14), with high follicle-stimulating hormone (FSH) levels, low inhibin B concentration, low ovarian volume and low antral follicle count indicating a reduced reproductive potential (15).

Since 2005, measurement of serum levels of anti-mullerian hormone (AMH) has emerged as another useful marker of ovarian reserve, which has been shown to be more sensitive than FSH and inhibin B or ultrasound markers in assessing chemotherapy-induced ovarian follicle loss (16). Moreover, it may also be of value in children where FSH and inhibin B are not useful (17), as AMH is detectable in girls of all ages and rises through childhood. Moreover, prospective studies have demonstrated that pretreatment AMH could predict post-treatment ovarian recovery (18). This could potentially allow for the development of ovarian damage prediction tools that would combine chronological age and AMH concentration (19).

4 Fertility Preservation Strategies for Women

Strategies for mitigating the effects of gonadotoxic treatment on female fertility have been evolving in response to the increasing societal trend to postpone procreation until the end of reproductive years, when the incidence of diseases requiring gonadotoxic treatment is increasing, and the current focus is on quality survival.

Available fertility preservation methods range from well-established techniques, such as embryo and mature oocyte cryopreservation, to experimental techniques, such as ovarian tissue cryopreservation. Currently, the National Institute for Health and Clinical Excellence (NICE) only supports the use of embryo and mature oocyte cryopreservation

following ovarian stimulation as the option of choice for fertility preservation (20).

4.1 Embryo Cryopreservation

Embryo cryopreservation is a well-established technique with proven safety and effectiveness. Indeed, embryo cryopreservation is routinely performed in assisted reproductive technique centres worldwide for many different clinical indications such as to store surplus embryos or to prevent ovarian hyperstimulation syndrome (21). Long-term outcome data on the health of children born after frozen embryo transfer have been generally reassuring (22, 23). Embryo cryopreservation can, thus, be safely used to preserve fertility in women who have gone through puberty and have an available partner or are willing to use donor sperm. However, embryo cryopreservation cannot be used for prepubertal girls or women where the timing of initiation of cancer treatment is critical.

Limitations of embryo cryopreservation include the need for controlled ovarian stimulation which requires time, involves risks that could further delay initiation of cancer treatment – such as the risk of ovarian hyperstimulation syndrome – and could potentially negatively affect the prognosis for women with oestrogen-sensitive cancer due to high oestrogen levels (24). Apart from the clinical challenges posed by embryo cryopreservation for cancer patients, complex legal and ethical issues need to be taken into consideration too. These include ownership rights for the frozen embryos and each partner's rights to their use. In the United Kingdom, cryopreserved embryos are the joint property of the woman and her partner and this could lead to difficult ethical dilemmas and legal decisions regarding their utility or disposition in case of intra-couple disagreement (25) or death of either partner.

4.2 Mature Oocyte Cryopreservation

Mature oocyte cryopreservation could be considered as an alternative to embryo cryopreservation for patients seeking fertility preservation options and who can delay cancer treatment. Indeed, outcomes of cryopreserved-thawed oocytes have significantly improved since the introduction of vitrification and they now appear to be similar to those obtained with fresh oocytes (26). Current evidence has proven that vitrification of mature oocytes yields a high oocyte survival rate when compared with slow freezing and enhances the development of the resultant embryo(s) (27). However, these promising results are coming from mature oocyte vitrification in egg donation programmes and hence caution needs to be applied when using these outcomes to advise cancer patients. Outcome data on oocyte cryopreservation in cancer patients are limited due to the fact that oocyte cryopreservation in this population group is a relatively new approach while treatment and follow-up requirements of cancer patients mandate complete remission of the disease before considering use of cryopreserved oocytes.

Another limiting factor of oocyte cryopreservation is its low final yield. It is thought that around 20 vitrified mature oocytes are required to achieve a live birth with the quoted optimum live birth rate per vitrified oocyte in egg donation programmes being 5.7% (26). The above response to controlled ovarian stimulation protocols may prove challenging for the majority of cancer patients as a recent meta-analysis of retrospective studies showed that cancer patients had lower numbers of both total and mature oocytes in comparison to healthy, age-matched control individuals (28).

4.3 Ovarian Transposition

In ovarian transposition, the ovaries and their vessels are carefully mobilized through an open or laparoscopic approach and transplanted usually to the anterolateral abdominal wall a few centimetres above the umbilicus. Even though ovarian transposition has been shown to preserve ovarian function in the large majority of patients (88.6%–90%) (29), the risk of ovarian failure after pelvic radiotherapy varies from 15% to 40% (30, 31). This risk is further increased if radiotherapy is combined with chemotherapy (6). Moreover, as gynaecologic cancers can coexist, the risk of ovarian involvement in the presence of pelvic cancer should be assessed prior to proceeding to ovarian transposition.

4.4 Ovarian Tissue Cryopreservation

Ovarian tissue cryopreservation with subsequent transplantation has been suggested as a possible fertility preservation option for any female patient undergoing gonadotoxic treatment. Ovarian tissue containing immature follicles has been successfully cryopreserved in several animal and human models

and the first successful application of this technology in humans was reported in 2004 (32). During these last fifteen years of clinical progress in ovarian tissue cryopreservation, 30 live births after orthotopic reimplantation of cryopreserved ovarian tissue have been reported (33).

Ovarian tissue cryopreservation is currently the only option available for prepubertal girls and for women who cannot significantly delay cancer treatment (34). However, major limitations still exist that prevent ovarian tissue cryopreservation from being recognized as a proven fertility preservation option. The efficiency of ovarian tissue cryopreservation and reimplantation is difficult to establish because the number of reimplantations performed worldwide remains unknown. Unpublished data, however, from the Donnez group indicate a low success rate (10% reported success rate). Moreover, as the primordial follicle pool and, therefore, the efficacy of ovarian tissue cryopreservation is age dependent, there is the need to define optimal age limits for the use of this fertility preservation technique. There have been several attempts worldwide to set the upper age limit but no recommendations have been made regarding the lower age limit yet as there is no consensus on the age at which reproductive potential is actually reached. The longevity of orthotopic ovarian tissue reimplantation is another issue. Current data supports that this procedure offers a limited window of opportunity to achieve a pregnancy for cancer survivors as the quoted mean duration of ovarian function after transplantation is 4–7 years (35). Moreover, fertility outcomes among women with proven complete restoration of ovarian function after cryopreserved-thawed ovarian tissue reimplantation have been variable. Lastly, the risk of reimplanting malignant cells remains a serious concern related to the use of cryopreserved-thawed ovarian tissue in cancer survivors. A recent review (36) classified malignant diseases into three categories based on the risk of ovarian involvement: the high risk group, which includes malignancies such as leukaemia, neuroblastoma and Burkitt lymphoma, has an estimated risk of ovarian metastasis of 11%; the moderate risk group, which includes malignancies such as non-Hodgkin lymphoma, Ewing sarcoma, has a risk of ovarian metastasis between 0.2% and 11%; and the low risk group, which includes malignancies such as Hodgkin lymphoma, Wilms' tumour, has a $<0.2\%$ risk.

4.5 GnRH Analogues

Gonadotrophin-releasing hormone agonists (GnRHa) have been proposed as adjuvant treatment to minimize the chemotherapy-induced gonadotoxicity and were first tested more than three decades ago (37). The proposed fertility preserving mechanism of action is thought to be based on the hypogonadotrophic state that GnRHa generate. The GnRHa-induced hypogonadotrophic state causes pituitary desensitization and, thus, prevents the increase in FSH, which subsequently interrupts the vicious cycle of chemotherapy-induced follicular demise, supraphysiologic FSH levels and recruitment of further follicles (38). A recent meta-analysis showed that temporary ovarian suppression with GnRHa reduces the risk of premature ovarian insufficiency in breast cancer patients but not in ovarian or lymphoma patients. Moreover, these cancer survivors' ultimate reproductive ability was unclear (39).

5 Future Fertility Preservation Strategies

A number of well-established and experimental fertility preservation options that are currently available for women exposed to gonadotoxic treatments have been described earlier. However, each one of them has significant limitations and, therefore, research is focused on developing future fertility preservation strategies that would reduce the off-target effects of oncological or non-oncological treatments on the ovaries while minimizing the treatment burden for patients.

For women in whom cryopreserved-thawed ovarian tissue reimplantation is not advisable due to increased risk of reimplanting malignant cells, use of isolated ovarian follicles has been proposed as a safer alternative. In vitro follicle culture aims to develop culture systems that can support complete growth of oocytes from early primordial stages through to maturity. Complete follicle development in vitro from primordial stages has only been achieved in mice (40). However, the success of complete murine in vitro oocyte development has worked as proof of concept and has driven the development of methods to be applied to other species and particularly to humans. Indeed, in recent years a great deal of progress has been made in developing in vitro follicle culture systems for humans, which could have a revolutionary impact on reproductive medicine (41).

Despite advances in in vitro follicle culture, there is still much to do before isolated ovarian follicles can be used successfully as a strategy for obtaining competent oocytes. An alternative approach would, thus, be the development of an artificial ovary by transferring isolated ovarian follicles onto a scaffold that would be able to support the growth and maturation of follicles in vivo. The first step in developing an artificial ovary was accomplished in 2012 with the creation of a biodegradable scaffold consisting of an alginate matrigel matrix onto which isolated preantral follicles were grafted (42). Moreover, an artificial ovary that allowed survival and growth of isolated murine ovarian follicles has recently been achieved using a fibrin scaffold (43).

In the past decade, the isolation of oogonial stem cells in the human ovary (44) raises the possibility of using these stem cells to produce new oocytes to replace the ovarian reserve destroyed by gonadotoxic treatment. Indeed, a number of studies have shown that oogonial stem cells can be isolated, cultured and subsequently developed into oocytes under certain conditions, even though more research is needed to improve the efficacy of oogonial stem cell isolation and development into oocytes. Alternatively, it has been hypothesized but not yet proved that induced pluripotent cell-derived stem cells from embryonic stem cells, the bone marrow or peripheral blood could provide an alternative route for ovarian reserve restoration.

Alternative mitigation strategies for gonadotoxic treatments that have been proposed and assessed in animal models (45) include targeted delivery of chemotherapeutic agents by encapsulating them in nanoparticles with special affinity to cancer cells or the use of agents that inhibit the apoptotic effects of chemotherapy or radiotherapy on primordial follicles.

6 Conclusion

Advances in reproductive medicine and cryobiology have led to the development of various fertility preservation techniques that could help mitigate the risks of gonadotoxic treatments and address the reproductive health needs of women with an oncological or non-oncological diagnosis. The availability of fertility preservation options, thus, represents a strong incentive to make counselling about the risks of gonadotoxicity and available fertility preservation options an integral part of the care of women exposed to gonadotoxic treatment.

References

1. National Center for Biotechnology Information. Fertility preservation 2012 [cited 2015 January 14]. Available from: www.ncbi.nlm.nih.gov/mesh/?term=fertility+preservation.

2. Mersereau JE, Goodman LR, Deal AM, Gorman JR, Whitcomb BW, Su HI. To preserve or not to preserve: how difficult is the decision about fertility preservation? *Cancer.* 2013; 119(22):4044–50.

3. NCIN. Macmillan-NCIN work plan - Segmenting the cancer population: All cancers combined, 20-year prevalence at the end of 2010, UK 2013 [cited 2015 July 7]. Available from: www.ncin.org.uk/about_ncin/segmentation.

4. Gidoni Y, Holzer H, Tulandi T, Tan SL. Fertility preservation in patients with non-oncological conditions. *Reproductive Biomedicine Online.* 2008; 16(6):792–800.

5. Green DM, Kawashima T, Stovall M, Leisenring W, Sklar CA, Mertens AC, et al. Fertility of female survivors of childhood cancer: a report from the childhood cancer survivor study. *Journal of Clinical Oncology: Official Journal of the American Society of Clinical Oncology.* 2009;27(16):2677–85.

6. Wallace WH, Thomson AB, Kelsey TW. The radiosensitivity of the human oocyte. *Human Reproduction.* 2003;18(1):117–21.

7. Wallace WH, Thomson AB, Saran F, Kelsey TW. Predicting age of ovarian failure after radiation to a field that includes the ovaries. *International Journal of Radiation Oncology, Biology, Physics.* 2005;62(3):738–44.

8. Meirow D, Biederman H, Anderson RA, Wallace WH. Toxicity of chemotherapy and radiation on female reproduction. *Clinical Obstetrics and Gynecology.* 2010;53(4):727–39.

9. Wallace WH, Shalet SM, Crowne EC, Morris-Jones PH, Gattamaneni HR. Ovarian failure following abdominal irradiation in childhood: natural history and prognosis. *Clinical Oncology (Royal College of Radiologists (Great Britain)).* 1989;1(2):75–9.

10. Signorello LB, Cohen SS, Bosetti C, Stovall M, Kasper CE, Weathers RE, et al. Female survivors of childhood cancer: preterm birth and low birth weight among their children. *Journal of the National Cancer Institute.* 2006;98(20):1453–61.

11. Critchley HO, Wallace WH, Shalet SM, Mamtora H, Higginson J, Anderson DC. Abdominal irradiation in childhood; the potential for pregnancy. *British Journal of Obstetrics and Gynaecology.* 1992;99(5):392–4.

12. Templeton A, Morris JK, Parslow W. Factors that affect outcome of in-vitro fertilisation treatment. *Lancet.* 1996;348(9039):1402–6.

13. te Velde ER, Pearson PL. The variability of female reproductive ageing. *Human Reproduction Update.* 2002;8(2):141–54.

14. Larsen EC, Muller J, Schmiegelow K, Rechnitzer C, Andersen AN. Reduced ovarian function in long-term survivors of radiation- and chemotherapy-treated childhood cancer. *The Journal of Clinical Endocrinology and Metabolism.* 2003;88(11):5307–14.

15. Speroff L, Fritz M. *Clinical Gynecologic Endocrinology and Infertility.* Philadelphia: Lippincott Williams & Wilkins; 2005.

16. Anderson RA, Themmen AP, Al-Qahtani A, Groome NP, Cameron DA. The effects of chemotherapy and long-term gonadotrophin suppression on the ovarian reserve in premenopausal women with breast cancer. *Human Reproduction.* 2006; 21(10):2583–92.

17. Kelsey TW, Wright P, Nelson SM, Anderson RA, Wallace WH. A validated model of serum anti-mullerian hormone from conception to menopause. *PloS One.* 2011;6(7):e22024.

18. Dillon KE, Sammel MD, Prewitt M, Ginsberg JP, Walker D, Mersereau JE, et al. Pretreatment antimullerian hormone levels determine rate of posttherapy ovarian reserve recovery: acute changes in ovarian reserve during and after chemotherapy. *Fertility and Sterility.* 2013;99(2):477–83.

19. Anderson RA, Rosendahl M, Kelsey TW, Cameron DA. Pretreatment anti-Mullerian hormone predicts for loss of ovarian function after chemotherapy for early breast cancer. *European Journal of Cancer.* 2013;49(16):3404–11.

20. National Institute for Health and Care Excellence (NICE). Fertility assessment and treatment for people with fertility problems (CG 156) 2013 [cited 2014 2 June]. Available from: http://guidance.nice.org.uk/CG156.

21. Herrero L, Martinez M, Garcia-Velasco JA. Current status of human oocyte and embryo cryopreservation. *Current Opinion in Obstetrics and Gynecology.* 2011;23(4):245–50.

22. Bedoschi GM, de Albuquerque FO, Ferriani RA, Navarro PA. Ovarian stimulation during the luteal phase for fertility preservation of cancer patients: case reports and review of the literature. *Journal of Assisted Reproduction and Genetics.* 2010;27(8):491–4.

23. Oktay K, Buyuk E, Libertella N, Akar M, Rosenwaks Z. Fertility preservation in breast cancer patients: a prospective controlled comparison of ovarian stimulation with tamoxifen and letrozole for embryo cryopreservation. *Journal of Clinical Oncology: Official Journal*

of the American Society of Clinical Oncology. 2005;23(19):4347–53.

24. Azim AA, Costantini-Ferrando M, Lostritto K, Oktay K. Relative potencies of anastrozole and letrozole to suppress estradiol in breast cancer patients undergoing ovarian stimulation before in vitro fertilization. *The Journal of Clinical Endocrinology and Metabolism.* 2007;92(6):2197–200.

25. Bankowski BJ, Lyerly AD, Faden RR, Wallach EE. The social implications of embryo cryopreservation. *Fertility and Sterility.* 2005;84(4):823–32.

26. Cobo A, Garcia-Velasco JA, Domingo J, Remohi J, Pellicer A. Is vitrification of oocytes useful for fertility preservation for age-related fertility decline and in cancer patients? *Fertility and Sterility.* 2013;99(6):1485–95.

27. Edgar DH, Gook DA. A critical appraisal of cryopreservation (slow cooling versus vitrification) of human oocytes and embryos. *Human Reproduction Update.* 2012;18(5):536–54.

28. Friedler S, Koc O, Gidoni Y, Raziel A, Ron-El R. Ovarian response to stimulation for fertility preservation in women with malignant disease: a systematic review and meta-analysis. *Fertility and Sterility.* 2012;97(1):125–33.

29. Barahmeh S, Al Masri M, Badran O, Masarweh M, El-Ghanem M, Jaradat I, et al. Ovarian transposition before pelvic irradiation: indications and functional outcome. *The Journal of Obstetrics and Gynaecology Research.* 2013;39(11):1533–7.

30. Bisharah M, Tulandi T. Laparoscopic preservation of ovarian function: an underused procedure. *American Journal of Obstetrics and Gynecology.* 2003;188(2):367–70.

31. Morice P, Juncker L, Rey A, El-Hassan J, Haie-Meder C, Castaigne D. Ovarian transposition for patients with cervical carcinoma treated by radiosurgical combination. *Fertility and Sterility.* 2000; 74(4):743–8.

32. Donnez J, Dolmans MM, Demylle D, Jadoul P, Pirard C, Squifflet J, et al. Livebirth after orthotopic transplantation of cryopreserved ovarian tissue. *Lancet.* 2004; 364(9443):1405–10.

33. Donnez J, Dolmans MM, Pellicer A, Diaz-Garcia C, Sanchez Serrano M, Schmidt KT, et al. Restoration of ovarian activity and pregnancy after transplantation of cryopreserved ovarian tissue: a review of 60 cases of reimplantation. *Fertility and Sterility.* 2013;99(6):1503–13.

34. Donnez J, Jadoul P, Squifflet J, Van Langendonckt A, Donnez O, Van Eyck AS, et al. Ovarian tissue cryopreservation and transplantation in cancer patients. *Best Practice & Research: Clinical Obstetrics & Gynaecology.* 2010; 24(1):87–100.

35. Kim SS. Assessment of long term endocrine function after transplantation of frozen-thawed human ovarian tissue to the heterotopic site: 10 year longitudinal follow-up study. *Journal of Assisted Reproduction and Genetics.* 2012;29(6):489–93.

36. Dolmans MM, Luyckx V, Donnez J, Andersen CY, Greve T. Risk of transferring malignant cells with transplanted frozen-thawed ovarian tissue. *Fertility and Sterility.* 2013;99(6):1514–22.

37. Glode LM, Robinson J, Gould SF. Protection from cyclophosphamide-induced testicular damage with an analogue of gonadotropin-releasing hormone. *Lancet.* 1981; 1(8230):1132–4.

38. Blumenfeld Z. GnRH-agonists in fertility preservation. *Current Opinion In Endocrinology, Diabetes, and Obesity.* 2008; 15(6):523–8.

39. Del Mastro L, Ceppi M, Poggio F, Bighin C, Peccatori F, Demeestere I, et al. Gonadotropin-releasing hormone analogues for the prevention of chemotherapy-induced premature ovarian failure in cancer women: systematic review and meta-analysis of randomized trials. *Cancer Treatment Reviews.* 2014; 40(5):675–83.

40. Eppig JJ, Wigglesowrth K, O'Brien MJ. Comparison of embryonic developmental competence of mouse oocytes grown with and without serum. *Molecular Reproduction and Development.* 1992;32(1):33–40.

41. Telfer EE, Zelinski MB. Ovarian follicle culture: advances and challenges for human and nonhuman primates. *Fertility and Sterility.* 2013;99(6):1523–33.

42. Vanacker J, Luyckx V, Dolmans MM, Des Rieux A, Jaeger J, Van Langendonckt A, et al. Transplantation of an alginate-matrigel matrix containing isolated ovarian cells: first step in developing a biodegradable scaffold to transplant isolated preantral follicles and ovarian cells. *Biomaterials.* 2012; 33(26):6079–85.

43. Luyckx V, Dolmans MM, Vanacker J, Legat C, Fortuno Moya C, Donnez J, et al. A new step toward the artificial ovary: survival and proliferation of isolated murine follicles after autologous transplantation in a fibrin scaffold. *Fertility and Sterility.* 2014;101(4):1149–56.

44. Zuckerman S. The number of oocytes in the mouse ovary. *Recent Progress in Hormone Research.* 1951;6:63–108.

45. De Vos M, Smitz J, Woodruff TK. Fertility preservation in women with cancer. *Lancet.* 2014; 384(9950):1302–10.

Donor Recruitment

Jane A. Stewart

1 Introduction

Sperm donation in the United Kingdom was first described as a treatment in 1945 in Mary Barton's article in the *British Medical Journal* (BMJ) [1]. Before and since that publication, innumerable children have been born as a result of either formal or informal sperm donation. Sperm freezing has been undertaken in animal work e.g. cattle for many years, and advances in the reliability of freezing and thawing techniques paved the way for the formation of sperm 'banks'. In the United Kingdom in 1990, the storage of human gametes became a licensable activity through the Human Fertilisation and Embryology Act regulated by the Authority (HFEA) [2].

Registration of all donors and recording of all treatment cycles using those donors has given a unique record of the generation of donor-conceived families in the United Kingdom, and around 40,000 children have now been born as a result of licensed treatment using donated gametes or embryos.

Regulations initially restricted donor use to the conception of 10 children, later to be extended to include genetic siblings i.e. 10 families rather than individuals [3]. This is most relevant for sperm donors since a series of donations will readily supply enough sperm to meet that number. HFEA data confirms that sperm (and egg) donors have been registered at a steadily increasing rate over some years [4]. Egg donors may be used to treat more than one recipient in any one treatment cycle but are unlikely to undertake sufficient successful cycles to meet the 10-family limit. Altruistic egg donors are generally in short supply; the shortfall being made up by known donors and so-called egg sharers, if possible siblings are catered for by embryos frozen in the same cycle.

Sperm donors may limit their donation to a single known family or withdraw their consent before the quota is reached whilst others may simply not be selected by that many recipients over the duration of their donation storage. Moreover, there is a mismatch in the numbers of donors and recipients in some racial groups resulting in a scarcity of suitable sperm. It is therefore the experience of many treatment centres and patients that there is not enough sperm to meet demand or not enough choice to satisfy need. Many patients arrange the import of sperm from abroad or travel abroad for treatment. Others may resort to online resources for sperm donors which can be risky in terms of safety and health as well as legally, including for the donor. Some such websites and services have operated illegally and been closed down.

There have been a number of initiatives over recent years which have been considered to have an effect on donor recruitment either as a primary factor or as a secondary result.

Much anxiety was generated in 2004 when the move was made to ensure that all UK registered donors (gametes or embryos) could be identifiable to offspring when those children reached their age of maturity at 18 [5]. The experience of our clinic [6] was that sperm donors in fact continued to be recruited at a similar rate but their demographics changed – they were older, more likely to be in a relationship and more likely to have children of their own. The immediate effect of the removal of anonymity was that donors recruited prior to the legal changeover could no longer be used for first pregnancies, reserved only for sibling treatments to allow completion of families. Unfortunately, shelving those previous donors (a bank built up over the course of 20 years) left a significant shortfall which has taken a further 10 years to recoup [7].

It has been argued that there should now be a lesser demand for sperm donation since intracytoplasmic sperm injection (ICSI) introduced in the early 90s greatly improved in vitro fertilization (IVF) outcomes for couples where there was a significant male factor problem. More recently, sophisticated surgical techniques for sperm retrieval have made IVF with

ICSI accessible to azoospermic men including some in whom spermatogenesis is extremely limited and resulting in respectable chances of pregnancy and live birth. This change in demand has been offset, at least in part, by the increasing numbers of women either single or in same-sex relationships who come forward for licensed treatment not only because of the legal and quality assurance of the regulated centre but also because for some, and in some areas only, there is a recognition that NHS funding is appropriate in these situations thus allowing better access.

It remains true, however, that since donor sperm insemination is a low tech, minimally invasive and arguably a more natural treatment than the complexity of IVF for a woman who has no fertility problem of her own, the use of donor sperm remains a first-line choice for some heterosexual couples also.

Egg donation has been available since the first IVF cycles were undertaken since the uterus can accept an embryo whatever its parental makeup. Thus, eggs donated by another woman can be fertilized with the male partner's sperm and placed into the recipient woman's uterus with rates of success that mirror those attributes of the donor rather than the recipient. Egg donors are relatively hard to come by and many egg donors donate specifically for someone they know (including a family member) rather than as a so-called altruistic donation to an unknown individual. Egg sharing, a well-established strategy, has facilitated egg donation for many years but is essentially limited to those women who are paying for their own treatment. It was anticipated that those women would be deterred from donating when the anonymity of donors was withdrawn since there became then the possibility of contact from genetic offspring whom they had never parented, with the distinct possibility that they may themselves remain childless. This is offset of course by the attraction of potentially affordable treatment that might otherwise be beyond their reach in a culture where state funding for fertility treatment remains rationed. Thus careful counselling of such donors is required to ensure they have fully considered the potential ramifications of their choice to donate both for their current situation and also for their long-term future.

With changes in patient pathways – blastocyst and single embryo transfer – and improvements in freezing technologies, increasing numbers of embryos are being stored for later use. With legal storage of up to at least 10 years it is unsurprising that many embryos are abandoned or destroyed. Donation to research makes use of a proportion of those embryos where couples are willing. A smaller number are donated to treat others. Given that the decision to donate is usually made some time after the embryos have been stored and often nearing the storage consent limits, the cost effectiveness of taking a couple through the counselling, screening and consents to allow for embryo donation is in doubt if there is not already an identified recipient. Few couples have an absolute need for embryo donation i.e. where there is both a female egg problem (usually age) and an insurmountable sperm problem. Embryo recipients may however, include single, older women and older women in same-sex relationships where the chances of pregnancy are age limited. Of course whilst the principle of using embryos that have already been created is hugely attractive both ethically and financially, the drawback of such treatment for them is little freedom in the selection of characteristics of the gamete providers in combination, which may mean that embryos are rejected.

2 Recruitment of Donors

It is clear then, that there will continue to be a need for donated gametes and/or embryos to fulfil couples' or individuals' family aspirations, including the potential for a woman to carry her own child. It is also clear that in the United Kingdom the need has yet to be fully met with shortfalls in both egg and sperm donations and the limitations relating to embryo donation. Good and effective donation programmes are required to support that need. In Europe, successful donation – particularly sperm donation – is centred in donor banks where the core business is recruitment and management of donors. In the United Kingdom there is an increasing awareness that such an approach is valuable; however, there must be an aspiration that such banks sit within the NHS as part of a fully resourced, fully funded fertility service. Sadly that is not likely and donation is already being exploited by private markets – sperm banks, recruitment agencies etc. An attempt to provide a state-run sperm donor service failed after two years in 2016 [8]. Fresh oocyte donation is currently the usual method although with improvement in vitrification techniques the idea of an oocyte bank is becoming more attractive for more efficient use of eggs and fairer distribution. Agencies managing embryo 'adoption' have developed in the United States and may alter the way embryo donation is managed in the United Kingdom in time. The steps to developing a functional national service is outwith the remit of this chapter; however, whatever the setting, good donor recruitment practice is key.

Donor recruitment requires consideration of what makes a good donor and also how best to look after those men and women who come forward to be donors.

2.1 What Makes a Good Donor?

Whilst not addressing all areas of donor recruitment and assessment, the joint paper [9] published on behalf of the British Fertility Society (BFS) and Royal College of Obstetricians and Gynaecologists (RCOG) in conjunction with the British Andology Society (BAS) and Association of Clinical Embryologists (ACE) and the Association of Biomedical Andrologists (ABA) remains the authoritative document for donor screening and is referred to by HFEA in its Code of Practice [10].

2.1.1 A Suitable Donor

There are some basic requirements to ensure that a gamete donor will provide the best chance of success for treated recipients (Box 31.1).

For cost effectiveness and success and to limit the risk of a child with problems, both egg and sperm donors will be selected on the basis of age (recommended under 36 years for egg donation; recommended under 41 years for sperm and the equivalent at the time of storage for each for embryo donors). Egg quality relates to age but efficient treatment requires a number of eggs to be available which can be retrieved

Box 31.1 Basic considerations for gamete and embryo donation recruitment

Egg donor	A good ovarian reserve
	Accessible ovaries
	Age limit
Sperm donor	Normal semen analysis
	Good freeze/thaw parameters
	Age limit
Embryo donors	Good quality embryos
	Age limits at the time of
	storage

easily; hence, egg donors need to have a good ovarian reserve and have ovaries that are readily accessible for oocyte retrieval. Sperm quality should be good (normal WHO parameters [11]) but also survive the freeze and thaw in good condition. A decision to accept a donor whose sperm could only be used through ICSI would be considered controversial. Clearly where gametes or embryos have been stored an effective and successful freeze programme is necessary.

2.1.2 A Safe Donor (Table 31.1)

2.1.2.1 Genetic Safety

Best practice dictates that all donors provide a good account of their family history in order to pick out any thread of an inheritable disorder. A specific concern should be further explored with them, including the possibility of genetic referral for further evaluation of the family. By way of screening a simple karyotype excludes sex chromosome duplications and will pick up significant translocations. Depending on the population of origin, common specific recessive disorders are sought (typically in the United Kingdom, Caucasian population cystic fibrosis as a minimum).

Genetic review cannot be comprehensive and many genetic conditions arise de novo in an embryo to cause problems for the individual in life however screening the donor as described will limit the risk of significant avoidable transmission of disease.

2.1.2.2 Infection Safety

The risk of transmitting infection from a donor to the birth mother and/or offspring depends on the treatment involved. Penetrative sexual intercourse is the significant factor for sexually transmitted infection e.g. Chlamydia and gonorrhoea, it is also well known as a route of transfer of blood-borne viruses (BBVs) such as HIV, Hepatitis B, Hepatitis C and HTLV.

The use of washed sperm for intrauterine insemination and all of the steps involved for IVF prior to embryo transfer means that that risk is almost certainly modified if not removed completely. Some studies have shown that the attachment to sperm of infective agents may play a role in transmission but firm evidence for the transmission of infection through gamete and embryo donation is lacking.

Whilst screening cannot be comprehensive, there is a duty to ensure that any risk is minimized. The starting point must be to ensure that the donor is free of significant infection at least at the time of donation.

Table 31.1 Screening tests for donors

Genetic	"Test" undertaken	Specifics	Notes
	Family and personal history	History and questionnaire GP corroboration	Questionnaire and personal interview carried out by a qualified and trained healthcare professional
	Karyotype	Chromosomal abnormalities Translocations	
	Autosomal recessive conditions	Cystic fibrosis (Caucasian) α- and β-Thalassaemia (Mediterranean, Middle Eastern, Indian subcontinent) Sickle cell disease (African, afro-carribean) Tay-Sachs (Eastern European Jewish)	
Infection	Examination	Herpes, warts	
	Bacterial screen	Syphilis Gonorrhoea Chlamydia	Validated test algorithm for T.pallidum Chlamydia & Gonococcus - NAT test of urine
	Blood borne viruses	HIV 1&2 HTLV 1&2 Hep B Hep C	Serum or plasma negative for anti-HIV 1&2, HbsAg, Anti- HBc Anti-HCV-Ab HTLV-1&2 when from or partner from high risk area. Consider malaria and T. cruzi
	Travel risk	eg Zika	Defer or decline
Matching	Blood group	Rhesus status	
	CMV		
Quarantine	sperm	180 days	Or NAT test for viral particles BBVs

A comprehensive medical and social history, taking into account sexual orientation and behaviours as well as travel history, will give information in relation to risk as well as histories of herpes or warts outbreaks. Current UK guidelines [9] dictate that prospective donors are screened for STIs including syphilis and BBVs including HTLV in risk populations.

Traditionally, screening is undertaken at the time of recruitment with relevant examination. For sperm donors screening is undertaken immediately prior to commencing sperm storage, at the end of the storage process and after six months quarantine period. Donors are asked to confirm that they have had no relevant exposure or symptoms on each occasion they attend.

It is considered acceptable (HFEA Licence condition T52 [10]) to undertake nucleic acid amplification testing (NAT) assessment for BBVs which gives a more immediate reassurance (excluding current viraemia) and which, combined with antibody testing, obviates the need for a prolonged quarantine period. This is particularly useful e.g. where there is a known sperm donor, who may be geographically distant from the treating centre, producing a limited number of ejaculates for immediate use.

Egg donors generally provide eggs that are donated fresh for immediate use although cryopreservation of eggs has improved considerably over recent years making more feasible the possibility of eggs being banked. Egg donors therefore are screened at recruitment and again immediately prior to oocyte retrieval. NAT assessment could be used appropriately in this setting.

All couples storing gametes will have been screened for BBV and, therefore, the battery of infection screening undertaken for embryo donation involves the exclusion of past or current infection by way of risk assessment since it is unlikely that they will have considered this option before completion of their own treatment and active extensive STI screening is not necessarily prerequisite to fertility treatment.

Cytomegalovirus (CMV) screening has caused much debate in the past. CMV may be transmitted by a number of routes but may be shed in semen by a donor who is immune. New and recurrent infections in pregnant women are a source of significant fetal and neonatal morbidity as well as long-term issues for affected offspring. Apparent immunity does not prevent shedding and in the woman does not prevent further infection. The uncertainty and the effect of high rates of CMV positivity and high rates of community acquisition, means that recommendations have ranged from only recruiting CMV negative donors (restrictive on donor recruitment) to ignoring the perceived risk on the basis that it may be no higher than that of community acquisition (the risk is almost certainly significantly less in egg and embryo donation). An updated review of this discussion is awaited.

The importance of reviewing a donor's travel history has been highlighted recently through the understanding of the risk of sexual transmission of Zika virus. Recommendations are that sperm donors travelling in a risk area (or who have had sex with a man who has travelled to a risk area) should be deferred from further donation for an extended period of time (or until NAT testing excludes Zika RNA in semen, or NAT test is negative for Zika virus in those who were asymptomatic). The risk of using samples already in store where this consideration has not been made is considered to be sufficiently small to allow their continued use. For any such recommendation, up to date advice on areas of risk and abstinence periods should be consulted.

2.1.3 A Matched Donor

Matching donors is an interesting topic since it raises a number of questions. In the United Kingdom, where couples are encouraged to tell children of their origins and where the genetic differences are therefore understood and accepted, attempting to 'hide' those differences by matching appearances seems rather disingenuous. It is important for children, however well informed, to feel that they 'fit in' and so although potentially at least related directly to one family parent, having a donor matched in general terms (hair colour, eye colour, build), may be of benefit. Blood group, the

old 'give-away' of illegitimacy, being less openly scrutinized is probably now effectively redundant (other than perhaps the benefits of taking rhesus status into account). Explicit in HFEA guidance is the understanding that ethnic origin need not dictate donor selection although clearly matching general characteristics will take this into account at least in part.

2.1.4 A Responsible and Informed Donor

Part of the process of donor recruitment must include counselling for the implications of what is proposed. This includes ensuring that the donor understands the nature and purpose of the history-taking and the screening tests, their limitations and their implications for them as an individual as well as potentially for their own family and future offspring in case of an unexpected positive result.

A donor needs to fully understand the process of donation. It is a big commitment not only physically to undergo ovarian stimulation and oocyte retrieval but also to attend over a period of some months to store sufficient sperm for use.

Donors also need to understand the legal implications of being a donor including their rights and responsibilities in relation to the recipients and their offspring. In the United Kingdom, donors give up any parental rights and responsibilities; they need to be able to be identified to genetic offspring but can receive no identifying information themselves. They are entitled only to know how many children have been born, the years of their birth and the sex of those children.

The most important area of information and counselling for gamete and embryo donors is psychosocial.

Donors may put restrictions on how their donation may be used but in practice such restrictions are rarely made. They must accept, therefore in principle, that they have no role in deciding who may be treated including the ethnic origin, sexual orientation, past history, age, socio-economic group etc. of recipients and therefore can have no influence over the 'nurture' of their genetic offspring which may be at odds with their own preference. Moreover, they may meet such a child who will ultimately be related to their own children and the rest of their own genetic family. This can sit uncomfortably with some and donation in that setting is better avoided. Many donors have not completed or perhaps not started their own family, or may not foresee having their own children and need to consider carefully what it would mean to them, and their current or future life partner, to be contacted by a child who is genetically related to them when they may not have offspring of their own.

There are numerous potential scenarios to consider which are individualized in an in depth discussion around the donor's motivation to donate and what they understand by what it would mean to them.

An emotionally engaged donor will have thought of the various scenarios which may affect them; the possibility that the donation may fail (more relevant where resource is limited e.g. egg and embryo donation); that they themselves will remain childless whilst their genetic children exist and may or may not contact them (a particularly poignant consideration for egg sharers); how they may tell partners and children including those that may not yet exist; how contact from a donation conceived child may affect them in time to come.

All donors in the United Kingdom are offered therapeutic counselling in addition to donor implications counselling in order to ensure that they have fully considered their actions and had the opportunity to review and revise their thoughts before giving consent and proceeding.

2.1.5 A Motivated and Well-Meaning Donor

Donors in the United Kingdom are generally considered to donate altruistically, in other words for no great gain to themselves (other than in the case of gamete – usually oocyte – sharers where some costs of private treatment may be offset by donation – considered to be treatment in kind). Review of donor compensation through the SEED report [3] and then in a 2011 consultation [12] took into account public and professional views on this, allowing currently up to a maximum of £750 compensation of donors without specific account of the costs incurred being required. Above this amount, proper account of the compensation given must be provided to the regulator.

2.1.6 A Valued Donor

In the setting of altruism it is clear that the sacrifice and consideration required to take the step of becoming a gamete or embryo donor should be cherished. On behalf of those recipients who need the help of these individuals it is important that donors are valued for their contributions.

With regard to the donation process this should be undertaken in as effective and efficient a manner as possible, allowing for flexibility of appointments and self-determination of the pace of the process. Donors

Box 31.2	
Perspective	
Clinic	Committed
	Sincere
	Honest/frank
	Motivated
	Reasonably 'normal'
	Passes the 'tests'
Recipient	Characteristics
	Which ones?
	• Appearance
	• Academic success
	• Sporting prowess
	• Interests
	• Match
	Pen portraits
	Success rates
	Integrity
Donor conceived child [12]	Curious about donor looks
	To learn about ancestry
	To learn about medical history
	So donor can learn about child
	To establish a relationship with the donor

should feel supported and be able to maintain contact with professionals involved, including counselling facilities, both during and after completion of their donation period.

Compensation is allowed and it is important that that is provided as agreed.

Finally there needs to be support both nationally and through centres for donors at a time when offspring may be acquiring identifying information about a donor. The responsibility for this process has been delegated by the HFEA to an external agency which will oversee introductions ensuring that they are undertaken in a sensitive and supportive fashion.

In summary the idea of a good donor comes from a variety of perspectives (Box 31.2).

3 Other Issues

3.1 Limiting Consent

Donors may limit their consent in a number of ways; they may reduce the number of families that may be produced from their donations (particularly pertinent for sperm donors where the legal limit 10 families is likely to be met, and known donors who are likely to consent only for their named recipient). They may also add qualification to the nature of the recipient (specific religious beliefs, sexuality, single women – may be considered by donors) although in practice this is rarely an issue and care needs to be taken to avoid frank prejudice against protected groups defined by the Equality Act 2010 [13].

Donors may also limit the use to which their donations are put e.g. sperm donors may decline for the sperm to be used through the IVF process but soley for insemination. Whilst the provision is made in the consent forms used, again, in practice it is rarely an issue.

Donors may withdraw or change their consent at any time. In the United Kingdom, this means that in principle any ongoing treatment would be cancelled, any embryos in store would be disposed of and there would be no opportunity to continue to treat the same family for siblings. Donors need to be aware of the potential implications of their decision to withdraw consent and whilst that decision is ultimately theirs to make it would be good practice to meet with them to ensure that they are clear about complete withdrawal or whether or not for example they might allow retention of already stored embryos or sibling treatments.

3.2 Known Donors

In some circumstances, in part because of recruitment issues, known donors come forward to donate for an individual or family. These may be family members, friends or acquaintances who want to help. The principles of screening and consent are the same. With regard to decision-making and consent there are of course some additional discussions to be had. Known donors will have a different relationship with the recipient and ultimately any child resulting from their donation. Whilst they may not be intimately involved in the family they do need to consider how that relationship would work and what their feelings might be if it changed – including in the event of no child, or a baby with problems.

3.3 Importing Donated Sperm

Whilst practice in other countries is beyond the remit of this chapter, it is important to note that Persons Responsible (those individuals responsible for the legal compliance of a licenced centre) are obliged to vouchsafe that any reproductive material brought to their centre for treatment purposes has been procured in a fashion that would match the legal and Code of Practice requirements of the United Kingdom (10). This includes assurances regarding donor payment.

3.4 Informal Sperm Donation

By nature of their procurement oocytes and embryos destined for donation will always originate in a licensed centre in the United Kingdom. Over years however a number of different mechanisms for sperm donation have been used. The growth of the internet has allowed contact networks of donors and recipients to develop and companies tapping into those networks have appeared and disappeared over time.

There is a fine line between the potentially ill-advised private recruitment of a donor in this way and the illegal activity of unlicensed procurement and distribution. In both situations however, the donor may find himself legally liable for costs relating to a child that is genetically his. Registration of a donor through a licensed centre devolves his parental rights over, and responsibilities for, a child; he is no longer the legal parent of any child born following the use of his donated sperm. In practice this then means that the child has no rights of inheritance (including nationality) from the donor and the donor has no financial or other parental responsibilities to the child or its mother. In the case of informal donation however that is not the case and whilst men may believe that they have separated themselves by some form of written agreement, it is not clear that that would provide the expected protection if challenged in court. They also may have a right of access to a child conferred upon them through the courts which is highly unlikely to be supported for a registered donor except in exceptional circumstances (e.g. a known donor otherwise closely involved in the family).

4 Conclusion

The recruitment of gamete and embryo donors is a complex process not least for the relative scarcity of such individuals. There are significant steps to be taken to ensure they are suitable candidates both in terms of effectiveness and safety and also in relation to their own expectations. It is important that donors are well informed, well motivated, valued and supported.

In this way the integrity of the relationship between the donor and donor-conceived offspring can be upheld ensuring the most satisfying and satisfactory outcome for all.

References

[1] Barton, M, Walker, K and Wiesner BP. (1945) Artificial insemination. *BMJ* 1, 40–43.

[2] Human Fertilisation and Embryology Act 1990. HMSO London.

[3] HFEA. (2005) *SEED Report – a report on the Human Fertilisation and Embryology Authority's review of sperm, egg and embryo donation in the UK.* London.

[4] HFEA. (2014) *Egg and sperm donation in the UK: 2012–2013.* London.

[5] Human Fertilisation and Embryology Authority (Disclosure of Donor Information) Regulations 2004. HMSO London.

[6] Paul, S, Harbottle, S and Stewart, JA (2006) Recruitment of sperm donors: the Newcastle upon Tyne experience 1994–2003. *Hum Reprod* 21; 150–158.

[7] Gudipati, M, Pearce, K, Prakash, A et al. (2013) The sperm donor program over 11 years at Newcastle Fertility Centre. *Hum Fertil* 16; 258–265.

[8] www.bbc.co.uk/news/uk-37786576.

[9] Association of Biomedical Andrologists, Association of Clinical Embryologists, British Andrology Society, British Fertility Society and Royal College of Obstetricians and Gynaecologists. (2008) UK Guidelines for the medical and laboratory screening of sperm, egg and embryo donors (2008). *Hum Fert* 11, 201–210.

[10] HFEA. (2016) *Code of practice.* 8th Edn. HFEA. London.

[11] World Health Organisation. (2010) *WHO laboratory manual for the examination and processing of human sperm.* 5th Edn. WHO Press. Switzerland. ISBN 978 92 4 154778 9

[12] Beeson, D, Jennings, P and Kramer, W. (2011) Offspring searching for their sperm donors: how family type shapes the process. *Hum Reprod* 26, 2415–2124.

[13] Equality Act 2010. HMSO London.

Gamete Donation

Alison Taylor

1 Introduction

1.1. Types of Treatment Using Gamete Donation

Assisted conception techniques using donated gametes includes the use of donated sperm in donor insemination (DI) or in vitro fertilisation (IVF) with donor sperm (DIVF), egg donation or embryo donation.

1.1.1 Donor Sperm

Use of donor sperm has fallen dramatically since the introduction of intracytoplasmic sperm injection (ICSI) for severe male factor fertility and the ability to surgically retrieve sperm directly from the testis or epididymis for men with azoospermia (Figure 32.1). This trend may be reversing slightly since 2010: 4,452 cycles of DI were performed in 2012 in the United Kingdom compared to 4,101 in 2011, and 3,878 in 2010. This recent increase reflects an increasing demand for the use of donor sperm from single women and same-sex couples [1].

1.1.2 Egg Donation

The majority of egg donation cycles are anonymous with a smaller proportion of cycles using a known donor such as a relative or friend. Anonymous donors may be altruistic non-treatment seeking donors or egg-sharing donors who donate eggs as part of their own IVF treatment cycle. The demand for egg donation increases in women over 40 years, and in women over 45 years more treatment cycles are now performed using donor eggs than using their own eggs (Figure 32.2) [2].

1.1.3 Embryo Donation

Embryo donation is not commonly performed, but may be an option for couples or individuals who need both donor eggs and donor sperm to conceive.

Embryos are normally donated by couples who have frozen embryos following their own treatment, and no longer wish or need to keep them for their own use.

1.2 Proportion of ART Cycles Using Donated Gametes in the United Kingdom

In 2013, there were 48,477 fresh IVF cycles and 4,611 DI cycles in the United Kingdom. 5% of these fresh IVF cycles used donated sperm, 4% used donated eggs and less than 1% used both donated eggs and sperm, or donated embryos (Figure 32.3). Therefore, in total, just under 1 in 10 IVF cycles used donated gametes. 2% of the 13,353 frozen embryo transfer cycles in 2013 used donated embryos [1].

1.3 Proportion of Patients Having Fertility Treatment with Donated Gametes Who Are Single or in a Same-Sex Partnership

Of the 6,285 patients accessing fertility treatment with donated gametes in 2013, almost two-thirds registered with a male partner, 15% had no registered partner and 21% registered with a female partner. Women in same-sex partnerships may choose to donate eggs to each other (Figure 32.4) [1].

2 Screening Gamete Donors

Screening of gamete donors is addressed in Chapter 31.

3 Counselling

3.1 HFEA Requirements

Under the HFEA Code of Practice [3] it is obligatory for clinics in the United Kingdom to offer implications counselling to potential gamete donors, and also to individuals or couples seeking to use donated gametes or embryos in their treatment. Specific

Number of cycles started each year.

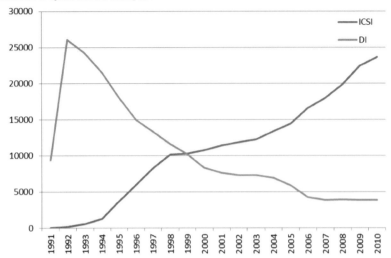

Fig. 32.1 Number of cycles of DI and ICSI in UK 1991–2010 (source HFEA)

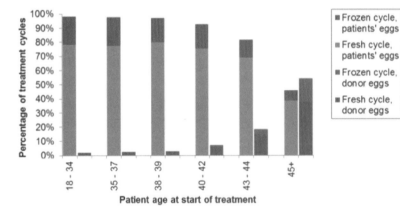

Fig. 32.2 The distribution of different treatment types by age (source HFEA 2012)

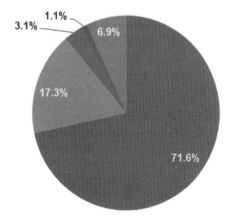

Fig. 32.3 Proportion of IVF and DI cycles started in UK (source HFEA data 2012)

Table 32.1 Cycles of DIVF and DI in women registered with a female partner

Year	Number of DIVF cycles	No. Live births	No. DI cycles	No. Live births
2010	568	177 (31.2%)	1028	141 (13.7%)
2011	766	223 (29.1%)	1271	148 (11.6%)

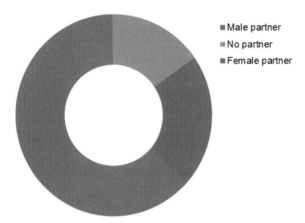

■ Male partner
■ No partner
■ Female partner

Fig. 32.4 Partnership status of donor gamete recipients in UK (source HFEA 2013)

counselling about the use of donated gametes or embryos should be separate from the implications counselling of treatment in general and should take place before treatment starts.

3.2 Scope of Counselling

Counselling will normally discuss issues such as legal aspects, rights and responsibilities for donors and recipients, as well as exploring how individuals may feel, who to tell, whether or not to tell a child he or she was born as a result of use of donated gametes and if so when, what information will be available about a donor to parents of a donor-conceived child and to the child him- or herself at the age of 18.

4 Sperm Donation

4.1 Indications for Sperm Donation

4.1.1 Azoospermia

Non-obstructive azoospermia with no sperm found in testicular biopsies or for those men unwilling or unable to go through surgical sperm retrieval.

4.1.2 Severe Oligoasthenoteratozoospermia (OATs)

Most couples will normally choose to try using the male partner's sperm with ICSI, but a small proportion of couples may elect to use donor sperm or resort to use donor sperm if IVF/ICSI is repeatedly unsuccessful.

4.1.3 Single Women

In the last two decades there have been an increasing number of single women seeking help to conceive using donor sperm. In 2013, 943 (15%) of the patients using donor gametes in the United Kingdom were single women.

4.1.4 Women Registered with a Female Partner

An increasing number of IVF and DI cycles are being performed for women who register for treatment with a female partner (Table 32.1). In 2011 there was a 36% increase in IVF cycles with donor sperm performed compared to 2010 and a 24% increase in the number of DI cycles to these women.

4.1.5 Other Indications

Other indications include avoiding transmission of genetic risk to children, severe forms of ejaculatory failure refractive to treatment and rarely where there has been severe Rhesus isoimmunisation.

4.2 Sources of Donor Sperm

All sperm donors used in UK licensed clinics are registered with the HFEA and have to undergo appropriate screening tests (see Chapter 31) before the sperm can be used. Sperm is cryopreserved while these tests are completed. Most donor sperm is used anonymously, but some individuals or couples will choose to use a known donor. Many clinics in the United Kingdom import sperm from one of the sperm banks abroad, such as those in Denmark or the United States, because the cost, time and resources required to recruit donors themselves is too high. [1]. Sourcing sperm abroad may help meet the need for specific matches for particular ethnic groups. The number of imports of donor sperm has increased steadily since 2004 and now accounts for approximately a third of donor sperm used in the United Kingdom (Figure 32.5).

Table 32.2 DIVF and DIUI Live birth rates national data cycles 2012 (HFEA)

Age (years)	IVF own eggs with donor sperm	IVF own eggs with partner's sperm	DIUI (unstimulated)	DIUI (stimulated)
<35	40.3%	32.2%	14.9%	19.7%
35–37	30.5%	27.4%	11.6%	14.1%
38–39	26.9%	19.9%	7.7%	10.5%
40–42	16.7%	13.4%	3.8%	5.7%
43–44	6.6%	5.1%		
45+		0.8%		

Number

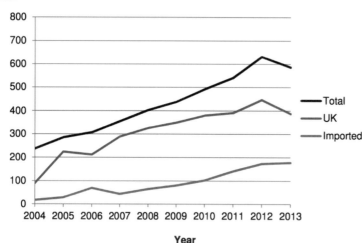

Fig. 32.5 Number of newly registered sperm donors in UK 2004–2013 (source HFEA data)

4.3 Factors Affecting Success of Treatment with Donor Sperm

4.3.1 Female Age

As with other types of assisted conception treatment, increasing female age adversely affects the chances of a successful outcome (Table 32.2). National data for live birth rates following IVF for 2012 demonstrate that for each age group, use of donor sperm rather than partner sperm was associated with at least as good as, if not better, chance of a successful outcome.

4.3.2 Number of Cycles

Cumulative pregnancy rates over a number of cycles of DIUI are similar to the pregnancy rate expected for couples trying to conceive naturally over several months to a year for each age group [4] (Figure 32.6).

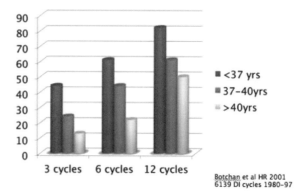

Botchan et al HR 2001
6139 DI cycles 1980-97

Fig. 32.6 Cumulative live birth rates for DIUI by age groups

4.3.3 Fresh Versus Frozen Sperm

Prior to concerns about viral transmission with donated sperm, and quarantining by freezing while screening for HIV, hepatitis B and C, donor sperm was used fresh rather than frozen. Historical data suggest that pregnancy rates using fresh sperm were higher than when frozen thawed sperm was subsequently used [4]. However safety concerns mean licensed clinics now only use frozen screened donor sperm.

4.3.4 Intracervical Versus Intrauterine Insemination

A Cochrane review demonstrated a significantly higher chance of a live birth per woman treated with cryopreserved donor sperm by intrauterine insemination compared to intracervical insemination with an odds ratio of 1.98 (1.02, 3.86 95% CI) [5].

4.3.5 Stimulated Versus Natural Cycles for DIUI

Pregnancy rates in cycles using ovarian stimulation give higher live birth rates than in natural cycles (Table 32.2). 75% of the 3,334 cycles of DIUI performed in the United Kingdom in 2013 were with stimulation, 25% without [2]. The risks of multiple pregnancy need to be considered when using stimulation, and some women may prefer to minimise this risk by using natural cycles.

5 Egg donation

5.1 Definitions: Egg Donation and Egg Sharing

Egg donation: Altruistic donation of all eggs resulting from a stimulation cycle to one or more recipients.
Egg sharing: A woman undergoing IVF treatment who donates some of her eggs to a recipient and keeps the remainder for her own use. The egg sharer's treatment is normally highly subsidised or free.

5.2 Indications

Indications for the use of donor eggs include ovarian failure (primary and secondary, premature or physiological), reduced ovarian reserve, poor quality eggs, repeated failed IVF especially in older women and a small number of women who wish to avoid passing on a genetic risk to their child(ren).

5.3 Should Patients With Low Ovarian Reserve Only Be Offered Egg Donation?

Many patients with a low ovarian reserve are excluded from eligibility for NHS-funded IVF using their own eggs because a high FSH level or low AMH level is used to exclude offering treatment. These patients are often told that their only option for conception is with donor eggs, as the likelihood of a successful outcome using their own eggs is negligible. However, some patients, particularly those who are younger, may still have a reasonable chance of conception even with a limited number of eggs at egg collection and will normally prefer to try using their own eggs before moving on to egg donation. It may feel easier to accept the use of donor eggs if they have been allowed to try using their own eggs first. Reduced numbers of eggs in young patients does not necessarily mean the eggs are always poorer in quality. It will mean the chances of pregnancy in one cycle are less than those women with normal or high ovarian reserve as these women will have a larger number of embryos from which to choose for transfer, but cumulative data using the same number of eggs over more than one cycle give the same chances of a live birth.

Data from Lister Fertility Clinic 2005–2014 showing live birth rate per egg collection by number of eggs obtained and age group can be seen in Figure 32.7. Even with very limited numbers of eggs at egg collection (1–2 eggs) the chance of a live birth in women under 38 years is 15%. With 3–4 eggs, the likelihood of live birth increases to 25–28%. Many of these patients with low ovarian reserve have been denied treatment elsewhere and recommended egg donation.

5.4 The Demand for Donor Eggs

It is difficult to quantify the total demand for donor eggs in the United Kingdom, as an unknown number of couples seek treatment abroad for reasons such as the following:

- Long waiting lists
- Shortage of specific ethnic /racial matches
- To avoid the possibility of children born following treatment being able to find out the identity of the donor later
- For more information about the donors, including pictures, available in some countries e.g. USA

Following the change in compensation for egg donors in the United Kingdom in 2012, the number of new non-egg-sharing donor registrations increased to approximately 1,100 in 2013 compared to approximately half this number between 2004 and 2008 [1]. Increased public awareness of the need for egg donors may also have contributed to the rise in new donors. In the United Kingdom 2,148 cycles of egg donation were performed in 2013, a third of these using egg-sharing donors [2]. In Europe the number of egg donation

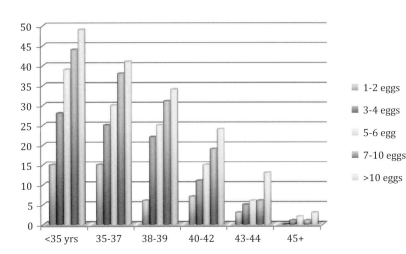

Fig. 32.7 Live birth rate per egg collection by age group and number of eggs collected (source Lister Fertility Clinic 2005–2014, 20,003 egg collections)

Legend:
- 1-2 eggs
- 3-4 eggs
- 5-6 egg
- 7-10 eggs
- >10 eggs

cycles rose from 15,028 in 2007 to 24,517 in 2010 and represents approximately 4% IVF cycles performed. In the United States the proportion of cycles using donor eggs is higher at approximately 12%.

5.5 Risks for Egg Donors

Egg donors need to be carefully counselled about potential risks of donating eggs before they consent to proceed to treatment. These risks include

- Risks of ovarian stimulation
  - Side effects of medication used for superovulation
  - Ovarian hyperstimulation syndrome (severe 1–2%)
- Risks of egg collection [10]
  - Pelvic infection (0.3–0.6%)
  - Ovarian torsion (0.1%)
  - Injury to blood vessels or other pelvic organs (0.03–0.5%)
  - Risks from GA / sedation (1 in 10,000 adverse reaction)
- Psychological/emotional factors including discussion about preparing for the possible future contact or lack of contact from a child born as a result of their donation, how they might feel if they experience difficulty conceiving themselves.

5.6 Expenses for Egg Donors

In 2012 regulations changed in the United Kingdom to allow expenses of up to £750 per cycle of egg donation, with the provision to claim for additional expenses to cover higher costs such as travel, childcare or accommodation. Donors coming from overseas to the United Kingdom are entitled to the same expenses as those living in the United Kingdom but are not entitled to cover excess expenses for overseas travel.

5.7 Assessment of Potential Egg Donors/Sharers

Figure 32.8 shows the pathway used to assess potential egg donors or egg sharers at the Lister Fertility Clinic. Regular optional patient information evenings are held for women interested in becoming an egg sharer or donor. All patients have an initial blood test for anti-mullerian hormone (AMH) and an ultrasound scan, following which three appointments are made:

1. Clinical: with a doctor to review medical, gynaecological, obstetric and family histories, discuss what is involved in going through a cycle of ovarian stimulation and egg collection with potential problems and risks, number of eggs needed for egg sharing, what happens if fewer eggs are obtained at egg collection and the chances of a successful outcome if doing egg sharing.
2. Counselling: with a counsellor for implications counselling regarding donation of their eggs
3. Nursing: With a member of the dedicated egg donation nursing team to have the opportunity to discuss practicalities of a treatment cycle, the waiting list and for the nursing team to record matching details.

If there are any concerns raised at any of these appointments regarding suitability to be an egg

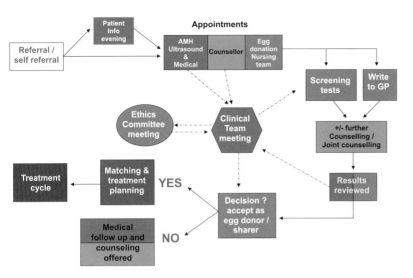

Fig. 32.8 Assessment of a potential egg donor or egg sharer at Lister Fertility Clinic

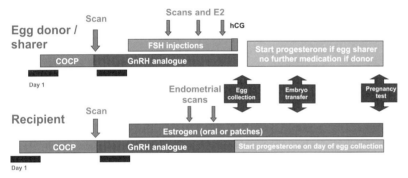

Fig. 32.9 Synchronisation of egg donor/ sharer with egg recipient

donor, it may be referred to a clinical team meeting for case discussion. If proceeding, the egg donation nursing team organises the screening tests, and a letter is sent to the patient's GP to confirm medical history and ensure they are not aware of any reasons why the individual should not donate. Further counselling sessions are available if required by the potential donor and are mandatory for any couples considering known donation, where individual counselling sessions are followed by joint counselling sessions before treatment begins. Results of the screening tests, and response to the GP letter, are reviewed by the clinical teams and any concerns are referred back to a clinical team meeting. Occasionally, cases may be referred to the Ethics Committee for consideration, such as requests for inter-generational familial donation. If the potential egg donor is accepted for treatment, the nursing team matches the donor with a recipient and initiates synchronisation of their cycles for a treatment cycle. If information suggests it would not be appropriate to proceed with egg donation, a

doctor's consultation and further counselling support are offered to discuss their options.

5.8 Synchronising Cycles and Endometrial Preparation

Most egg donation cycles use fresh eggs, so the recipient's endometrium needs to be prepared for embryo transfer in synchrony with the donor's stimulation cycle. If not contraindicated, the oral contraceptive pill can be used for both parties to help with synchronisation (Figure 32.9). Alternatively, GnRH analogues may be used to help with synchronising the start of stimulation for a donor and start of endometrial preparation for a recipient. Recipients who are postmenopausal on hormone replacement therapy (HRT) can continue their normal HRT until just before the donor is ready to begin stimulation, when a withdrawal bleed is initiated before beginning endometrial preparation. Oral or transdermal oestrogen may be used for the recipient's endometrial preparation.

Table 32.3 HFEA data 2011–2012 live birth rates by age comparing own eggs and donor eggs

Age (years)	IVF own eggs 2011–2012	No. cycles own eggs	IVF donor eggs 2011–2012	No. cycles with donor eggs
<35	32.5%	41,075	33.6%	464
35–37	27.3%	21,017	37.1%	693
38–39	20.3%	14,931	33.9%	657
40–42	13.2%	12,430	34.8%	1263
43–44	4.3%	3,991	33.3%	913
45+			34.1%	1431

Table 32.4 National data for egg-sharing donors 2011–2012 HFEA

	Egg-sharing donors	Egg-sharing recipients	All egg donation cycles
Cycles	1,773	1,625	5,421
Live Birth rate	38.1%	36.1%	34.5%

5.9 Luteal Phase Support and Hormonal Support for Early Pregnancy

In an egg donation pregnancy, the recipient has no corpus luteum to provide hormonal support for the luteal phase and early pregnancy, so exogenous oestrogen and progesterone are required to 12 weeks gestation. After the donor's egg collection, the recipient continues oestrogen and adds progesterone, either as vaginal pessaries (e.g. cyclogest, utrogestan) or injectable progesterone (e.g. gestone, lubion).

5.10 Use of Frozen Donor Eggs

The use of frozen stored eggs for egg donation has the advantage of removing the need to synchronise donor and recipient's cycles. Thawed eggs can be inseminated with the partner's sperm and replaced in the recipient, whose endometrium can either be prepared with a natural ovulatory cycle if she has regular cycles or using an HRT protocol if not.

Recently published national data for egg donation cycles performed in 2013 in the United States has, for the first time, given success rates for fresh and frozen donor oocytes. In 2013, 8,922 cycles of egg donation with fresh donor oocytes were performed with a live birth rate of 49.6% per recipient cycle started. In the same year 2,227 cycles of egg donation using banked donor oocytes were performed with a live birth rate of 43.2% per recipient cycle started [6].

5.11 Success Rates of Egg Donation in the United Kingdom

Data from the HFEA (Table 32.3) shows the age-related drop in live birth rate per cycle started for women using their own eggs in 2011–2012. For recipients of donor eggs, the age of the recipient does not affect the outcome with similar live birth rates through all age groups.

5.11.1 Is the Chance of Pregnancy for Egg-Sharing Donors and Recipients Compromised?

When considering egg sharing, it is important to ensure that the chances of pregnancy and live birth for egg-sharing donors and their recipients is not significantly compromised by the sharing of eggs. National data from the HFEA for 2011–2012 shows the chance of live birth for egg-sharing donors is no different to that for recipients and that both are as good as, if not better than, for all egg donation cycles, and better than the live birth rate for women under 35 years undertaking IVF with their own eggs (Tables 32.3 and 32.4)

5.12 Risks of Egg Donation Pregnancies

Several studies confirm the increased risk of both pregnancy-induced hypertension (PIH) and pre-eclampsia (PE) in egg donation pregnancies, irrespective of the age of the recipient [7,8]. The risk of PIH in egg donation pregnancies is 18–23%, and pre-eclampsia is 11%. Some studies also suggest there may be an increase in first trimester bleeding in egg donation pregnancies, and one study reported a 12% risk of postpartum haemorrhage [8]. Operative delivery rates are often high in these women [12]. Older women may have a higher incidence of the co-morbidities that could increase obstetric risk such as obesity, hypertension and diabetes. Careful medical assessment is needed for older women undergoing egg donation treatment to identify risk factors for complications in pregnancy. For some women referral to an obstetric physician may be appropriate for pre-pregnancy counselling and assessment to plan care for pregnancy. Women with Turner's syndrome may also have significant congenital cardiac disease and need specific cardiological assessment prior to pregnancy.

5.13 Known Egg Donation

In known egg donation the recipient knows the identity of the donor, who is usually a family member or friend. Some patients prefer to know the person donating the eggs, as they will know more about their characteristics and personality than with an anonymous donor, and, where a family member is used such as a sister, there will be shared genetic background. Known egg donation needs careful consideration and counselling of all parties concerned, to ensure there is no coercion of the donor and that everyone (including the partners of the recipient and donor) are comfortable to proceed. This normally involves separate medical and counselling appointments for the recipient and donor, followed by joint counselling sessions with the donor, recipient and their partners. Specific issues that need exploration include how both parties might feel if the treatment is successful or unsuccessful, if there is a miscarriage or a fetal abnormality detected in pregnancy, who else will know within their circle of family and friends, what information a child born as a result of treatment might be told and what the relationship between the child and donor might be.

5.14 Ethical Issues/Controversies

Egg donation means that pregnancy is possible for women who have passed the physiological menopause. This raises the issue of whether there should be an upper age limit for the recipients of donor eggs, whether the age of their partner, or whether they have a partner at all, should be taken into account, and how these factors might impact on the welfare of any child(ren) born following treatment, when deciding whether to offer treatment. Requests for inter-generational gamete donation within the same family

such as daughter-to-mother egg donation, or a father wanting to donate sperm to his son and partner may provoke interesting discussions within clinical teams, and sometimes referral to an Ethics Committee before deciding whether to proceed or not with treatment.

6 Legal Issues of Gamete Donation

Legal aspects of gamete donation in the United Kingdom are described in the Human Fertilisation and Embryology Act (1990) and subsequent amended Act 2008 [9].

A woman who gives birth to a child following treatment with donor gametes, is the legal mother of the child and her husband or partner is the legal father, unless he can show he did not consent to treatment. A donor must be of legal age (i.e. 18 years or over) and donors have no legal rights or responsibilities to child(ren) born as a result of their donation. The Human Fertilisation and Embryology Authority (HFEA) keeps a register of donors, and outcomes of all treatment cycles using donated gametes. Donor anonymity is no longer protected in the United Kingdom, several other European countries and Australia [11], and all donors must consent to identifying information being made available to children born following treatment once they are adults. A donor may withdraw their consent to the use of their gametes at any time before gametes or embryos are replaced into a recipient and a recipient may not freeze embryos unless the gamete donor has given consent. If a donor withholds significant information about their medical or family history that results in a medical problem for a child born after treatment, they could be sued. No more than 10 families can be created within the United Kingdom from one donor [11].

7 Useful Sources of Information and Support for Patients, Donors and Donor-Conceived Individuals

7.1 HFEA: www.hfea.gov.uk

The HFEA is a useful source of information for gamete donor, gamete recipients, parents of donor-conceived children and donor-conceived individuals themselves. Parents can find out how to apply for non-identifying information about a donor for their child. Donor-conceived people can find out how to apply for non-identifying information about the donor at 16 years of age and identifying information about the donor at 18 years of age.

7.2 Donor Conception Network: www.dcnetwork.org

The donor conception network provides support and information for individuals or couples considering use of donor gametes and for children born following treatment with donor gametes, using literature (for adults and children), workshops, counselling and support groups.

7.3 Daisy Network: www.daisynetwork.org.uk

The Daisy Network provides support and information for women who have experienced a premature menopause.

7.4 Donor Sibling Link: www.hfea.gov.uk/donor-sibling-link.html

The HFEA has also set up the Donor Sibling Link to enable donor siblings who were conceived after 1 August 1991 to find out information and potentially contact each other. Free counselling support is available via the HFEA for donor-conceived people who are considering applying for information about the donor or donor siblings.

7.5 Donor-Conceived Register: www.donorconceivedregister.org.uk

This register enables people conceived through donated sperm or eggs before 1991, their donors and half-siblings to exchange information and, where desired, to contact each other.

References

1. Egg and Sperm Donation in the UK 2012–2013 HFEA Report published 2014 www.hfea.gov.uk/docs/Egg_and_sperm_donation_in_the_UK_2012-2013.pdf.

2. Fertility Treatment in 2013: Trends and Figures HFEA Report published 2014 www.hfea.gov.uk/docs/HFEA_Fertility_Trends_and_Figures_2013.pdf.

3. HFEA Code of Practice 8th Edition 2015 www.hfea.gov.uk/docs/HFEA_Code_of_Practice_8th_Edtion_(Apr_2015).pdf.

4. Botchan A, Hauser R, Gamzu R et al. Results of 6139 artificial insemination cycles with donor spermatozoa. *Human Reproduction* 2001; 16: 2298–304.

5. Besselink DE, Farquhar C, Kremer JAM et al. Cervical insemination versus intra-uterine insemination of donor sperm for subfertility. *Cochrane Database of Systematic Reviews* 2008; Issue 2. Art. No.: CD000317. doi: 10.1002/14651858.CD000317.pub3.

6. SART data paper for frozen OD eggs in USA.

7. H Letur-Koenirsch et al. O-163 Pregnancies issued from egg donation are associated to a higher risk of hypertensive pathologies then control ART pregnancies. Results of a large comparative cohort study. Abstracts. ESHRE 2014.

8. Abdalla HI, Billet A, Kan AK et al. Obstetric outcome in 232 ovum donation pregnancies. *British Journal of Obstetrics and Gynaecology* 1998; 105(3): 332–7.

9. Human Fertilisation and Embryology Act 1990, amended 2008. http://webarchive.nationalarchives.gov.uk/20130107105354/http://www.dh.gov.uk/prod_consum_dh/groups/dh_digitalassets/@dh/@en/documents/digitalasset/dh_080206.pdf.

10. Sarhan A, Muasher SJ. Surgical complications of in vitro fertilisation. *Middle East Fertility Society Journal* 2007; 12: 1–6.

11. Gong D, Liu YL, Zheng Z et al. An overview on ethical issues about sperm donation. *Asian Journal of Andrology* 2009; 11: 645–52.

12. Kort DH, Gosselin J, Choi JM et al. Pregnancy after age 50: defining risks for mother and child. *American Journal of Perinatology* 2012; 29: 245–50.

Chapter 33

Training Opportunities in Reproductive Medicine

Ippokratis Sarris

Reproductive medicine is an exciting specialty. It encompasses both medicine and surgery. It brings together far-flung disciplines such as gynaecology, endocrinology, genetics, embryology, andrology, imaging and more. It deals with women, men and yet to be born individuals. It is a constantly evolving field as our understanding of the complex process of reproduction is enriched at a break-neck pace. It is a specialty within which there are numerous job opportunities and career paths. An area where both academic and clinical work can coexist. Nevertheless, it is not always clear what the best pathways to gain training are.

All the chapters up to this point have been aimed at conveying scientific and practical knowledge in the field of reproductive medicine and assisted conception. The purpose of this chapter is different, in that it aims to shed some light in to the different training pathways available to junior doctors contemplating training and a career in reproductive medicine in the United Kingdom.

When choosing a training programme, it should be one that is suitable to the needs of the trainee and matches their expectations.

1 Future Job Role – The Destination

It is beyond the scope of this chapter to try and predict the future job market, as this is in a constant state of flux. The Royal College of Obstetrics and Gynaecology (RCOG) is always in a process of looking at the needs of the profession. However, as national needs and funding priorities change, predicting the future is not possible. Although presently there appears to be a focus on primarily providing delivery suite cover and a reduction in the NHS funding for IVF, and with the current financial climate it is unlikely that this is going to improve in the near future, subfertility is increasing in the general population and more couples are seeking treatment. Nevertheless, the National Institute for Clinical Excellence (NICE) has made some robust recommendations regarding the ideal funding for couples requiring fertility treatment and patients are willing to turn to the private provision of care in clinics around the United Kingdom. Therefore, the need for trained doctors in the field of reproductive medicine and surgery will not necessarily diminish.

When looking at a training pathway, traines should first start by looking at the type of job they would like to have in the future. Job requirements are specific to the needs that the person employed in them will undertake. These requirements differ according to the knowledge and skills required to fulfil them. Jobs in stand alone IVF units deliver specialised tertiary services. Jobs in a clinic or unit within a hospital setting tend to deliver secondary with or without tertiary services. In the NHS setting, emphasis is placed either in secondary or tertiary services and this is reflected in the types of NHS consultant posts. These tend to be either subspecialist consultant posts in reproductive medicine or general obstetric and gynaecology consultant posts with a special interest in reproductive medicine or subfertility.

In broad terms the differences between these posts can be summarised in Table 33.1.

A subspecialist consultant is more likely to be dealing with the medical, surgical and assisted conception management of tertiary subfertility patients and complex cases. In addition, they are expected to take on a leadership role in the field, be active in research and contribute to teaching.

A consultant with a special interest in subfertility is more likely to be dealing with the secondary-level management of patients and perhaps be involved with the running of a satellite unit for an assisted conception unit. Complex cases or those requiring tertiary level services, such as IVF, are usually referred on. Although this distinction might be relatively clear within their NHS consultant job plan, on occasion consultants who are not accredited subspecialists might still be employed to work at a private IVF unit outside of their NHS contractual obligations.

Table 33.1 Differences between type of NHS consultant posts

Subspecialist Consultant	Consultant with special interest
Mainly will be working in a tertiary teaching hospital	Mainly will be working in a district general hospital
More than 50% of the work load will be related to subfertility	Will have a significant work load related to general O&G duties
No (usually) or minimal obstetric workload	Will have some clinics for secondary subfertility care
	Might or might not work as a satellite for an external IVF unit

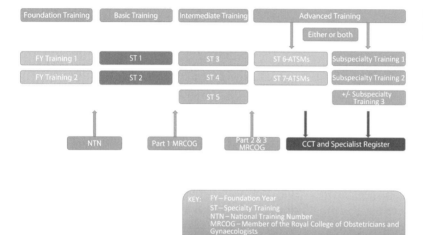

Fig. 33.1 Schematic layout of GMC accredited training in Obstetrics and Gynaecology

These two different types of posts require a different skill set to fulfil and consequently different training opportunities.

2 Training Programmes – The Pathway

In the United Kingdom there are two potential ways to train in reproductive medicine. One of them is accredited by the GMC and the other one is not. The GMC accredited pathway involves completion of either a Subspecialty Training (SST) Programme or an RCOG Advanced Training Study Module (ATSM). However, training can be gained through non-GMC accredited fellowships and the British Fertility Society (BFS) offers the opportunity to apply and gain certifications in modules relevant to practicing in the field.

2.1 GMC Accredited Training

The two GMC accredited training programmes, subspecialty training and RCOG ATSM, have very distinct and different objectives, entry criteria, structure and curriculum. These different training objectives reflect the different types of career pathways intended for those completing them. Subspecialist trained doctors are usually expected to take up subspecialist consultant posts, whilst ATSM trained doctors usually take up general consultant posts with a special interest in fertility. This is reflected by a recent RCOG survey that found that of those that remained in the United Kingdom and place of work was known, over 75% of trainees completing subspecialty training had moved in to a pure subspecialist consultant post.

2.1.1 Entry Criteria

The entry criteria for both subspecialty training and ATSM can be found on the RCOG website. Both are undertaken at the earliest during the last two years of the general core training programme, and once all the intermediate training competencies have been achieved (Figure 33.1). Trainees are expected to have passed all their membership exams (MRCOG). Applicants should usually hold a National Training Number (NTN) and should have completed satisfactorily year 5 before registering (i.e. be at a level of ST6/7, SpR 4/5 or on equivalent LAT). However, both types of training programmes can be entered and completed by non-training grade doctors. The ATSM can be completed by SAS doctors and consultants as long as they have completed the equivalent of the intermediate competences, have completed a minimum of 5 years in O&G or hold a UK CCT or CESR and are entered on the UK Specialist register in O&G. Subspecialty training programmes can be completed by candidates who hold a UK CCT or CESR and are entered on the UK Specialist register in O&G.

2.1.2 How to Apply

All applications and registrations are prospective. Although previous experience can contribute to the development of competence, the assessment of competence can only be performed following registration.

To register for the ATSM in subfertility and reproductive health, one has to apply directly to the RCOG. However, the support from those involved in this specific ATSM is required. This includes:

- The ATSM Educational Supervisor
- The ATSM Preceptor with responsibility for that module
- The deanery director of ATSMs

Advanced planning is recommended and NTN holders are usually given priority for ATSM training.

The RCOG does not organise subspecialty training posts or programmes. For these, one has to apply directly to the Deaneries/Trusts as set out in individual adverts, all of which are found in the BMJ or the NHS jobs website.

It is expected that during the training period trainees will be working in the United Kingdom for the duration of the ATSM or subspecialty training programme (or have sought prospective approval for recognition of overseas training if the applicant is a NTN holder).

2.1.3 Expected Length of Time to Complete Training

Allocated training sessions for the completion of ATSMs are timetabled within a trainee's otherwise normal weekly workload. A trainee should expect to be able to attend one to two sessions per week. Depending on the frequency of these sessions, the training opportunities within the unit where the training is taking place and the prior experience and aptitude of the individual trainee, the ATSM should be completed within 12–18 months. Completion of the theoretical course is mandatory for the award of the ATSM and attendance must take place no more than three years before the ATSM is completed.

SST can be undertaken either full time (part time for a flexible trainee) or as part of a mixed clinical/research job, such as a Clinical Lecturer (CL) post, meaning that 50% of the trainee's time is for clinical training and 50% for research. If done on a full-time basis, SST programmes are two or three years in length, depending on if the successful applicant fulfils the research requirement of the SST curriculum. Although prior research experience is not an absolute requirement, having what is referred to as 'research exemption' tends to be desirable as the training programmes can then be two years of equivalent full time clinical training and the third year is not required. Research exemption has to be prospectively approved by the RCOG on a trainee-by-trainee basis. It is usually granted if the applicant has a higher research degree such as a PhD or an MD (a master's degree does not qualify) or two first-author original papers or meta-analysis (not review) in citable, refereed journals in a relevant field. The research component of SST may now be satisfied by completion of the RCOG Advanced Professional Module (APM) in clinical research either during a three-year SST Programme or prospectively (two- year programme).

Clinical Lecturer posts tend to be four-year posts, incorporating the equivalent of two years of full-time clinical training and two years of research, and it is usually an essential requirement that applicants already hold a higher research degree such as a PhD or an MD (or at least have the thesis for such a degree submitted by the time of the interview).

2.1.4 Training Programmes' Curriculum Differences

2.1.4.1 Differences in Training Objectives

The differences in the two types of training programmes reflect the different skills required for the type of consultant jobs expected to be taken up by the trainees after they have completed their training as highlighted previously. These can be summarised in Table 33.2.

2.1.4.2 Differences in the Training Structure

ATSMs are undertaken alongside general training. However, as SST programmes are entirely dedicated to the field of reproductive medicine and surgery, no general training is incorporated. Therefore, before starting subspecialty training, trainees are expected to have completed all the intermediate and any advanced core competences of the O&G specialty that lie outside the subspecialty field. If these have not been achieved there is only limited scope to either plan for them to be achieved early within the subspecialty training, or to delay the start date of the training. There is no provision to complete those core skills after SST.

In general, in subspecialty training programmes there is

- Protected training with little or no service commitment (except on-call) – an average week for a subspecialty trainee may look something like that in Table 33.3
- No general obstetrics and gynaecology training although it is expected that skills will be maintained.

Table 33.2 Summary of skills expected to be attained through training

	SST	ATSM
Clinical skills:	Tertiary management	Secondary management
Non clinical skills:	Leadership	Leadership
	Research skills	Clinical governance
	Clinical governance	Management
	Management	

- Competency-based modules with potential further specialised training in area of interest

In general, in advanced training study module programmes

- Competencies are attained during the general training programme
- Individuals continue to train in both obstetrics and gynaecology
- There is a wide selection of ATSMs to choose from
- The choice of ATSM to undertake is decided based on the likely consultant posts to be available
- A trainee can complete multiple ATSMs. Completion of two ATSMs is a mandatory requirement for the award of a CCT or CESR(CP) unless subspecialty training has been undertaken.

2.1.4.3 Differences in the **Curriculum**

Subspecialist training offers a comprehensive programme that is based on discreet modules (see Box 33.1), with emphasis on tertiary management of cases. There is also an essential research component. Its purpose is to ensure and demonstrate competency in the design and execution of a research study of sufficient quality to meet internationally agreed standards. The curriculum also integrates aspects of management, clinical governance and leadership training specific to the field.

ATSM training places an emphasis on secondary management of cases, trainees have a personal choice of choosing two or more modules (ATSMs) to fit their career path and the non-clinical skills required

Table 33.3 Example of what an average week for a subspecialty trainee might entail

	a.m.	p.m.
Monday	Scanning for treatment cycle tracking	Fertility Clinic / Embryo transfers
Tuesday	Gynaecology operating	Fertility Clinic
Wednesday	Egg collections	Complex reproductive medicine clinic
Thursday	Specialised session (such as andrology operating or clinic, genetics clinic, endocrinology clinic)	Specialised session (such as andrology operating or clinic, genetics clinic, endocrinology clinic)
Friday	Gynaecology operating	Meetings (such as teaching, (quality management, unit management)
Weekend	Reproductive medicine unit cover (either physical or over the phone) General out-of-hours on-call commitment	

Box 33.1   Subspecialist training curriculum modules

Clinical
- *Female Reproductive Endocrinology*
- *Endometriosis*
- *Reproductive Surgery*
- *Subfertility and Assisted Conception*
- *Andrology*
- *Early Pregnancy Problems*

Non-clinical

Includes: *Research, clinical governance, management, and teaching*

---

of any doctor are expected to be gained through their general training.

2.1.4.4 Differences in the **Supervision**

An ATSM is undertaken under the supervisions of one or more ATSM Educational Supervisors under the auspice of the ATSM Preceptor and the deanery ATSM director. Once all of the components of the ATSM have been completed to the satisfaction of the Educational Supervisor and Preceptor, the relevant completed form is sent to the RCOG.

In subspecialty training there will be a large number of trainers as the curriculum covers a wide breath of specialised areas. All of this is undertaken under the overall supervision of the Subspecialty Training Programme Supervisor (STPS). Two subspecialists nominated by the RCOG's subspecialty committee undertake a formal annual assessment. They will then make recommendations regarding the progress towards or attainment of subspecialist accreditation to the RCOG subspecialist committee and the Head of School (who acts on behalf of the Postgraduate Dean) that will form part of the evidence required at the trainee's ARCP/RITA process. Once the subspecialty programme has been completed, the trainee can register with the GMC a subspecialty accreditation alongside their primary specialty. The provision of training from the training centre towards the trainee is also reviewed.

2.2 Non-GMC accredited training

2.2.1 **Fellowships**

Fertility units in the United Kingdom frequently offer the opportunity to work and train within them as a

Clinical Fellow (CF). Some will be purely aimed at provision of supervised clinical work (either directly or indirectly depending on the level of experience of the person employed in the post). The service provision that goes with this type of job forms the basis for training and gaining experience in the particular field. Learning is therefore self-directed. Other jobs, such as Clinical Research Fellow (CRF) positions, have a mix of both service provision and research. The emphasis on each will depend on the priorities and funding for each post. These can often lead to the attainment of a higher research degree, such a PhD or MD, given the right circumstances. In these instances, a research supervisor, which might not necessarily be the same person as the clinical supervisor, will help and guide the CRF in their academic pursuit. Once more, by the nature of higher degrees, research is self-guided. Compared to CF posts, in CRF jobs there is often a competition between time required for clinical service provision and time needed for academic research work. A delicate balance has to be struck and factors such as funding, workload etc. come in to play. However, often the bulk of the research work is done in one's spare time. CRF jobs can be very demanding but potentially extremely rewarding as well. Therefore, CF posts by and large tend to be one to two years in duration whilst CRF posts tend to be two to three years to allow for completion of a higher degree.

2.2.2 **BFS Certification Modules**

The BFS offers currently six certification modules in key areas of reproductive medicine. These can be found in Box 33.2. One has to be a BFS member in order to register and complete these.

Each module has a logbook that has to be completed and a corresponding study day(s) associated with it. Attendance at this specific study day is a mandatory part of the certification process.

The average module completion time is usually 6–12 months and depends not only on the size and capacity of individual training centres but also on the exposure and available training opportunities that each trainee has available to them. Each module has to be completed within 18 months of attendance to the associated study day.

Training can begin once the BFS Training Subcommittee has approved the relevant application. The study day can be attended prior to starting the module, as long as the training is completed within 18 months. Training is meant to be prospective.

Box 33.2 BFS Certifications

Theoretical
- Assisted conception
- Management of the infertile couple
- Fertility preservation and creating modern families

Practical
- Pelvic ultrasound
- Embryo transfer / IUI
- Quality management of a fertility service
- Male fertility

However, although not recommended, it is up to the discretion of the BFS trainer along with the trainee to decide if retrospective sign off of competencies can be included in the logbook. Each module requires regular appraisal meetings with the trainer, which has to be done prospectively.

It is the responsibility of the prospective trainee to approach a BFS certified trainer within a certified training centre. It can be challenging for such opportunities to become available for individuals not already working within a fertility unit. However, those undergoing fellowships usually do so in units that have been accredited by the BFS for the provision of some, if not all, BFS training modules. As such, trainees employed as fellows are often able to achieve the competencies required for certification.

3 Job Market for Training – The Competition

Competition for training posts will depend to an extent on which training pathway one chooses to follow. There is limited number of centres around the country and not all are certified to provide training, GMC accredited or not. As most GMC accredited training tends to occur within NHS hospitals and in combination with local postgraduate deaneries, national funding is an important factor in availability of recognised posts. Funding is required not only to pay for the salary and training of a trainee, but also for NHS-funded in vitro fertilisation (IVF) treatments which will sustain the workload that will provide the training opportunities. As the latter is becoming more limited, fewer centres are able to support the training requirements. ATSMs

are relatively immune to this as the curriculum is set up for secondary-level management and trainees undertake these as part of their general training within weekly, allocated slots. For subspecialty training however, posts tend to be supernumerary in nature and without a significant service provision component. Therefore, as NHS-funded tertiary-level fertility treatment is becoming more limited, it may become harder for new centres to gain accreditation and for existing ones to maintain their existing subspecialty programmes. Also, funding for these subspecialty training posts is not always guaranteed as deaneries may choose to divert this to other areas of training within the general field of O&G. Therefore, there is a smaller number of registered trainees than there are approved centres with training programmes available.

Nevertheless, the need for trained doctors in the field of reproductive medicine will not necessarily diminish as subfertility is increasing in the general population and more couples are seeking treatment. Therefore, units are willing to offer job and training opportunities to trainees as fellows. Funding for such posts is local, in contrast to funding for ATSM and SST jobs that in its majority comes from central deanery training budgets. Therefore, as workload for some units increase they may have the flexibility to offer employment and therefore training opportunities through fellowships within them.

As competition for any job that offers good training is high, it is always wise to plan ahead in order to improve the chances of getting it. When applying for a post, having prior experience in an IVF clinic is useful. However, this is not always possible as many times the aim of applying is in fact exactly to gain such experience in an assisted conception unit. Nevertheless, having allied skills such as ultrasound is very useful. Having done (or be in the process of doing) research, audits, case reports or a review article shows commitment to the field and generic skills. As many available posts can be a number of years in duration (anywhere from one to four) looking ahead and tailoring your training time to apply for the right job is essential. Finally, reproductive medicine is a small specialty, so getting known by attending conferences (such as the BFS annual conference) and courses is a good way for trainers to know that someone is interested and committed long term to the field.

4 Further Information – References

For further information on GMC accredited training programmes, such as entry criteria for ATSM and SST posts and training centres, visit the RCOG website at www.rcog.org.uk and look for the relevant sections in the curriculum pages which can be found under the careers and training section.

For further information on BFS certification modules, training centres and accredited trainers visit the BFS website at www.britishfertilitysociety.org.uk and look under the education and training subsection.

Most fellowship jobs and subspecialty training posts will be advertised in the BMJ (http://careers.bmj.com) and/or on the NHS jobs website (www.jobs.nhs.uk), and setting up a regular alert for relevant jobs is a useful way to ensure that one does not miss an opportunity.

Index